Third Edition

Appleton & Lange's Review of
GENERAL PATHOLOGY

Third Edition

Appleton & Lange's Review of
GENERAL PATHOLOGY

Martin Gwent Lewis, MB, BS, MD, FRC (Path)
Clinical Professor
Department of Pathology and Laboratory Medicine
University of South Florida
Tampa, Florida
and
Department of Pathology
Palms of Pasadena Hospital
St. Petersburg, Florida

Thomas K. Barton, MD
Clinical Assistant Professor
Department of Pathology and Laboratory Medicine
University of South Florida
Tampa, Florida
and
Department of Pathology
Palms of Pasadena Hospital
St. Petersburg, Florida

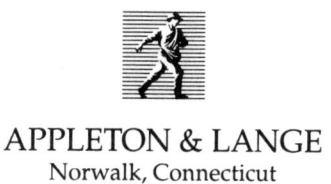

APPLETON & LANGE
Norwalk, Connecticut

0-8385-0161-3

Notice: The author(s) and the publisher of this volume have taken care to
make certain that the doses of drugs and schedules of treatment are correct
and compatible with the standards generally accepted at the time of
publication. Nevertheless, as new information becomes available, changes in
treatment and in the use of drugs become necessary. The reader is advised to
carefully consult the instruction and information material included in the
package insert of each drug or therapeutic agent before administration.
This advice is especially important when using new or infrequently used drugs.
The publisher disclaims any liability, loss, injury, or damage incurred as
a consequence, directly or indirectly, of the use and application of any of
the contents of this volume.

Copyright © 1993 by Appleton & Lange
Simon & Schuster Business and Professional Group
Copyright © 1989 by Appleton & Lange
A Publishing Division of Prentice Hall
Copyright 1981 by Arco Publishing, Inc.

All rights reserved. This book, or any parts thereof, may not be used or
reproduced in any manner without written permission. For information,
address Appleton & Lange, 25 Van Zant Street, East Norwalk, Connecticut 06855.

95 96 97 / 10 9 8 7 6 5 4

Prentice Hall International (UK) Limited, *London*
Prentice Hall of Australia Pty. Limited, *Sydney*
Prentice Hall of Canada, Inc., *Toronto*
Prentice Hall Hispanoamericana, S.A., *Mexico*
Prentice Hall of India Private Limited, *New Delhi*
Prentice Hall of Japan, Inc., *Tokyo*
Simon & Schuster Asia Pte. Ltd., *Singapore*
Editora Prentice Hall do Brasil Ltda., *Rio de Janeiro*
Prentice Hall, *Englewood Cliffs, New Jersey*

Library of Congress Cataloging-in-Publication Data

Lewis, Martin Gwent
    Appleton & Lange's review of general pathology / Martin Gwent
  Lewis, Thomas K. Barton.—3rd ed.
      p. cm.
    Includes bibliographical references.
    ISBN 0-8385-0161-3
    1. Pathology—Examinations, questions, etc. I. Barton, Thomas K.
II. Hoffman, Howard, M.D. III. Title. IV. Title: Appleton and
Lange's review of general pathology. V. Title: Review of general
pathology. VI. Title: General pathology.
    [DNLM: 1. Pathology—examintion questions. QZ 18 L675g 1993]
RB119.L485 1993
616.07'076—dc20
DNLM/DLC   93-2667
for Library of Congress   CIP

Acquisitions Editor: Jamie L. Mount
Production Editor: Sondra Greenfield
Designer: Penny Kindzierski

PRINTED IN THE UNITED STATES OF AMERICA

Contents

Preface vii

Introduction ix

   1. Cell Inury and Death 1
      Answers and Explanations 10

   2. Inflammation, Healing, and Repair 21
      Answers and Explanations 35

   3. Hemodynamic, Fluid, and Acid-Base Alterations:
      Thrombosis, Embolism, and Infarction 49
      Answers and Explanations 57

   4. Immunopathology 67
      Answers and Explanations 76

   5. Infectious Diseases 85
      Answers and Explanations 93

   6. Genetic, Metabolic, and Environmental Pathology 105
      Answers and Explanations 114

   7. Neoplasia and Abnormalities of Growth 121
      Answers and Explanations 140

   8. Photographic Exercises 149
      Answers and Explanations 171

   9. Practice Test 179
      Answers and Explanations 189

Practice Test Subspecialty List 197

Practice Test Answer Grid 199

Preface

The purpose of this book is to provide a format for review and revision of general pathology and both practice and self-assessment of knowledge required for the successful approach to examinations such as the United States Medical Licensing Examination.

It is not in any way intended to be a replacement for standard and more extensive and comprehensive textbooks of pathology but rather as a supplement, and to be used with the understanding that it is not an introduction to pathology but rather a book to be used by students who have already completed courses in pathology and read the more extensive texts.

At the end of the book, a practice test is presented so that in the final instance the readers can actually test their abilities and knowledge in the style and time frame that will be expected of them in the performance of the actual examination. Answers and explanations are also provided with the practice test, as are some hints and advice on the best method of approaching such an exam from a practical point of view.

Illustrated photographic questions are also included in each chapter, and, in addition, a separate chapter devoted entirely to such photographic questions is provided to give practice and experience. This particular approach is being used more and more frequently in a number of professional examinations in pathology.

Finally, in addition to reviewing pathology and practicing examintaion techniques, it is hoped that the readers will be stimulated to a greater study of pathology with particular emphasis on its clinical application.

General pathology or the general principles of disease is not the province of medical students or medical practitioners alone, but is also important to students of science, particularly those entering careers in biomedical research. It is hoped that these exercises will be a value to all who study disease for whatever reason.

Introduction

This book has been designed to help you review general pathology for your course and the United States Medical Licensing Examination (USMLE) Step 1 and Step 3. This 896-question, comprehensive review of general pathology contains multiple-choice questions, written in the new question format of the USMLE. Each question is referenced to a core textbook and has a paragraph-length explanation for the answer. In addition, the last chapter contains questions from all areas of general pathology arranged as an integrated practice test for self-assessment purposes. The exact exam-type questions, and internal design will help you to both assess your areas of strength and weakness and become familiar with the question types and presentation of material in general pathology that you will encounter on the USMLE Step 1.

ORGANIZATION OF THIS BOOK

This book is divided into nine chapters. Seven chapters provide a review of the major areas of pathology. The eighth chapter provides practice with pattern identification. The last chapter is a Practice Test, which integrates all of these areas into one simulated examination.

The format is arranged to facilitate review by providing a brief summary of basic facts and concepts at the beginning of each chapter and somewhat more extensive review of those basic facts at the end of each chapter to amplify the individual answers to the questions presented.

The style and presentation of the questions have been fully revised to conform with the USMLE. This will enable you to familiarize yourself with the types of questions to be expected and provide practice in recalling your knowledge in that particular form. Following the answer to each question, a reference to a particular and easily available text is provided for further reference and reading.

This introduction provides specific information on the USMLE Step 1, information on question formats, question answering strategies, and various ways to use this review.

THE UNITED STATES MEDICAL LICENSING EXAMINATION STEP 1

The USMLE Step 1 is a two-day examination consisting of approximately 800 questions to test your knowledge in the basic sciences. It contains multiple-choice questions organized within three dimensions. Each dimension is weighted, however, the projected percentages for these dimensions is subject to change from exam to exam. The three dimensions are: (1) System, (2) Process, and (3) Organizational Level. The application materials illustrate the percentage breakout, and offer you a detailed content outline to aid in your review.

Question Formats

There are three question format types used: (1) one best answer-single item, (2) choosing/matching and, (3) extended choosing/matching. Within these formats you will encounter varying levels of difficulty. There are rote questions (although minimal in comparison to past exams), memory questions that require understanding of the problem, and questions that require both understanding and judgement. In view of the changes made in the examination format and perspective, this text has been written with emphasis on the judgement-type question. Clinical application and critical thinking questions are offered as the standard in this examination.

One best answer-single item questions. The majority of the questions are posed in the A-type, or "one best answer-single item" format. This is the most popular question format in most exams. It generally contains a brief statement, followed by five options of which only ONE is entirely correct. The options on the USMLE are lettered A, B, C, D, and E. Although the format of this question type is straightforward, the questions can be difficult because some of the distractors may be partially right. The instructions for this type of question will generally appear as below:

DIRECTIONS: Each of the numbered items or incomplete statements in this section is followed by an-

swers or by completions of the statement. Select the ONE lettered answer or completion that is BEST in each case.

An example of this question type is:

1. An obese 21-year-old woman complains of increased growth of coarse hair on her lip, chin, chest, and abdomen. She also notes menstrual irregularity with periods of amenorrhea. The most likely cause is

    (A) polycystic ovary disease
    (B) an ovarian tumor
    (C) an adrenal tumor
    (D) Cushing's disease
    (E) familial hirsutism

In the question above, the key word is "most." Although ovarian tumors, adrenal tumors, and Cushing's disease are causes of hirsutism (described in the stem of the question), polycystic ovary disease is a much more common cause. Familial hirsutism is not associated with the menstrual irregularities mentioned. Thus, the most likely cause of the manifestations described can only be "(A) polycystic ovary disease."

STRATEGIES FOR ANSWERING ONE BEST ANSWER-SINGLE ITEM QUESTIONS

1. Remember that only one choice can be the correct answer.
2. Read the question carefully to be sure that you understand what is being asked. Pay attention to key words like "most" or "least."
3. Quickly read each choice for familiarity. (This important step is often not done by test takers.)
4. Go back and consider each choice individually.
5. If a choice is partially correct, tentatively consider it to be incorrect. (This step will help you eliminate choices and increases your odds of choosing the correct answer.)
6. Consider the remaining choices and select the one you think is the answer. At this point, you may want to quickly scan the stem to be sure you understand the question and your answer.
7. Fill in the appropriate circle on the answer sheet.
8. If you do not know the answer, make an educated guess. Your score is based on the number of correct answers, not the number you get incorrect. Do not leave any blanks.
9. The actual examination is timed for an average of 50 seconds per question. It is important to be thorough to understand the questions, but it is equally important for you to keep moving.

One Best Answer-Matching Questions. This format presents lettered options followed by several items generally related to a common topic. The directions for this question type will generally appear as follows:

DIRECTIONS: Each set of matching questions contains lettered options, followed by several items. For each item, select the one best lettered option that is most closely associated with it. <u>Each lettered heading may be selected once, more than once, or not at all.</u>

Below is an example of this type of question:

For each adverse drug reaction listed below, select the antibiotic with which it is most closely associated.

(A) Tetracycline
(B) Chloramphenicol
(C) Clindamycin
(D) Cefotaxime
(E) Gentamicin

2. Bone marrow suppression

3. Pseudomembranous enterocolitis

4. Acute fatty necrosis of liver

Note that, unlike the single item questions, the choices in the matching sets PRECEDE the actual questions. However, as with the single item questions, only one choice can be correct for a given question.

STRATEGIES FOR ANSWERING ONE BEST ANSWER-MATCHING QUESTIONS

1. Remember that the lettered choices are followed by the numbered questions.
2. As with single item questions, only one answer will be correct for each item.
3. Quickly read each choice for familiarity.
4. Read the question carefully to be sure that you understand what is being asked. Pay attention to key words like "most" or "least."
5. Go back and consider each choice individually.
6. If a choice is partially correct for a particular item, tentatively consider it to be incorrect. (This step will help you eliminate choices and increases your odds of choosing the correct answer.)
7. Consider the remaining choices and select the one you think is the answer.
8. Fill in the appropriate circle on the answer sheet.
9. if you do not know the answer, make an educated guess. Your score is based on the number of correct answers, not the number you get incorrect. Do not leave any blanks.
10. Again, the actual examination allows an average of 50 seconds per question.

Extended Choosing/Matching Questions. The USMLE Step 1 utilizes a new type of matching question that is similar to the one above, but can contain up to 26 lettered options followed by several items. The directions for this type of question will generally read as follows:

DIRECTIONS: Each set of matching questions in this section consists of a list of up to 26 lettered options

followed by several numbered lists. For each numbered item, select the one lettered option that is most closely associated with it.

An example of this type of question is:

(A) sarcoidosis
(B) tuberculosis
(C) histoplasmosis
(D) coccidiomycosis
(E) amyloidosis
(F) bacterial pneumonia
(G) mesothelioma
(H) carcinoma
(I) fibrosing alveolitis
(J) silicosis

627. A right lower lobectomy specimen contains a solitary 1.2 cm diameter solid nodule. The center of the nodule is fibrous. The periphery has granulomatous inflammation. With special stains multiple 2 to 5 cm budding yeasts are evident within the nodule. Acid-fast stains are negative.

628. A left upper lobectomy specimen is received containing a 4.6 cm nodule with central cystic degeneration. Microscopically, the nodule is composed of anaplastic squamous cells. Similar abnormal cells are seen in a concomitant biopsy of a hilar lymph node.

629. After a long history of multiple myeloma, a 67-year-old male is noted to have abundant acellular eosinophilic deposits around the pulmonary microvasculature at autopsy. A congo red special stain demonstrates apple green birefringence.

630. A large pleural-based lesion is found on chest x-ray of an asbestos worker. Electron microscopy of the biopsy shows abundant long microvilli.

Note that, like other matching sets, the lettered options are listed first.

STRATEGIES FOR ANSWERING EXTENDED MATCHING/CHOOSING-TYPE QUESTIONS

1. Read the lettered options through first.
2. Work with one item at a time.
3. Read the item through, then go back to the options and consider each choice individually.
4. As with the other question types, if the choice is partially correct, tentatively consider it to be incorrect.
5. Consider the remaining choices and select the answer.
6. Fill in the appropriate circle on the answer sheet.
7. Remember to make a selection for each item.
8. Again, the test allows for 50 seconds per item.

ORGANIZATION OF THIS REVIEW

Basic Chapter Layout

This book is divided into seven subtopic chapters that consist of short summaries, questions, answers, and explanations. The questions are grouped together, followed by an answer/explanation section. The answer section provides the answer to each question, gives an explanation and review of why the answer is correct, explains why the other choices are incorrect, offers background information on the subject matter, and cites references to core textbooks for further study. You are urged to use the reference material to further your understanding.

Practice Test

Chapter 9 contains the 153-question Practice Test and reviews all the topics covered in Chapters 1 through 7. The questions are grouped according to question type with the subject areas integrated. Specific instructions on how to take the Practice Test are given on page 179.

The Practice Test is followed by a subspecialty list, which will enable you to analyze your areas of strength and weakness. This can help you focus your review on specific areas. For example, by checking off your incorrect answers, you may find that you have missed a fair number of immunopathology questions. This would indicate that immunopathology may be an area of weakness. In this case, you could note all the references (in the Answers and Explanations section) for your incorrect answers and read those sources. You might also want to purchase an immunopathology text or review book to do a much more thorough review.

HOW TO USE THIS BOOK

There are two logical ways to get the most value from this book. We will call them Plan A and Plan B.

In **Plan A,** you go straight to the Practice Test and complete it according to the instructions given on page 179. Using the subspecialty list, analyze your areas of strength and weakness. This will be a good indicator of your initial knowledge of the subject and will help to identify specific areas for preparation and review. You can now use the first seven chapters of the book to help you improve your relative weak points.

In **Plan B,** you go through Chapters 1 through 7 checking off your answers, and then comparing your choices with the answers and discussions in the book. Once you have completed this process, you can take the Practice Test and see how well prepared you are. If you still have a major weakness, it should be apparent in time for you to take remedial acton.

In Plan A, by taking the Practice Test first, you get quick feedback regarding your initial areas of strength and weakness. You may find that you have a good command of the material, indicating that perhaps only a cursory review of the first seven chapters is necessary. This, of course, would be good to know early in your exam preparation. On the other hand, you may find that you have many areas of weakness. In this case, you could then focus on these areas in your review—not just with this book, but also with textbooks.

It is, however, unlikely that you will not do some studying prior to taking the National Boards (especially since you have this book). Therefore, it may be more realistic to take the Practice Test after you have reviewed the first seven chapters (as in Plan B). This will probably give you a more realistic type of testing situation since very few of us just sit down to a test without studying. In this case, you will have done some reviewing (from superficial to in-depth), and your Practice Test will reflect this studying time. If, after reviewing the first seven chapters and taking the Practice Test, you still have some weaknesses, you can then go back to the first seven chapters and supplement your review with your texts.

SPECIFIC INFORMATION ON THE UNITED STATES MEDICAL LICENSING EXAMINATION STEP 1.

The offficial source of all information with respect to the USMLE Step 1 is the National Board of Medical Examiners (NBME), 3930 Chestnut Street, Philadelphia, PA 19104. Established in 1915, the NBME is a voluntary, nonprofit, independent organization whose sole function is the design, implementation, distribution, and processing of a vast bank of question items, certifying examinations, and evaluative services in the professional medical field.

In order to sit for the Step 1 examination, you must be either an officially enrolled medical student or a graduate of an accredited U.S. or Canadian medical school. It is not necessary to complete any particular year of medical school in order to be a candidate for Step 1. Neither is it required to take Step 1 before Step 2.

In applying for Step 1, you must use forms supplied by the NBME. Remember that registration closes *10 weeks* before the scheduled examination date.

Scoring

Because there is no deduction for wrong answers, you should **answer every question.** Your test is scored in the following way:

1. The number of questions answered correctly is totaled. This is called the raw score.
2. The raw score is converted statistically to a "standard" score on a scale of 200 to 800, with the mean set at 500. Each 100 points away from 500 is on standard deviation.
3. Your score is compared statistically with the criteria set by the scores of the second-year medical school candidates for certification in the June administration during the prior four years. This is what is meant by the term, "criterion-referenced test."
4. A score of 500 places you around the 50th percentile. A score of 380 is the minimum passing score for Step 1; this probably represents about the 12th to 15th percentile. If you answer 50% or so of the questions correctly, you will almost certainly receive a passing score.

Remember: You do not have to pass all seven basic science components, although you will receive a standard score in each of them. A score of less than 400 (about the 15th percentile) on any particular area is a real cause for concern as it will certainly drag down your overall score. Likewise, a 600 or better (85th percentile) is an area of great relative strength.

Physical Conditions

The NBME is very concerned that all their exams be administered under uniform conditions in the numerous centers that are used. Except for several No. 2 pencils and an eraser, you are not permitted to bring anything (books, notes, calculators, etc.) into the test room. All examinees receive the same questions at the same session. The questions, however, are printed in different sequences in several different booklets, and the booklets are randomly distributed. In addition, examinees are removed to different seats at least once during the test. And, of course, each test is monitored by at least one proctor. The object of these maneuvers is to discourage cheating or even the temptation to cheat.

The number of candidates who fail Step 1 is quite small; however, individual students as well as entire medical school programs benefit when scores are high. No one wants to squeak by with a 350 when a little effort might raise that score to 450. That is why you have made a wise decision to use the self-assessment and review materials available in this, the 3rd edition of *Appleton & Lange's Review of General Pathology.*

CHAPTER 1

Cell Injury and Death

> The chief point in this application of Histology and Pathology is to obtain a recognition of the fact, that the cell is really the ultimate morphological element in which there is any manifestation of life, and that we must not transfer the seat of real action to any point beyond the cell.
> —Rudolph Virchow (1858)

There are basic responses of cells to various forms of insult. Injury is produced by physical, chemical, microbial, immunologic, or even genetic means; the effects of ionizing radiation have been selected to be discussed in depth in this chapter. With injury, there is stress on the dynamic nature of the cells' response to injury, ie, the ability of cells to adapt to varying levels of injury. Characteristic morphologic alterations of a degenerative nature arise in response to sublethal injury, with sequential changes in both morphology and biochemistry.

When the ability of cells to regulate their metabolism is exceeded by excessively large, persistent, or unusual forms of injury, the process of necrosis is initiated. The characteristic morphologic changes of cell death and the underlying biochemical basis are examined in this chapter, and comparison is made between methods of coping with widespread tissue injury and normal physiologic processes involving cell replacement. Emphasis is placed on the effects of inflammation and repair, which various forms of cell death initiate.

The detailed treatment of radiobiology and radiation pathology is aimed at familiarizing the reader with the basic forms of ionizing radiation and the major syndromes that may be initiated by various absorbed doses. The organs and cells most at risk are indicated.

BASIC FACTS AND CONCEPTS

Many forms of injuries result in a series of adaptive processes on the part of the cell that returns the cell to a state of equilibrium with its environment. Some stimuli cause such drastic changes that a return to the normal steady state is impossible, and a series of irreversible changes leads to cell death (Fig 1–1).

Subsequent additional events following these forms of necrosis include saponification, mummification, calcification, ossification, and acute inflammation and resulting fibrosis in some cases (see Chapter 2). Table 1–1 provides a more detailed summary of the main features, and Table 1–2 shows a comparison between the varieties of cell injury and responses. Figure 1–2 is a schematic representation of a typical mammalian cell.

ABNORMAL ACCUMULATION OF VARIOUS SUBSTANCES WITHIN CELLS

There are two basic types of accumulation: (1) excess of substances normal to the particular cell and (2) abnormal substances, and three basic mechanisms: (1) decrease in normal metabolic removal, (2) inability to metabolize the substance, and (3) deposition of abnormal exogenous substance in which the cell has no mechanism to metabolize it.

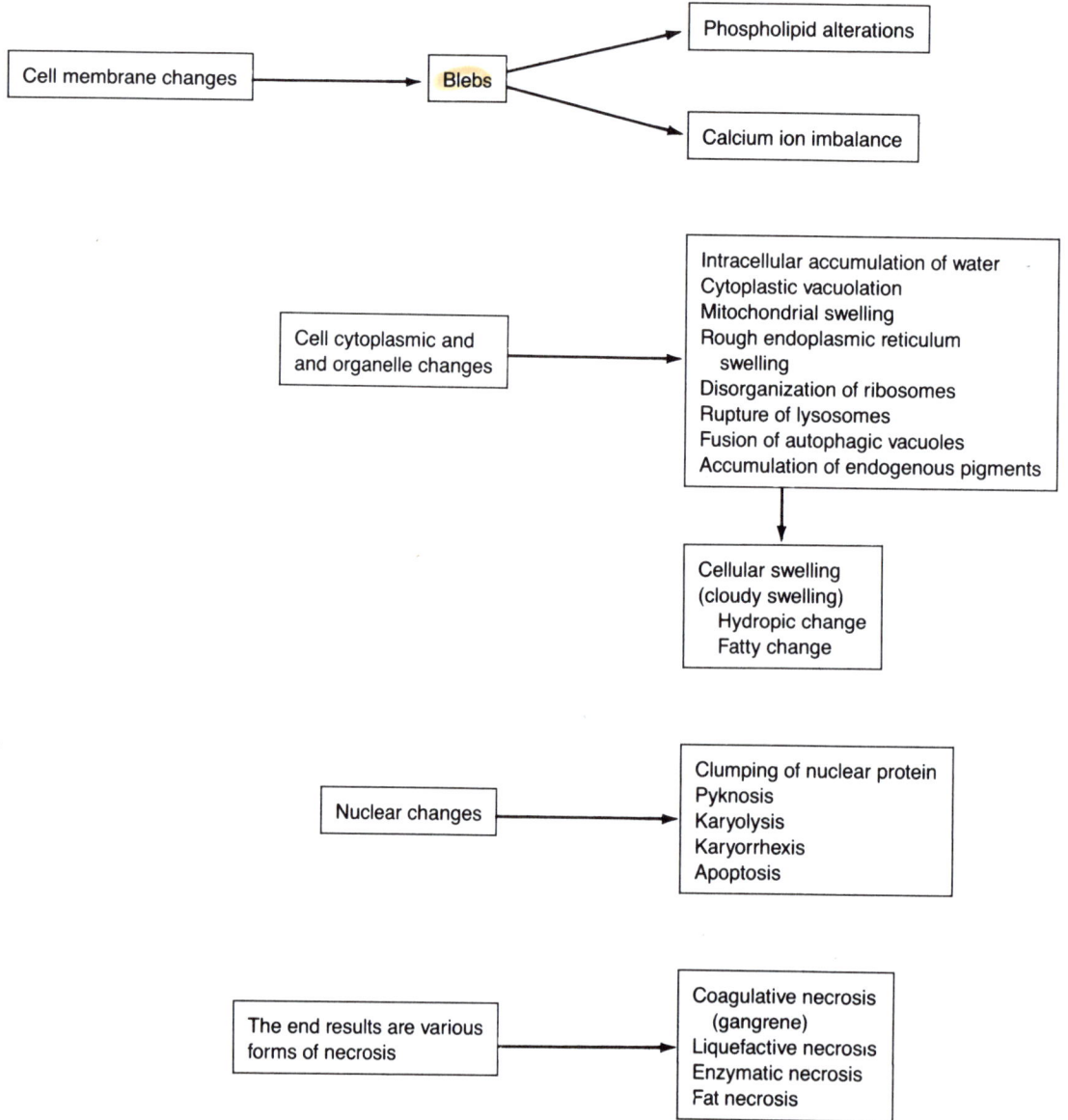

Figure 1-1. Types and modes of change follow irreversible damage to cells.

TABLE 1-1. SALIENT FEATURES OF CELL INJURY AND DEGENERATION

Condition	Microscopic Findings
Hydropic degeneration	Accumulation of intracellular fluid. Cells have a pale appearance of cytoplasm with distortion of nucleus. Cytoplasm is less granular than usual. Typically seen in proximal tubules of kidney
Hyaline degeneration	Homogeneous pink and ground-glass appearance, often the blurring hyaline obliteration of nuclear structure. Seen typically in small blood vessels or in the islets of Langerhans in diabetes
Fatty degeneration	Accumulation of lipids gives cells an empty appearance due to removal of lipids during normal processing of tissue. Seen typically in liver cells in response to a variety of insults
Amyloid deposition	Pink-staining material with a smudge-out appearance. Seen typically in interstitial tissue in spleen, liver, and the like or in the glomeruli of the kidney
Colliquative necrosis	Amorphous material, often bluish staining due to the nuclear protein present. Seen in an abscess and in brain infarcts where the staining is complicated by lipid
Fat necrosis	Breakdown of fat cells with a pale-staining appearance. Often complicated by deposition of calcium salts (staining dark blue) or alkaline change (saponification)
Dystrophic calcification	Deposition of calcium salts in tissues secondary to previous degenerative changes. As mentioned, fat necrosis may be one such predisposing abnormality

TABLE 1-2. COMPARISON OF VARIOUS FORMS OF CELL INJURY AND DEGENERATIONS

Condition	Degeneration	Infiltration	Breakdown of Cells	Inflammatory Response	Attraction of Calcium Salts
Hyaline degeneration	Yes	Yes	Not usually	Late or infrequent	Variable
Hydropic degeneration	Yes	No	No	No	No
Fatty degeneration	Yes	No	Late	Usually not or late	No
Amyloidosis	Yes	Yes	Variable or secondary response to pressure	Yes	
Colliquative necrosis	Yes	Yes	Yes	Yes	Variable
Fat necrosis	Yes	Yes	Yes		Yes

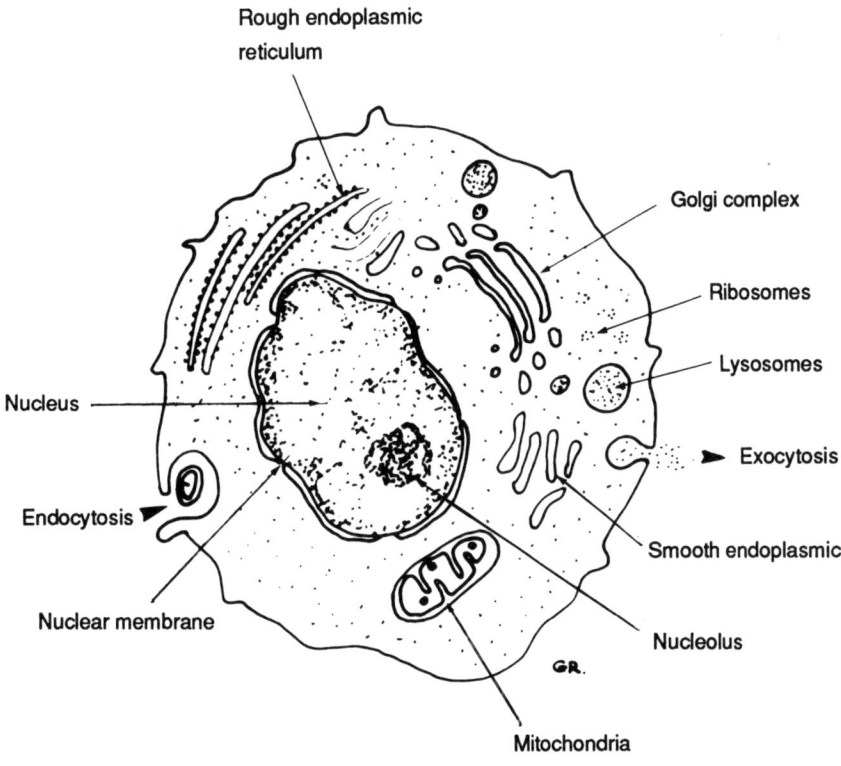

Figure 1-2. This is a schematic representation of a typical mammalian cell with the more important organelles, structures, and physiologic processes labeled.

Questions

DIRECTIONS (Questions 1 through 34): Each of the numbered items or incomplete statements in this section is followed by answers or by completions of the statement. Select the ONE lettered answer or completion that is BEST in each case.

1. Autolysis involves which organelle system as a major factor?

    (A) Golgi complex
    (B) nucleus
    (C) rough endoplasmic reticulum (RER)
    (D) lysosomes
    (E) nucleolus

2. Liquefaction, or colliquative necrosis, is seen especially in

    (A) lungs
    (B) kidney
    (C) brain
    (D) heart
    (E) liver

3. Gas gangrene is a form of necrosis associated with

    (A) mycotic infections
    (B) emphysema
    (C) tuberculosis
    (D) infections with *Clostridium*
    (E) muscle trauma

4. Atrophy in the thyroid epithelium in Hashimoto's disease results from

    (A) autoimmunity
    (B) pituitary malfunction
    (C) malnutrition
    (D) pressure caused by adjacent neoplasm
    (E) excessive thyroid-stimulating hormone (TSH)

5. Mitochrondria contain enzymes involved in

    (A) activation and synthesis of some amino acids
    (B) glycolysis
    (C) oxidative phosphorylation
    (D) fatty acid synthesis
    (E) phosphogluconate pathway

6. The unit of exposure for health physics purposes is

    (A) roentgen equivalent physical (rep)
    (B) roentgen equivalent mammal (rem)
    (C) curie
    (D) relative biologic effectiveness (rbe)
    (E) microcurie

7. The cell type most likely to be damaged by ionizing irradiation is

    (A) glial cell
    (B) erythrocyte
    (C) intestinal crypt cell
    (D) melanocyte
    (E) cartilage

8. The most likely cause of death following exposure to 700 rads is

    (A) bone marrow syndrome
    (B) central nervous system (CNS) syndrome
    (C) gastrointestinal syndrome
    (D) respiratory failure
    (E) skin exfoliation

9. The LD_{50} for humans is approximately

    (A) 100 rads
    (B) 500 rads
    (C) 750 rads
    (D) 1000 rads
    (E) 5000 rads

10. In the bone marrow syndrome, the most significant cause of nonterminal anemia is

    (A) frank hemorrhage
    (B) leakage from the circulation
    (C) lysis of circulating erythrocytes
    (D) deficiency of erythropoiesis
    (E) leukemic transformation

11. In death resulting from the gastrointestinal syndrome, the mean survival time is measured in

    (A) hours
    (B) days

(C) weeks
(D) months
(E) years

12. The main cellular target for the action of radiation is

    (A) DNA
    (B) cell membrane
    (C) mitochondria
    (D) ribosomes
    (E) lysosomes

13. The principal action of ionizing irradiation on cellular DNA is considered to be

    (A) pyrimidine dimers — from UV radiation
    (B) addition products } from ionizing radiation
    (C) organic peroxides
    (D) single-strand breaks
    (E) gene deletion — long term

14. Which of the following radiations is most penetrating to human tissue?

    (A) alpha — most damaging
    (B) beta
    (C) gamma
    (D) x-ray
    (E) protons

15. Which of the following radiations is most damaging to human tissue, given equal penetration?

    (A) alpha
    (B) beta
    (C) gamma
    (D) x-ray
    (E) protons

16. Which of the following cell types has been shown to be most sensitive to low doses of irradiation in the mouse?

    (A) lymphoblasts
    (B) megakaryocytes
    (C) small lymphocytes — exception to rule
    (D) normoblasts
    (E) keratinocytes

17. A bone-seeking isotope, such as strontium-90, produces damage to the hemopoietic system via emitted

    (A) beta particles — most import. in the bone marrow
    (B) alpha particles
    (C) x-rays
    (D) gamma particles
    (E) protons

18. Which of the following lists of tissue is in the correct order of radiosensitivity?

    (A) red cell precursors, neurons, lymphocytes, muscle fibers, small intestinal epithelial cells, fibroblasts, keratinocytes
    (B) lymphocytes, red cell precursors, intestinal epithelial cells, neurons, keratinocytes, fibroblasts, muscle fibers
    (C) intestinal epithelium, neurons, lymphocytes, fibroblasts, muscle
    (D) neurons, muscle, fibroblasts, lymphocytes, keratinocytes
    (E) keratinocytes, muscle, neurons, red cell precursors, fibroblasts

19. The most likely nuclear change associated with cell injury is

    (A) cloudy swelling
    (B) hydropic change
    (C) pyknosis
    (D) fatty change
    (E) membrane blebs

20. Which of the following is LEAST associated with nuclear change in cell injury?

    (A) pyknosis
    (B) karyolysis
    (C) karyorrhexis
    (D) apoptosis
    (E) swelling of rough endoplasmic reticulum (RER)

21. The response to injury that produces cellular swelling, referred to as either cloudy swelling or hydropic change, is LEAST characteristic of

    (A) mitochondrial swelling
    (B) rough endoplasmic reticulum (RER) swelling
    (C) disorganization of ribosomes
    (D) karyorrhexis
    (E) lysosomal rupture

22. Which of the following microscopic descriptions is most characteristic of hyaline degeneration?

    (A) homogeneous ground-glass, pink-staining appearance in cells
    (B) accumulation of lipids in cells
    (C) presence of calcium salts with destruction of cellular detail
    (D) pyknotic densely stained nucleus
    (E) total amorphous appearance with no cell membrane discernable

23. The cellular change associated with cell injury that is LEAST LIKELY to lead to recovery is

    (A) hyaline change
    (B) hydropic change
    (C) fatty change
    (D) colliquative necrosis
    (E) cloudy swelling

24. Which of the following cellular responses to injury is the most reversible?

    (A) amyloid deposition
    (B) fat necrosis
    (C) colliquative necrosis
    (D) hydropic change
    (E) apoptosis

25. Which of the following cell changes associated with injury is most likely to be accompanied by disruption of the cell membrane?

    (A) cloudy swelling
    (B) hydropic change
    (C) apoptosis
    (D) coagulative necrosis
    (E) pyknosis

26. Dry gangrene is best described microscopically by

    (A) enzymatic fat necrosis
    (B) coagulative necrosis
    (C) swelling of rough endoplasmic reticulum (RER)
    (D) cell membrane blebs
    (E) caseous necrosis

27. In glycogen storage disorders, which of the following causes is most accurate?

    (A) accumulation of abnormal amounts of a normal substance
    (B) deposition of exogenous abnormal substance in the cells
    (C) deposition of abnormal amounts of lipid in the cells
    (D) deposition of mucopolysaccharides in the cells
    (E) accumulation of immunoglobulin in the cells

28. Which of the following is NOT involved in the cellular accumulation of materials via the lysosomal system?

    (A) endocytosis
    (B) autophagosomes
    (C) primary lyosomes
    (D) apoptosis
    (E) phagosomes

29. Accumulation of metabolic products in the cytoplasm of cells is LEAST related to

    (A) endocytosis
    (B) exocytosis
    (C) autophagosomes
    (D) apoptosis
    (E) residual bodies

30. Which of the following is most likely to result in calcium salt deposition in the tissues affected?

    (A) amyloid change
    (B) hyaline degenerative change
    (C) colliquative necrosis
    (D) fat necrosis
    (E) hydropic change

31. Which of the following LEAST directly involves nuclear changes in the cell?

    (A) pyknosis
    (B) karyolysis
    (C) autophagic vacuole fusion
    (D) karyorrhexis
    (E) apoptosis

Questions 32 through 34. Refer to Figure 1–3.

32. The area numbered 1 represents

    (A) mitochondrion
    (B) nucleolus
    (C) Golgi complex
    (D) lysosome
    (E) rough endoplasmic reticulum (RER)

33. The area numbered 6 represents

    (A) smooth endoplasmic reticulum
    (B) nucleus
    (C) polyribosomes
    (D) mitochondrion
    (E) Golgi complex

34. The area numbered 7 represents

    (A) mitochondrion
    (B) Golgi complex
    (C) nuclear membrane
    (D) polyribosomes
    (E) rough endoplasmic reticulum (RER)

DIRECTIONS (Questions 35 through 89): Each group of items in this section consists of lettered headings followed by a set of numbered words or phrases. For each numbered word or phrase, select the ONE lettered heading that is most closely associated with it. Each lettered heading may be selected once, more than once, or not at all.

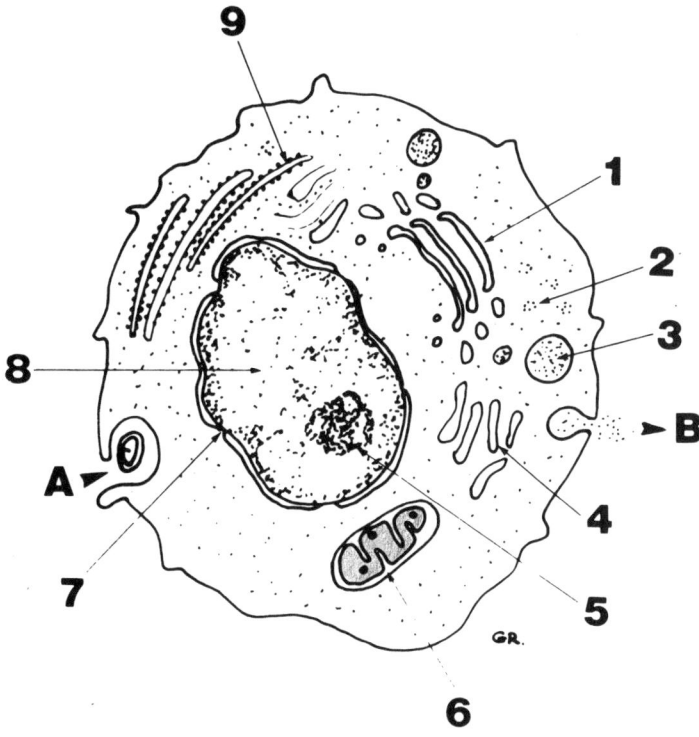

Figure 1–3. This is a schematic representation of a typical mammalian cell with the more important organelles and structures indicated by the numbers 1 through 9, and two physiologic processes labeled A and B.

Questions 35 through 38

(A) curie
(B) rad
(C) roentgen
(D) roentgen equivalent mammal (rem)

B 35. Unit of absorbed dose

D 36. Unit of dose equivalent (absorbed dose × quality factor)

A 37. Unit of activity (3.7×10^1) nuclear transformation/sec)

C 38. Unit of exposure for x-rays or gamma rays

Questions 39 through 41

(A) whole body exposure to 10,000 rads
(B) whole body exposure to 3000 rads
(C) whole body exposure to 700 rads

A 39. Vomiting

A 40. Seizures

B 41. Diarrhea

Questions 42 through 46

(A) fatty degeneration
(B) cloudy swelling
(C) coagulation necrosis
(D) caseous necrosis
(E) fibrinoid necrosis

A 42. The liver after carbon tetrachloride uptake

A 43. Choline deficiency

D 44. Loss of tissue architecture, with a cheesy appearance and consistency

B 45. Reduction in both oxidative phosphorylation and mitochondrial activity

E 46. Classically seen in blood vessels, with loss of architecture and incorporation of plasma proteins into the vessel wall

Questions 47 through 49

(A) heterophagy
(B) pyknosis
(C) autophagy
(D) karyolysis
(E) exocytosis

47. Envelopment of damaged endogenous cellular elements and their digestion in the lysosomal system

48. Digestion in the lysosomal system of exogenous substances entering the cell through endocytosis

49. Cellular discharge of particular matter too large to diffuse through the cell membrane

Questions 50 through 53

(A) cloudy swelling
(B) karyorrhexis
(C) residual body
(D) saponification
(E) liquefaction necrosis

50. Salts deposited in necrotic fatty tissue

51. Lysosomal inclusion bodies

52. Reversible cellular change

53. Nuclear fragmentation

Questions 54 through 57

(A) caseous necrosis
(B) fat necrosis
(C) coagulation necrosis
(D) liquefaction necrosis
(E) dilation of the endoplasmic reticulum

54. Expected changes in the kidney after complete occlusion of the renal artery

55. Expected changes in the cerebral cortex after occlusion of the middle cerebral artery

56. Expected changes with infection by tubercle bacilli

57. Reversible cellular change

Questions 58 through 61

(A) melanin
(B) lipofuscin
(C) hemosiderin
(D) bilirubin
(E) ceroid

58. Increased content in tissues is termed "jaundice"

59. Lipochrome yellow-brown pigment that increases with aging

60. Aggregates of ferritin micelles

61. Brown-black pigment formed by the oxidation of tyrosine

Questions 62 through 65

(A) ribosomes
(B) mitochondria
(C) primary lysosomes
(D) cell membrane
(E) centriole

62. Major site of oxidative phosphorylation and energy production

63. Major site of protein synthesis

64. Intracellular bodies that organize mitotic division

65. Intracellular bodies containing hydrolytic enzymes necessary for the digestion of endogenous and exogenous substances

Questions 66 through 69

(A) Councilman bodies
(B) psammoma bodies
(C) Gandy-Gamna bodies
(D) Civatte bodies
(E) glycogen bodies

66. Intracellular accumulations seen with Pompe's disease

67. Apoptosis seen with lichen planus

68. Apoptosis seen with infectious or toxic hepatitis

69. Splenic scars containing calcium and hemosiderin

Questions 70 through 73

(A) single exposure of 25 rads
(B) single exposure of 150 rads
(C) single exposure of 250 rads
(D) single exposure of 800 rads
(E) single exposure of 1250 rads

70. Acute cerebral syndrome, 100% mortality

71. Acute hematopoietic syndrome, 20 to 50% mortality

72. No short-term effects, 0% mortality

73. Acute radiation syndrome, 0% mortality

Questions 74 through 77

(A) fibrinoid necrosis
(B) gangrenous necrosis
(C) enzymatic fat necrosis
(D) gummatous necrosis
(E) liquefactive necrosis

74. Frequently seen with acute pancreatitis C

75. Frequently seen with syphilitic infections D

76. Frequently seen with autoimmune disorders A

77. Frequently seen with ischemic distal extremities B

Questions 78 through 81

(A) cytokeratin
(B) factor VIII
(C) HMB-45
(D) desmin
(E) glial fibrillary acid protein

78. Intermediate filament present in astrocytes E

79. Intermediate filament present in all epithelial cells A

80. Intermediate filament present in smooth muscle cells D

81. Coagulation protein present in endothelial cells B

Questions 82 through 85

(A) Mallory body
(B) neurofibrillary tangle
(C) vimentin
(D) ankyrin
(E) pinocytosis

82. Cell membrane protein D

83. Increased with Alzheimer's disease B

84. Increased with alcoholic liver disease A

85. Intermediate filament present in all mesenchymal cells C

Questions 86 through 89

(A) inhibits cellular respiration
(B) protects protein synthesis
(C) inhibits cell division
(D) protects against radiation
(E) binds to protein sulfhydrals
(F) free radical formation
(G) protects mitochondria
(H) protects cytoskeleton

86. A 36-year-old male smelter experiences an accidental lethal exposure to mercuric gas. At autopsy his kidneys were swollen and demonstrate coagulative necrosis of the proximal tubular epithelial cells. What is the primary site of cellular injury occurring in mercury poisoning?

87. A 19-year-old commits suicide by ingesting sodium cyanide. At autopsy the characteristic findings of acute cyanide poisoning are present including a pervasive almond-like smell and acute hemorrhagic gastritis. By what method does cyanide poison cells? A

88. A 44-year-old is found to have an increased serum uric acid, increased urinary uric acid excretion, recurrent attacks of acute arthritis, and tophi. A diagnosis of gout is made. One of the medicines prescribed for the patient is colchicine. How does colchicine exert its beneficial effect? C

89. A 54-year-old male janitor is cleaning a soiled carpet with carbon tetrachloride in an enclosed room. He develops malaise, nausea, stomach pains, and convulsions. Several days later he dies. At autopsy there is marked fatty change in the liver, acute renal tubular necrosis, and cerebral edema. The cause of death is believed to be acute carbon tetrachloride poisoning. What is the primary mode of cellular injury in carbon tetrachloride poisoning? F

Answers and Explanations

1. **(D)** The lysosome system within the cell is a complex interaction and balance between endocytosis and pinocytosis and the primary lysosome system associated with the phagosomes versus the secondary lysosome and autophagosome side of the mechanism, which leads to exocytosis. This is summarized schematically in Figure 1–2. Although the Golgi apparatus and the RER contribute to this balance, it is the lysosome system itself with its release of hydrolases together with increased intercellular acidity that most favors tissue digestion and leads to autolysis rather than merely the accumulation of materials in the cells. *(3:28–30)*

2. **(C)** Liquefaction, or colliquative necrosis, is also important in one of the complications of acute inflammation (Chap 2). It is the breakdown of tissue as a result of severe injury resulting in a semifluid consistency. The degree of this type of necrosis in a particular tissue is partly determined by the inherent nature of the tissue concerned. The brain, which is in an almost semifluid state, is more easily broken down, and the lipid content added to the breakdown of the cellular components produces a particular kind of necrosis. Lungs, kidney, liver, and heart, which have a more solid cellular composition, undergo a different type of necrosis, and liquefaction is much rarer in these tissues (Table 1–2). *(1:16)*

3. **(D)** Gas gangrene is a form of tissue necrosis in which the underlying factor is ischemia, which leads to the necrosis. There is a superimposed production of gas, which is the by-product of anaerobic organisms that proliferate in the ischemic anaerobic conditions produced. The classic gas-producing organisms are *Clostridium* species. A mycotic infection is one in which a fungus is superimposed on a variety of different forms of tissue injury. Emphysema is a mechanical destructive process of the lung. Tuberculosis may produce caseous necrosis (Chap 2), but this is distinctly different from that of gas gangrene. Muscle trauma in and of itself will not produce this phenomenon, but necrotic dead muscle following tissue trauma may be complicated by gas gangrene if clostridial organisms are introduced into the tissue (Tables 1–1 and 1–2). *(1:17–19; 4–103)*

4. **(A)** Hashimoto's disease is an autoimmune disease in which the thyroid epithelium is damaged, leading to an atrophic or hypofunction of the thyroid gland. Pituitary malfunction may cause secondary changes in the thyroid, and malnutrition may result in some abnormalities. Pressure caused by an adjacent neoplasm may cause local problems. None of these, however, causes the diffuse destruction of the gland seen in Hashimoto's disease. Excess TSH, in fact, usually is secondary to the gland no longer functioning, and, therefore, the negative feedback control from TSH is altered but has nothing to do with initiation of the disease as far as can be determined. *(5:1138–1139)*

5. **(C)** The process of oxidative phosphorylation is a very important and vital step in energy production and transfer in most cells and is the function of the mitochondria and mitochondrial enzymes. The mitochondria have additional enzymatic functions. They also are involved in protein synthesis but not in the actual production of amino acid and fatty acid synthesis. Phosphogluconate pathways are of much less importance except under certain pathologic conditions in which lipid may accumulate as a result of malfunctioning of the mitochondrial mechanisms. *(2:2–9)*

6. **(B)** The unit of exposure used for health physics purposes in humans is the rem. All types of radiation have different propensities to interact with tissue and, therefore, have different rbe. The amount of radiation times its characteristic rbe equals its rem (radiation × rbe = rem). Such a calculation allows standard comparison of exposure for different types of radiation. The rep is not used for biologic systems. Other units, including curie and microcurie, are measurements of emission and are not used under these circumstances except in isotope work. *(2:505)*

7. **(C)** Intestinal epithelium, with its rapid turnover, is the most sensitive, particularly the crypt cells,

TABLE 1–3. RELATIVE SENSITIVITIES OF DIFFERENT CELL TYPES OF IRRADIATION

Cell Type	Radiosensitivity
Bone marrow Lymphoid Germ cells (testis, ovaries) Intestinal epithelium	Very sensitive
Epididymal and adnexal cells of skin Pharyngeal or esophageal Urothelium Gastric mucosa	Sensitive
Glial cells of CNS Connective tissue Endothelial Growing cartilage	Moderately sensitive
Mature cartilage and bone Mucous and serous glands Pulmonary Renal Hepatic Pancreatic Endocrine	Low sensitivity
Muscle Ganglion Neurons	Very low sensitivity

which are responsible for the continuous regeneration of the epithelium (Table 1–3). In general terms, the higher the turnover rate of the cells, the more likely they are to be radiosensitive. The glial cell has a particularly moderate sensitivity. The erythrocyte (mature), being a non-nucleated cell, has virtually no effect except in very high doses of radiation. The melanocyte is very sensitive to ultraviolet radiation but not ionizing radiation to the same extent, and cartilage cells have a relatively low sensitivity except in growing cartilage, which is moderately sensitive. *(3:256–270)*

8. **(A)** High doses of whole body irradiation in the range of 10,000 rads usually can cause sudden death thought to be from damage to all the systems, particularly the CNS. The gastrointestinal syndrome, in which the gastrointestinal tract is damaged, usually is an intermediate effect. The relatively lower doses of less than 1000 rads usually cause destruction of the bone marrow, with the concomitant effects of aplastic anemia. This is, therefore, a more prolonged rather than a sudden cause of death (Tables 1–3 and 1–4). *(3:270–273)*

9. **(B)** The LD_{50} for humans in terms of whole body irradiation is approximately 500 rads. Irradiation with 1000 rads or more would be rapidly fatal in most, if not all, patients, whereas 100 rads would produce a more prolonged effect and might not produce death. The effect would certainly vary among individuals. These are approximate figures. *(3:270–273)*

10. **(D)** Nonterminal anemia is usually the result of deficiency in erythropoiesis and is the most significant in terms of bone marrow damage. Although frank hemorrhage and leakage from the circulation may occur as a complication of other aspects or irradiation (eg, the effects on the gastrointestinal tract; Table 1–4), this usually is not a direct effect of the bone marrow. Lysis of the circulating erythrocytes can occur but requires enormous doses of irradiation, since mature erythrocytes can survive until they are deleted by natural events. It is the inability to replenish these erythrocytes that causes the nonterminal anemia of the bone marrow syndrome. Leukemic transformation is a very long-term effect in those individuals who survive the radiation. *(3:279)*

11. **(B)** The gastrointestinal syndrome following irradiation is a result of complete destruction of the sensitive, rapidly regenerating epithelium of the small intestine. There are protracted and violent diarrhea and loss of fluid. Death usually ensues in a matter of days and certainly within a week (Questions 8 through 10 and Tables 1–3 and 1–4). The central nervous system (CNS) syndrome, with death within a matter of minutes to hours, results from massive irradiation. The more protracted forms of irradiation effects that last weeks, months, or years are related to bone marrow and the more chronic effects of irradiation. *(1:175–178)*

12. **(A)** The main cellular target for the action of radiation is DNA and the alteration of cellular division. Although massive doses of irradiation can cause

TABLE 1–4. RADIATION EFFECTS

Tissue or Organ	Acute Radiation Effects	Chronic or Delayed Radiation Effects
Lung	Pulmonary edema and swelling of alveolar cells	Intestinal fibrosis, alveolar fibrosis, ischemic changes
Gastrointestinal tract	Death of small intestinal mucosa with widespread ulceration	Tortuosity of blood vessels, relative ischemia and submucosal fibrosis, chronic ulceration and strictures
Kidney	Acute proximal tubular necrosis with intestinal edema	Sclerosing of blood vessels, glomerular sclerosis, tubular ischemia and atrophy

damage to cell membrane, mitochondria, ribosomes, and indirectly the cytosome, these are not as characteristic as the effect on DNA, which is the cause of most of the cellular abnormalities in post-irradiation syndromes. *(2:505–507)*

13. **(D)** Pyrimidines are the primary products of ultraviolet irradiation. Additional products and peroxidation caused by the radiolysis of intracellular water by ionizing irradiation are secondary effects to the phenomenon of strand breakage. The translocation of gene loci is a long-term and more complex effect. *(2:505–507)*

14. **(C)** Electromagnetic radiations in the gamma range are more penetrating than x-rays, since they are of a higher energy (shorter wave length). Alpha and beta are particulate radiations and are, therefore, less penetrating, as are protons (Table 1–5). *(1:173–181)*

15. **(A)** Alpha particles have the highest linear energy transfer. They dissipate their energy in the shortest distance and are, therefore, the most damaging per unit length of penetration. Compare this with Question 14 and Table 1–5. *(1:173–181)*

16. **(C)** The small lymphocyte does not follow the usual principle that cells with high mitotic rates are more sensitive to irradiation. In the mouse, particularly, the small lymphocyte is highly radiosensitive and easily destroyed by irradiation. All of the other cells mentioned are, of course, affected by irradiation, usually when the entire bone marrow is destroyed, eg, in the bone marrow syndrome following irradiation. Small amounts of irradiation of the lymphocyte have been shown to be particularly effective when compared with that needed to destroy these other cells. *(2:508)*

17. **(A)** Beta particles are the most important factors in damage to the bone marrow in isotopes, such as strontium-90, that are concentrated in the bone. Although beta particles have a relatively low penetration of tissue, this is not an important factor, since the isotope has already been concentrated in the bone immediately adjacent to and surrounding the marrow. *(1:173–181)*

18. **(B)** The correct order of sensitivity of these tissues is lymphocytes followed by red cell precursors, intestinal epithelial cells, neurons, keratinocytes, fibroblasts, and finally, muscle fibers (Tables 1–3 and 1–4). *(3:257)*

19. **(C)** Pyknosis is a change in the nuclear protein in which the nucleus becomes more condensed before fragmentation, and dissolution of the nucleus is an end-stage and very severe form of cell damage. Cloudy swelling, hydropic change, fatty change, and membrane blebs all are associated with intracellular organelles or the cell membrane but are not nuclear events. *(2:4–16)*

20. **(E)** Swelling of the RER is associated with a number of injurious agents (Fig 1–1 and Table 1–6). All of the other events are nuclear changes and are much more serious and more permanent in nature. *(2:4–16)*

21. **(D)** Cloudy swelling or hydropic change is associated with swelling of the mitochondria and swelling and changes in the RER, with disorganization of ribosomes and, to a varying degree, lysosomal rupture. However, karyorrhexis is the phenomenon of disruption and breakdown of the nuclear protein and is a nuclear event that is a more advanced and serious consequence of cell injury (Table 1–6). *(5:5–6)*

22. **(A)** Hyaline degeneration is a complex series of cellular events. It has a particular appearance microscopically, with its ground-glass, pink-staining appearance and intact cell membrane. The accumulation of lipids, the presence of calcium salts, or the amorphous appearance of the cell with no discernible membranes as seen in amyloid are distinctly different. The pyknotic nucleus is not a characteristic of hyaline degeneration. (Tables 1–1 and 1–2). *(2:16–17,36–37; 5:29)*

23. **(D)** Hyaline change, hydropic change, fatty change, and cloudy swelling are intracellular events following injury that, theoretically, are reversible and can revert back to a normal-appearing cell. By definition, necrosis means death of the cell, and colliquative necrosis is merely a variant of this. Any form of necrosis clearly is not reversible. *(2:16–17; 5:5–6,29)*

24. **(D)** This is in a sense the reverse of Question 23. Hydropic change with the accumulation of materials in the cytoplasm can be altered if the stimulus is stopped. Amyloid deposition is a permanent state. Fat necrosis, with death of the cell, clearly is not reversible, nor is colliquative necrosis. Apop-

TABLE 1–5. SUMMARY OF EFFECTS OF IONIZATION IRRADIATION

Type of Ionization Irradiation	Tissue Penetration
X-rays	High (measured in feet)
Gamma rays	High (measured in feet)
Beta rays	Low (measured as 1.0 mm–1 cm)
Alpha rays	Very low (measured as <1.0 mm)
Protons	Intermediate (between gamma and beta)
Neutrons	High (measured in feet)

TABLE 1–6. COMPARISON OF MAIN SEQUENCES IN CELL DAMAGE PRODUCED BY CHEMICAL (TOXIC) AND ISCHEMIC INJURY

	Phase I	Phase II	Phase III
Chemical injury (carbon tetrachloride)			
— Endoplasmic reticulum		Lipid Peroxidation Membrane damage	→ Debris
→ Polysomes Mitochondria		Protein synthesis	Fatty change
→ Cell membranes		Alteration in sodium-potassium balance	→ Cell swelling
→ Lysosomes			→ Cell swelling
→ Cell sap			→ Alteration in pH
→ Nucleus			→ Clumping of chromatin → Karyolyisis → Debris
Ischemic injury			
→ Endoplasmic reticulum			→ Dilatation with detachment of polysomes and decrease in protein synthesis → Debris → Myelin forms
→ Mitochondria Decreased respiration			→ Swelling and loss of enzymes → Flocculation → Debris → Myelin forms
— Cell membranes Alteration in sodium-potassium balance			→ Release of cell enzymes CPK[a] SGOT SGPT
→ Lysosomes			→ Increased permeability Release of hydrolases
→ Cell sap		Increased glycosis	Decrease in pH
→ Cell nucleus			→ Clumping of nuclear protein → Karyolysis → Debris → Myelin forms

[a]CPK, creatine phosphokinase; SGOT, serum glutamic-oxaloacetic transaminase; SGPT, serum glutamic-pyruvic transaminase.

tosis is a phenomenon in which the cell nucleus becomes condensed and the cell membrane and cytoplasmic contents condense around the nuclear material, forming densely staining bodies known as apoptotic bodies. This again clearly is not a reversible situation. *(5:5–29)*

25. **(D)** The process of necrosis results in the final rupture of the cell and release of its contents into the surrounding media. Cloudy swelling and hydropic change, as noted in Questions 22 through 24, are reversible because the cell membrane remains viable. Pyknosis and apoptosis are nuclear events that are not reversible but in which the cell membrane remains intact and is, therefore, distinctly different from coagulation necrosis. *(2:16–17)*

26. **(B)** Swelling of the RER and cell membrane blebs are early changes in cell injury and may even be reversible (Tables 1–6 and 1–7). Fat necrosis and caseous necrosis are characteristically seen in certain tissues, such as fat, or are related to damage by the tubercle bacillus in the case of caseous necrosis. In coagulative necrosis, which is in some respects most similar to caseous necrosis, this is an ischemic event and related to the loss of blood supply. Gangrene characteristically is the result of this with a superimposed bacterial or fungal infection. *(2:16–19)*

27. **(A)** Glycogen storage disorders result from a variety of causes. There is accumulation of abnormal amounts of glycogen, which is a normal substance, and, therefore, this does not represent an exogenous amount of abnormal material or the deposition of lipids or mucopolysaccharides or immunoglobulins. There is a variety of reasons for glycogen to be stored abnormally in these cells (Table 1–7). *(2:23–24)*

TABLE 1–7. SUMMARY OF ACCUMULATION OF INTRACELLULAR MATERIAL

Type of Substance		Typical Disorder Produced	Typical Cells Involved
Lipids		Fatty change	Liver
			Heart
Proteins		Hyaline droplets	Proximal renal tubules
		Immunoglobulin (Russell bodies)	Plasma cells
Glycogen		Glycogen storage diseases	Liver, heart, muscle, renal
		Diabetes melitus	Liver, renal tubules, heart, islet
Complex substances		Gaucher's disease	Heart, liver kidney
Lipid, carbohydrates		Tay-Sachs disease	Cells of CNS,
Mucopolysaccharides		Niemann-Pick disease	Reticuloendothelial cells
Pigments		Lipofuscin	Liver, heart
		Melanin	Skin, tumors, macrophages
	Endogenous	Hematin	
		Hemosiderin	
		Hematin	Skin, connective tissue, cartilage
		Bilirubin	
		Homogentisic acid	
	Exogenous	Carbon	Histiocytes
		?	Macrophages

28. (D) Endocytosis, autophagosomes, primary lysosomes, and phagosomes (Fig 1–2) are the variations of the lysosomal system and its abnormalities in cell injury that result in accumulation of material. Apoptosis is a distinctly different phenomenon, in which the cell nuclear material becomes condensed and the cell literally shrinks around the nuclear material. *(2:26–28)*

29. (D) Apoptosis is not only a cellular phenomenon but a nuclear phenomenon, as well, and an end-stage of cell deletion without cell necrosis and disruption. The accumulation of metabolic products in the cytoplasm of cells usually is related to a balance between endocytosis and exocytosis with, in addition, a role played by autophagosomes and residual bodies (Fig 1–2). *(2:16–17)*

30. (D) When necrosis of fat cells occurs, the resultant pH changes and the formation of lipid soaplike materials are highly attractant to calcium ions, and calcium deposition is, therefore, a very characteristic phenomenon. In amyloid degeneration, hyaline degeneration, and hydropic change, no such calcium deposition is seen. Colliquative necrosis has in common with fat necrosis the disruption of cells and the breakdown and liquefaction of tissue. If this does not involve predominantly fat cells, calcium deposition is less likely (Tables 1–6 and 1–7). *(1:15–18)*

31. (C) Autophagic vacuole fusion is part of the lysosomal system (Fig 1–2) and is related to the balance between endocytosis and exocytosis and the by-product of cellular metabolism that may accumulate in certain types of damage. All of the other events—pyknosis, karyolysis, karyorrhexis, and apoptosis—are nuclear events. *(2:26–28)*

32. (C) This refers to the Golgi complex.

33. (D) The mitochondria are depicted.

34. (C) Number 7 refers to the nuclear membrane.

32 through 34. These questions recall information concerning recognition of organelles in the cytoplasm of cells (Fig 1–2). *(1:3)*

35. (B)

36. (D)

37. (A)

38. (C)

35 through 38. These questions concern definitions of various radiobiologic units. *(1:173–181)*

39. (A)

40. (A)

41. (B)

39 through 41. Whole body exposure to 10,000 rads is likely to produce a very rapid onset of severe central nervous system damage along with damage to multiple other systems. This will produce seizures and vomiting because of cerebral edema and raised intercranial pressure. Vomiting could also occur as a result of whole body irradiation to 700 rads, as can diarrhea, since the effect on the gastrointestinal tract may produce both. Whole body exposure to 700 rads is more likely to produce the later-onset clinical manifestations of bone marrow syndrome, which would not be applicable in these alternatives. Whole body exposure to 3000 rads would certainly produce the gastrointestinal syndrome and severe diarrhea (Table 1–4). *(1:173–181)*

42. **(A)**

43. **(A)**

44. **(D)**

45. **(B)**

46. **(E)**

42 through 46. Fatty degeneration can occur as a result of damage to the polysomes and mitochondria, particularly in toxic injury as seen in carbon tetrachloride poisoning of the liver. Choline deficiency may produce abnormal mitochondrial changes characteristic of fatty change and also further abnormal accumulation of fat because of deficient lipid metabolism in the liver cells. The picture of caseous necrosis is typically that of a loss of architecture with necrosis, with an appearance of a cheesy consistency. This usually is associated with necrosis associated with the lipid materials liberated from the tubercle bacillus. Cloudy swelling may occur as a result of both oxidative phosphorylation and mitochondrial and decreased activity but is a somewhat earlier change than that seen in fatty change in the same cells. A certain amount of overlap may occur. Fibrinoid necrosis is a breakdown of small blood vessels in which fibrin and other plasma proteins leak into the vessel wall and are trapped in the process, giving rise to a smudged-out and hyalinized appearance of the blood vessel walls (Fig 1–2, Tables 1–1, 1–2, and 1–7). The term "fibrinoid" is used to denote a fibrinlike staining characteristic that is not necessarily all fibrin. *(2:13; 4:103)*

47. **(C)**

48. **(A)**

49. **(E)**

47 through 49. Primary lysosomes are membrane-delimited structures containing a diverse mixture of hydrolytic enzymes. Fusion of a primary lysosome with membrane-bound exogenous material is called "heterophagy." The fusion of a primary lysosome with endogenous cellular material is called "autophagy." The enzymes within the primary lysosome are synthesized in the rough endoplasmic reticulum and packaged into vesicles in the Golgi structures. These enzymes are capable of accelerating the dissolution of most endogenous (DNA, RNA, proteins, lipids, and carbohydrates) cellular components as well as destroying exogenous materials, such as bacteria or viruses. The residual bodies are inclusions within the lysosomal vesicles composed of particular remnants that remain after autophagy or heterophagy. The residual bodies may be discharged from the cell through a process termed "exocytosis." In exocytosis the cell membrane of the phagosome fuses with that of the outer cell membrane, liberating the contents of the phagosome out into the extracellular space (Fig 1–4). *(2:26–28)*

50. **(D)**

51. **(C)**

52. **(A)**

53. **(B)**

50 through 53. Saponification is the process of converting fats into alkali salts. Saponification is commonly seen in areas of fat necrosis with subsequent calcium deposition, such as recurrent chronic pancreatitis. Pancreatitis releases the enzyme lipase into the adjacent fatty tissues, breaking down triglycerides to free fatty acids and glycerol. The fatty acids complex with plasma calcium to form soaps. Residual bodies are the insoluble debris which remain in secondary phagolysosomes after enzymatic oxidation. They are eventually discharged from the cell by the process of exocytosis (Fig 1–4). Cloudy swelling is an early reversible cellular change caused by alterations of the plasma membrane's ability to maintain the energy-dependent sodium pump with subsequent disordered cell water homeostasis. In cloudy swelling there is expansion of the cytoplasm, endoplasmic reticulum, and mitochondrium by an inflow of extracellular and intracellular water. Karyorrhexis is an irreversible change indicating death of the cell. Karyorrhexis is typified morphologically by progressive dissolution and disappearance of the nucleus. The nuclear dissolution is due to lysosomal enzymes, such as ribonuclease, which are liberated intracellularly during states of irreversible cell injury (Table 1–8). *(2:15–19)*

54. **(C)**

55. **(D)**

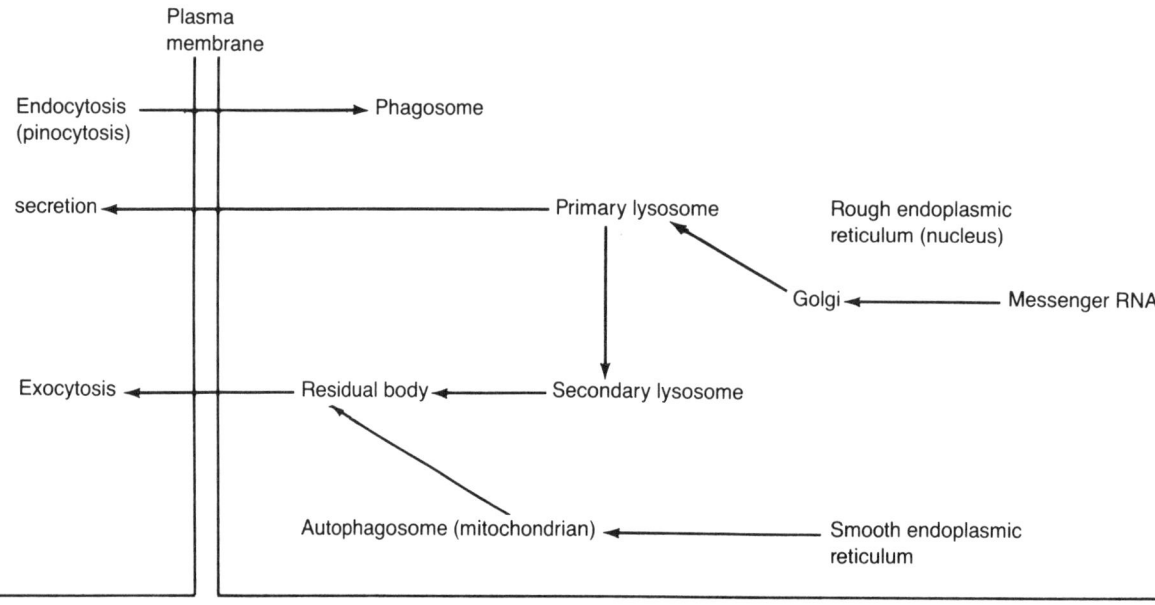

Cellular Accumulations: Result from an imbalance between endocytosis of materials, and their metabolism, and by-products removal through secretion or exocystosis. This also applies to normal by-products of cell organelle turnover and replacement (autophagy).

Apoptosis: This is a form of cell death without disruption of the plasma membrane. The cell simply shrinks about the condensed nucleus forming a dense staining body called an apoptotic body which may then be phagocytized by macrophages. The result is cell deletion without rupture of the cell contents into the surrounding tissues. This method of aging in tissues, and deletion of cells is seen in a wide variety of circumstances and is being increasingly recognized as an important mechanism also seen in neoplasms.

Figure 1-4. The lysosomal system.

56. (A)

57. (E)

54. through 57. Coagulation necrosis is most commonly caused by sudden cessation of blood flow to organs such as the heart, kidney, or spleen. Histologically, there is lack of staining in the affected tissues by routinely used hematoxylin and eosin dyes. This lack of dye uptake results in a characteristic faded ghost-like image of the normal archi-

TABLE 1-8. STRUCTURAL CHANGES IN CELL INJURY AND DEATH

Reversible Cell Injury	Irreversible Cell Injury
Blebs in cell membrane	Defects in cell membranes
Intramembraneous aggregations	Cell membrane myelin figures
Generalized cytoplasmic swelling	Lysosomal autolysis and rupture
Endoplasmic reticulum swelling	Endoplasmic reticulum rupture
Mitochondrial swelling with small densities	Mitochondrial swelling with large densities
Clumping of nuclear chromatin	Pyknosis, kayrorrhexis, karyolysis
Detachment of ribosomes	Rupture of ribosomes

tecture when the coagulated tissue is examined microscopically. Infarctions of the cerebral cortex, such as those following an occlusion of the middle cerebral artery, usually result in liquefaction necrosis. As the name implies, there is gross softening and rapid liquefaction of the brain tissue. The liquid tissues are composed of necrotic debris, numerous phagocytic microglial cells, a lack of granulation tissue, and an absence of collagen deposition. Infection by tubercle bacilli produces caseous necrosis and multinucleate Langhans' giant cells in individuals with intact delayed hypersensitivity. Dilation of the endoplasmic reticulum is a reversible cellular change. Other reversible cellular changes include cloudy swelling, fatty infiltration, ribosomal detachment, cytoplasmic blebs, and vacuole formation (Table 1-8). (2:4-5; 3:12-16)

58. (D)

59. (B)

60. (C)

61. (A)

58 through 61. Various pigments are found in cells in both normal and pathologic conditions. Bilirubin is

formed in the reticuloendothelial system through the normal catabolism of the hemoglobin porphyrin ring present in senescent erythrocytes. Newly formed bilirubin is then transported from the reticuloendothelial system into the liver. Once in the liver bilirubin is conjugated and excreted into the bile. Additional chemical alterations allow bilirubin to exit the body in urine (urobilinogen) or feces (stercobilinogen). A significant increase in the serum bilirubin is termed "jaundice." Jaundice may result from increased erythrocytic destruction (hemolysis), decreased uptake by the liver (hepatitis), or biliary tract obstruction (stones). Lipofuscin is a "wear-and-tear" pigment also called "lipochrome." It is found in the cytoplasm of many cells throughout the body, particularly with aging, malnutrition, or chronic disease. Hemosiderin is an aggregation of ferritin micelles. The iron molecules of hemosiderin impart a brownish-yellow hue to involved tissue. Hemosiderin is normally found in the histiocytes of the reticuloendothelial system. States of increased hemosiderin deposition are termed "hemosiderosis." Hemosiderosis may be either hereditary or acquired. Melanin is formed through the oxidation of tyrosine. Melanin pigment is brown-black and formed in melanosome organelles present in melanocytes. Once synthesized, melanin may be passed through melanocytic dendrites into adjacent keratinocytes. Melanin has a protective effect against actinic damage. *(1:9–10; 2:24–26)*

62. (B)

63. (A)

64. (E)

65. (C)

62 through 65. Reversible and irreversible cellular injuries may be morphologically correlated with corresponding alterations in the organelles, nucleus, cytoplasm, and cell membrane (Table 1–8). The cellular organelles each have distinct functions. The ribosomes are the site of protein synthesis as amino acid building blocks are strung together over the RNA template. Primary lysosomes are membrane-bound organelles containing hydrolytic enzymes. The primary lysosomes fuse with foreign or endogenous material to form phagolysosomes. The mitochondria are the major site of oxidative phosphorylation and energy production. Centrioles are intracellular organelles whose primary function is in organizing mitosis and chromosomal disjunction. The Golgi apparatus organelle packages enzymes into membrane-delimited structures. *(1:3)*

66. (E)

67. (D)

68. (A)

69. (C)

66 through 69. Pompe's disease is a hereditary glycogen storage disease (glycogenoses). Affected individuals are unable to fully metabolize glycogen due to a lack of the acid maltase enzyme. As a result, glycogen bodies accumulate in muscle cells throughout the body leading to cardiac failure in the infantile form of the disease. Apoptosis is the atrophic disappearance or dropping out of individual cells. In severe liver damage, such as with yellow fever or viral hepatitis, the apoptotic cells are called Councilman bodies. Civatte bodies are apoptotic cells from the basal epidermal layers seen with the dermatologic disorder of lichen planus. Both Councilman and Civatte bodies share a similar morphology being eosinophilic, anucleate, shrunken, and measuring about 10 microns in diameter. The Gandy-Gamna bodies are large (0.4 to 1.0 cm) multicellular collections of hemosiderin, scar tissue, and calcium in the spleens of individuals with portal hypertension and splenomegaly. *(5:747–748, 780,1226–1229,1409)*

70. (E)

71. (C)

72. (A)

73. (B)

70 through 73. Ionizing radiation is divided into particulate and waveform radiation. Alpha particles have minimal skin penetration potential and have a mass number of four. Beta particles can penetrate human tissue to a depth of about 1 cm and have negligible mass. X-rays and gamma rays are both waveform, nonparticulate radiations with high energies and deep tissue penetration abilities. An acute dose of 25 rads would produce no significant immediate effects. An exposure of 150 rads would produce an acute radiation syndrome with a 2- to 8-week latency period and the clinical features of nausea, vomiting, malaise, and fatigue. A single 250 rads exposure would produce a hematopoietic radiation syndrome with a latency period of 1 to 2 weeks and clinical symptoms of leukopenia and thrombocytopenia. An acute dose of 800 rads would produce a gastrointestinal radiation syndrome with a 1- to 14-day latency and clinical features of diarrhea, fluid loss, electrolyte imbalance, and gastrointestinal mucosal necrosis. A dose of 1250 rads would result in a cerebral syndrome characterized by ataxia, convulsions, delirium, coma, and death within 2 days. *(1:176–177)*

74. (C)

75. (D)

76. (A)

77. (B)

74 through 77. Cell death invariably results in necrosis. Different body sites and different pathologic processes may influence the morphologic pattern of necrosis. Acute pancreatitis, for example, may produce enzymatic fat necrosis characterized by the death of adjacent fat cells and enzymatically catalyzed (lipase) decomposition of triglycerides into free fatty acids. The released fatty acids then combine with calcium to form soaps (saponification). Syphilitic infections typically produce gummatous necrosis due to cell-mediated hypersensitivity to the infecting organisms. Most autoimmune disorders can cause fibrinoid necrosis characterized by acellular, strongly eosinophilic alterations in target organs. Gangrenous necrosis is a type of coagulative necrosis. It is common in the distal extremities of individuals with ischemia. The ischemic tissue dies and then becomes black, hard, and shrunken (dry gangrene). If there is superimposed bacterial infection, the tissue may liquefy or suppurate (wet gangrene). *(2:17–19)*

78. (E)

79. (A)

80. (D)

81. (B)

78 through 81. A number of intermediate cytoplasmic filaments are present in the cytoskeleton of cells. Cells usually synthesize only one or two kinds of intermediate filaments. For example, desmin is produced by smooth muscle cells, astrocytes make glial fibrillary acid protein, neurofilament is made by neurons, vimentin is found in mesenchymal cells, and mesothelial cells synthesize both keratin and vimentin. These filaments can serve as markers to identify the cell of origin in undifferentiated tumors. For example, undifferentiated carcinomas (malignant tumors of epithelial cells) will usually retain the ability to manufacture cytokeratin. By demonstrating the presence of cytokeratin in a tumor cell, we can usually assume that it arose from an aberrant epithelial cell line. In the practice of surgical pathology, a battery of several filaments are tested together as a panel. Most testing uses an immunologic method with a visible peroxidase endpoint (immunoperoxidase method). *(2:29–30)*

82. (D)

83. (B)

84. (A)

85. (C)

82 through 85. The cytomembrane skeleton of most cells contains the structural proteins of ankyrin and spectrin. In some cells, such as erythrocytes, the hereditary absence of membrane skeleton proteins may lead to deformed cells and hemolytic anemia. Intermediate filaments are present in the cytoplasm of cells. Different types of cells have different intermediate filaments. For example, vimentin is present in all mesenchymal cells, desmin in smooth muscle cells, and cytokeratin in epithelial cells. Mallory bodies, intracellular cytoplasmic eosinophilic inclusions, are usually seen scattered in hepatocytes of individuals with alcoholic liver disease. The Mallory bodies, also termed "alcoholic hyaline," are fibrillary degenerative concretions derived from the cell's cytoskeleton and contain the intermediate filament cytokeratin. Neurofibrillary tangles are seen with increased frequency in the cerebral neurons of Alzheimer's patients. They appear in the cytoplasm as agyrophilic complexes of interwoven paired helical protein filaments. *(1:648–649,945; 2:29–30)*

86. (E) Mercury poisons cells by binding to the sulfhydral moieties present in proteins. This binding usually inactivates a wide variety of enzyme systems throughout the cell via occupation of the enzymatic active site or by steric hindrance of the active site. Most accidental mercury poisonings are encountered in the mining or chemical industries. Inhalation is the usual route of poison exposure. Once inhaled, mercury is preferentially distributed to the kidneys. Binding to the sulfhydral groups of the proximal tubular cells results in cell death that displays a coagulative necrosis pattern. In lower doses, mercury intoxication exhibits principally neuropsychiatric features. *(3:200–203)*

87. (A) Cyanide poisons by inhibiting cellular respiration. Cyanide irreversibly binds to the enzyme cytochrome oxidase, the final enzyme in the respiratory chain, blocking respiration and oxygen-dependent energy production. Fatal intoxication can occur with the ingestion of only 0.1 mg of sodium cyanide. Most poisonings are suicidal in nature. However, some accidental intoxications result from exposure during the refining of gold and during laetrile therapy. *(1:190)*

88. (C) Colchicine inhibits cellular division. Colchicine is an alkaloid found in the seeds of the meadow saffron. Increased quantities of uric acid, a purine catabolite, is found in most individuals affected with gout and therapies are directed at reducing serum and urinary concentrations of uric acid. Colchicine is prescribed for patients with gout in an

attempt to reduce cellular mitosis and uric acid production. The clinical spectrum of gout usually includes podagra, tophus formation, and renal crystal deposition. Other anti-gout therapeutic agents used may include analgesics, anti-inflammatory drugs, and allopurinol (xanthine oxidase inhibitor). *(5:1381–1385)*

89. **(F)** Carbon tetrachloride damages cells through the formation of active-free radicals. Carbon tetrachloride is converted into toxic-free radicals by the smooth endoplasmic reticulum's mixed-function oxidase system. This system is designed to inactivate lipid soluble drugs. Once the formation of active-free radicals is begun the reaction becomes autocatalytic with rapid destruction of the endoplasmic reticulum, dissociation of polyribosomes, and cytoplasmic lipid accumulation. The cells of the liver, brain, and kidneys are prominently affected. *(2:13)*

REFERENCES

1. Chandrasoma P, Taylor CR: Concise Pathology, Norwalk, Appleton & Lange, 1991
2. Cotran RS, Kumar V, Robbins SL: Robbins Pathologic Basis of Disease, 4th edition, Philadelphia, Saunders, 1989
3. Kissane JM (ed): Anderson's Pathology, 9th edition, St. Louis, Mosby, 1990
4. Lewis MG, Rowden G: Histopathology: A Step by Step Approach, Boston, Little, Brown, 1987
5. Rubin E, Farber JL: Pathology, Philadelphia, Lippincott, 1988

CHAPTER 2

Inflammation, Healing, and Repair

> I consider inflammation as an increased action of that power which a part naturally possesses; and in healthy inflammation at least, it is probably attended with an increase in power; but in inflammations which terminate in mortification there is no increase in power, but on the contrary a diminution of it.
>
> —John Hunter (1794)

A central area in general pathology is covered extensively in this chapter. It is important to be able to identify the cardinal signs of inflammation and to understand the underlying mechanisms that produce these signs. The importance of an essentially vascular and microvascular response of the tissue to any injury must be appreciated, and the sequential events that result from injury must be understood.

The importance of fluid production in inflammation, including the differences between exudates and transudates (Table 2–1) is of considerable importance, and some understanding of the various chemical mediators of inflammation and their link with the complement system, and potentially with coagulation, should be appreciated. A good understanding of the processes of inflammation per se will permit evaluation of localized inflammatory response, with its own peculiarities, at any given site.

The various complications of the inflammatory response should be understood—the formation of pus, the abnormalities of the vasculature, and the production and manifestations of chronic inflammation that are related to the process of healing and repair. Although healing and repair are inevitable events after any injury in which inflammation has taken place, the degree of resolution with or without the formation of scar tissue depends on various factors, including complications. In addition, the relationship between acute inflammation, healing and repair, and chronic inflammation should be understood.

ACUTE INFLAMMATION

Basic Facts
Acute inflammation is an inevitable response of living vasculature to any injurious stimulus; a necessary precursor to healing and repair.

Cardinal Signs
- **Redness.** Increase in blood flow with stagnation and engorgement of blood vessels
- **Swelling.** Perivascular exudation of protein-rich fluid, the degree depending on the localization of the process and the severity of the response
- **Heat.** Variable, depending on increase in vascularity and proximity to body surfaces
- **Pain.** Complicated interaction of the physical and chemical components of the process
- **Loss of function.** Variable, depending on the site, severity, and extent

The process of acute inflammation is an extension and prolongation of the response to injury illustrated by the triple response of Lewis, as shown in Figure 2–1.

- **Chemical medication.** The controlled and regulated mechanism of enhancement of progressive incremental leukocytosis and phagocytosis
- **Systemic effects.** Include fever, increased erythrocyte sedimentation rate (ESR), and leukocytosis

Summary of Patterns and Modes of Acute Inflammation
- **Serous.** Collection of exudate in the simplest form of acute inflammation, often representing the earliest type of exudative process, with few leukocytes present
- **Fibrinous.** Exudation of fluid rich in fibrinogen, which on contact with body linings and surfaces deposits strands of fibrin
- **Catarrhal.** The process of inflammation involving mucus-secreting surfaces in which the fibrin and protein exudate is mixed with mucus
- **Suppurative.** Purulent exudate, containing fibrin and numerous neutrophils
- **Membranous (pseudomembranous).** A type of catarrhal inflammation with formation of a pseudomembrane exudate adherent to the underlying surface
- **Hemorrhagic.** Severe inflammatory exudate associated with damage to capillaries and consequent diapedesis and hemorrhage of red cells

TABLE 2–1. COMPARISON OF CHARACTERISTICS OF DIFFERENT TYPES OF EFFUSIONS (FLUIDS FROM BODY CAVITIES)

		Exudate due to inflammation		
	Transudate	Early or Mild	Moderate–Severe	Severe Suppurative
Protein	Low	Moderate	High, with fibrinogen	Very high, with fibrinogen and fibrin
Specific gravity	Low	Medium	High	High
Cellularity	Very low	Low	Moderate PMNs[a] a few monocytes	Many PMNs with toxic changes, dying and dead bacteria, RBCs[b] in some cases
Coagulability	No	Usually no	Yes	Variable, depending on enzymes released

[a] PMN, polymorphonuclear leukocyte.
[b] RBC, red blood cell.

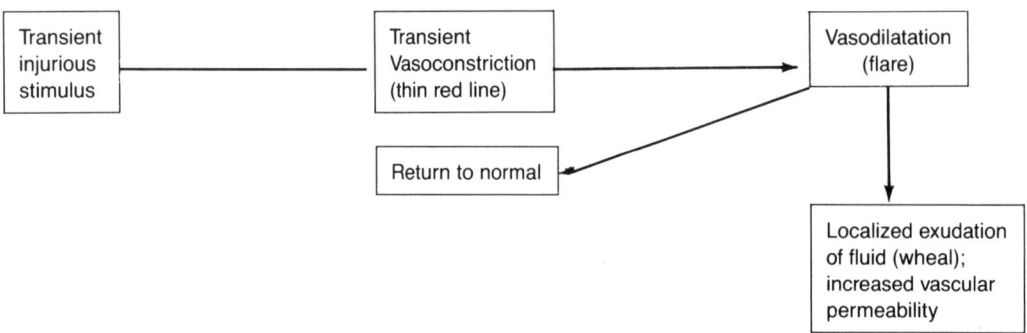

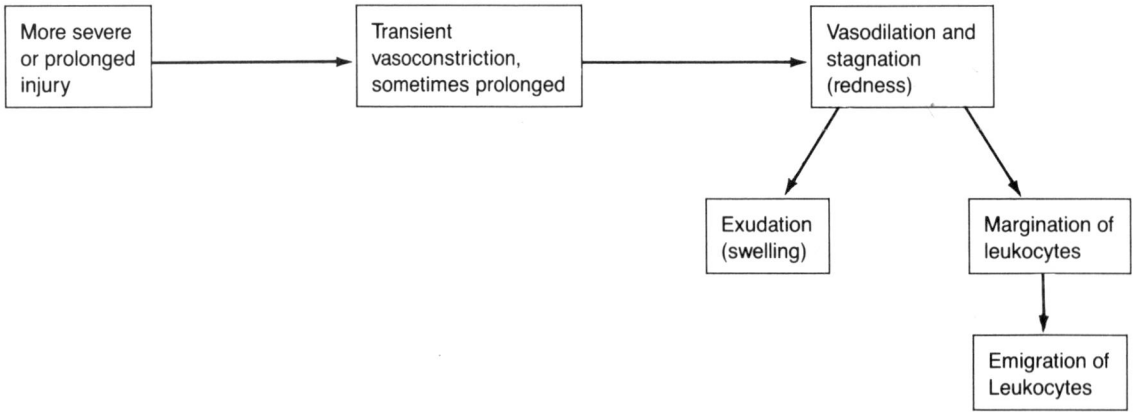

Figure 2–1. Triple response to injury (Lewis).

Further Modifications According to Type and Site

- **Effusions—body cavities.** Serous, fibrinous, purulent
- **Cellulitis—connective tissue.** If breakdown of tissue occurs, allows spread of exudate
- **Abscess.** Localized collection of dead and dying organisms and leukocytes with liquefaction necrosis of tissue
- **Ulceration.** Loss of continuity of surface of a tissue or organ, usually epithelial
- **Empyema.** A form of suppurative inflammation with collection of pus in the pleural cavity

Systemic Expression and Recognition in Acute Inflammation

- Fever
- Increased white blood cell count (leukocytosis) with increased proportion of band neutrophils (left shift)
- Elevated ESR
- Increased level of C-reactive protein in serum

CHRONIC INFLAMMATION

Basic Facts and Definitions
Chronic inflammation is a prolonged proliferative cellular response to injury, which may appear de novo or as a consequence of an initial acute inflammatory response (Figs 2–2, 2–3).

Characteristic Features
An accumulation in the tissues of lymphocytes, plasma cells, and monocytes and macrophages in various combinations. The end result is the production of collagen by stimulated fibroblasts. The appearance is often that of a combination of attempts at healing and repair in the presence of continued inflammatory response (Table 2–2).

Summary of Patterns and Modes of Chronic Inflammation

- **Chronic serous.** The persistence of serous exudation in a body cavity, usually with presence of varying numbers of lymphocytes
- **Chronic fibrous.** The continuation of injury and inflammatory response in the presence of attempts at healing, with resultant increased fibrosis, with variable numbers of lymphocytes
- **Chronic suppurative.** The response to large collections of pus (abscesses) that do not resolve or drain, present typically at the surrounding fibrous encapsulated areas
- **Granulomatous.** Characterized by the formation of granulomas, nodular proliferative lesions composed of monocytes forming sheets of cells (epithelioid histiocytes, some fusing to form multinucleated giant cells) surrounded by lymphocytes and fibroblasts, sometimes with areas of necrosis, such as caseation necrosis (as in tuberculosis) or gummatous necrosis (as in syphilis)

HEALING AND REPAIR

Definition
Healing is the replacement of lost tissue with collagen (scar tissue). This cannot be achieved by resolution or regeneration.

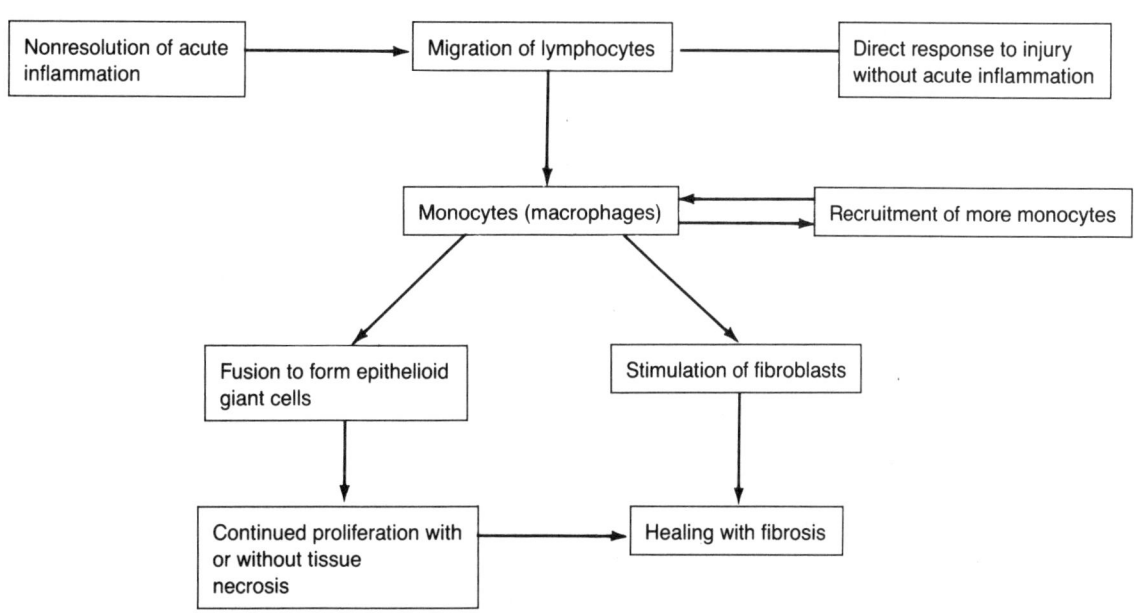

Figure 2–2. Schematic summary of sequential events in chronic inflammation.

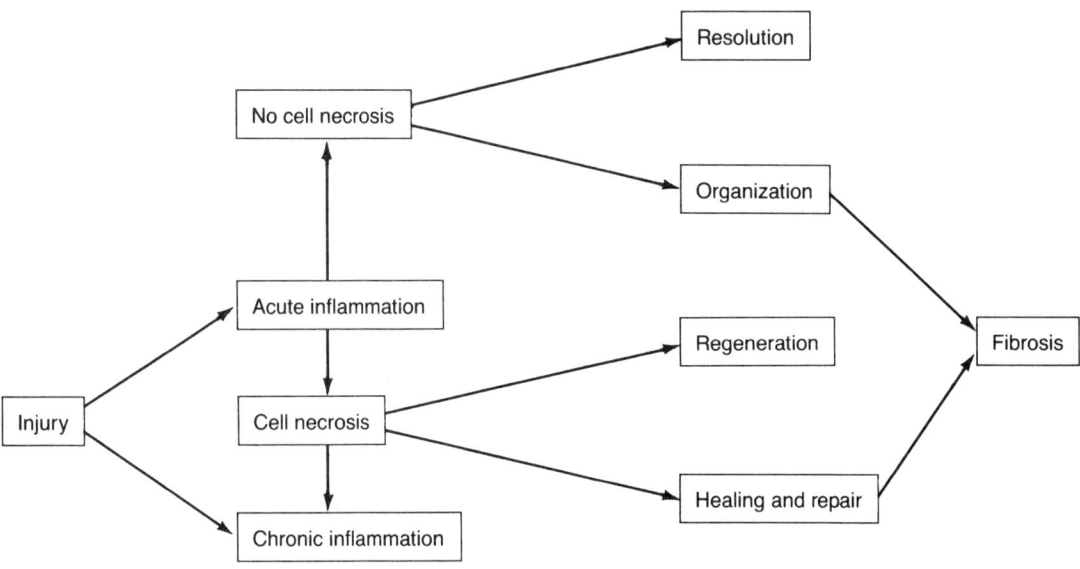

Figure 2-3. Summary of possible responses in injury.

TABLE 2-2. COMPARISON OF MAIN FEATURES OF ACUTE AND CHRONIC INFLAMMATION

	Acute Inflammation	Chronic Inflammation
Duration	Usually transient (hours to days), a rapid series of responses to injury (hours to days)	More slowly evolving, usually following acute inflammation that has not subsided (weeks to months)
Main tissue changes	Vascular response with increased permeability and exudation of proteinaceous fluid rich in fibrinogen	Increased collagen formation and proliferative vascular changes (eg, endarteritis obliterans in long-standing cases) not exudative
Characteristic cells	Polymorphonuclear leukocytes and occasional eosinophils (short-lived cells, recruited by chemotactic mediators)	Lymphocytes, monocytes, plasma cells, macrophages, including multinucleated giant cells (long-lived cells, recruited by chemotactic mediators)
Mediators	Sequential release of substances effecting vascular changes and chemotaxis	Products of inflammatory cells that further recruit other cells (including fibroblasts)
Usual outcome	Resolution with or without regeneration, or healing by repair with some fibrosis; may proceed to suppurative or chronic inflammation	Usually results in fibrosis and varying degrees of tissue replacement, rather than resolution or regeneration

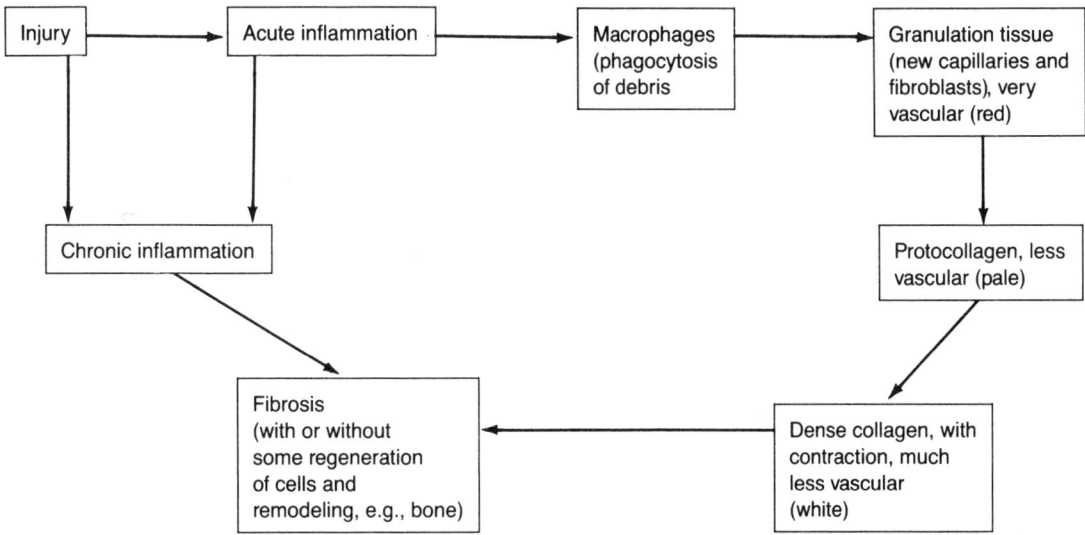

Figure 2-4. Summary of salient features and events in healing and repair.

Basic Facts

A summary of salient features and events in healing and repair is shown in Figure 2-4.

Summary of Patterns and Modes of Healing and Repair

- **Primary union.** Wound healing by first intention
- **Secondary union.** Wound healing by second intention

The basic events are the same, but the amount of granulation and, thus, scar tissue is greater in secondary union.

- **Fibrosis.** Fibrosis is the usual outcome of successful healing, but may result in lesions, some examples of which are shown in Table 2-3. In some severe cases, eventual superimposed calcification or ossification may occur

TABLE 2-3. EXAMPLES OF DETRIMENTAL ASPECTS OF HEALING BY FIBROSIS IN TISSUES AND ORGANS

Tissue or Organ	Detrimental Aspects of Healing
Lung	Peribronchial fibrosis and bronchiectasis Interstitial pulmonary fibrosis
Pleura	Pleural fibrosis and adhesions
Heart	Ventricular aneurysm formation due to replacement of necrotic myocardial wall by scar tissue
Pericardium	Constrictive pericarditis Pericardial adhesions
Peritoneum	Adhesions and fibrous bands (may cause intestinal obstruction)
Joints	Fibrosis, adhesions (may result in ankylosis)
Stomach	Fibrous stenosis of pylorus (following healing of gastric ulcer)
Brain	Gliosis (may cause hydrocephalus)

Questions

DIRECTIONS (Questions 1 through 50): Each of the numbered items or incomplete statements in this section is followed by answers or by completions of the statement. Select the ONE lettered answer or completion that is BEST in each case.

1. The cardinal sign(s) of acute inflammation is (are)

    (A) redness
    (B) swelling
    (C) heat
    (D) pain
    (E) all of the above

2. The manifestation of redness in acute inflammation is most likely the result of

    (A) edema of the tissues
    (B) margination of white blood cells in blood vessels
    (C) thrombosis of blood vessels
    (D) dilation of blood vessels
    (E) fibrin deposition in tissues

3. The cardinal sign of swelling associated with acute inflammation results from

    (A) arteriolar constriction
    (B) arteriolar dilatation
    (C) venous obstruction
    (D) outpouring of protein-rich fluid into tissues
    (E) proliferation of fibroblasts

4. Which of the following is most characteristic of a transudate?

    (A) increase in hydrostatic pressure
    (B) fluid with low specific gravity
    (C) fluid that does not clot on standing
    (D) little or no fibrinogen
    (E) all of the above

5. Which of the following is (are) most associated with an exudate?

    (A) altered vascular permeability
    (B) fluid with high specific gravity
    (C) fluid that clots on standing
    (D) presence of fibrinogen in the fluid
    (E) all of the above

6. Fluid removed from the peritoneal cavity has the following characteristics: high specific gravity, clots spontaneously on standing, turbid and yellow in color, contains fibrinogen. Which of the following does this most fully represent?

    (A) transudate caused by high portal vein pressure
    (B) transudate caused by right heart failure
    (C) exudate caused by peritoneal inflammation
    (D) fluid associated with starvation or protein loss
    (E) hemorrhage caused by ruptured aortic aneurysm

7. Pain associated with acute inflammation is thought to be caused by

    (A) pressure effects of exudate fluid
    (B) histamine
    (C) serotonin
    (D) kinins
    (E) all of the above

8. Which of the following are considered chemical mediators in the inflammatory response?

    (A) histamine
    (B) serotonin
    (C) kinins
    (D) prostaglandins
    (E) all of the above

9. Which type of inflammation commonly is characterized by collections of dead and dying polymorphs, dead and dying bacteria, and necrosis of tissue, all of which form a turbid or thick fluid in tissues?

    (A) catarrhal inflammation
    (B) phlegmonous inflammation
    (C) cellulitis
    (D) abscess formation
    (E) granulomatous inflammation

10. Which of the following events in acute inflammation occurs first?

    (A) phagocytosis
    (B) stasis
    (C) margination of leukocytes
    (D) emigration of leukocytes
    (E) lymphadenitis

11. Inflammation is best defined as

    (A) a reaction of the microcirculation in tissue to injury
    (B) a form of edema
    (C) chemotaxis of white cells to bacteria
    (D) a form of abnormal cell growth
    (E) cellular changes resulting in injury

12. Mediators of vascular permeability are thought to achieve their effects by

    (A) increased intravascular hydrostatic pressure
    (B) decreased intravascular hydrostatic pressure
    (C) contraction of endothelial cells and venules
    (D) dissolving capillary basement membrane
    (E) binding serum albumin to tissue

13. The immediate transient phase of vascular permeability in most types of tissue injury is mediated by

    (A) complement
    (B) Hageman factor
    (C) anaphylatoxin
    (D) histamine
    (E) serum albumin

14. Which of the following is most important in the early or exudative phase of acute inflammation?

    (A) lymphokines
    (B) leukotriene B4
    (C) histamine
    (D) prostaglandin D_2
    (E) interleukin I

15. Which chemical mediators of acute inflammation are NOT of cell membrane phospholipid origin?

    (A) leukotrienes
    (B) prostacyclins
    (C) histamine
    (D) prostaglandins
    (E) thromboxane

16. Which of the following substances is the best to REDUCE the effects of acute inflammation?

    (A) histamine
    (B) prostaglandin D_2
    (C) bradykinin
    (D) aspirin
    (E) eosinophilic chemotactic factor of anaphylaxis

17. Which cell types are most characteristic of tissue with acute inflammation?

    (A) plasma cells
    (B) foreign body giant cells
    (C) Langhans' giant cells
    (D) lymphocytes
    (E) polymorphonuclear leukocytes

18. Which cell types are most commonly seen in tissue undergoing chronic inflammation?

    (A) eosinophil leukocytes
    (B) mast cells
    (C) polymorphonuclear leukocytes
    (D) lymphocytes
    (E) platelets

19. The features, edema, presence of fibrin, dilatation, and vascular engorgement, are characteristic of

    (A) chronic inflammation
    (B) early acute inflammation
    (C) suppurative inflammation
    (D) late wound healing
    (E) granulation tissue

20. The features, monocytes, giant cells, fibroblasts, and lymphocytes, are characteristic of

    (A) acute inflammation
    (B) granulation tissue
    (C) wound healing
    (D) chronic inflammation
    (E) suppuration

21. The predominant cell seen in an inflammatory response to staphylococcal infection is

    (A) lymphocyte
    (B) monocyte
    (C) eosinophil
    (D) mast cell
    (E) polymorphonuclear leukocyte (PMN)

22. The predominant cell seen in inflammation resulting from viral infection is

    (A) lymphocyte
    (B) mast cell
    (C) eosinophil
    (D) polymorphonuclear leukocyte
    (E) plasma cell

23. The predominant cell seen in an inflammatory response to protozoal parasites is

    (A) lymphocyte
    (B) polymorphonuclear leukocyte
    (C) eosinophil
    (D) plasma cell
    (E) mast cell

24. The predominant cell seen in an inflammatory response to *Salmonella typhi* is

    (A) plasma cell
    (B) polymorphonuclear leukocyte
    (C) monocyte
    (D) mast cell
    (E) eosinophil

25. Granulation tissue is characterized by

    (A) proliferation of new capillaries with fibroblasts and new collagen formation
    (B) giant cells and fibroblasts
    (C) giant cells and lymphocytes
    (D) giant cells, plasma cells, and lymphocytes
    (E) neutrophils and necrotic tissue

26. The periphery of a hematoma is infiltrated by new capillaries, fibroblasts, and collagen; this process is described as

    (A) lysis of the clot
    (B) organization of the hematoma
    (C) recanalization
    (D) embolization
    (E) thrombosis

27. Which of the following are complications of acute inflammation?

    (A) suppuration
    (B) abscess formation
    (C) scar formation
    (D) organization with adhesions between mesothelial surfaces
    (E) all of the above

28. The proper formation of collagen in a healing wound requires

    (A) high levels of adrenocortical hormones
    (B) cholesterol
    (C) vitamin C
    (D) vitamin D
    (E) vitamin K

29. The modified form of granulation tissue containing new bone seen around a healing fracture is called

    (A) involucrum
    (B) laminated bone
    (C) fibrocartilage
    (D) callus
    (E) periosteal new bone

30. After injury with loss of cells, which of the following is (are) most likely to regenerate most completely?

    (A) neurons of the central nervous system (CNS)
    (B) liver parenchymal cells
    (C) skeletal muscle
    (D) heart muscle
    (E) neurons of the retina

31. Acute inflammatory exudate and saponification occur in

    (A) stromal fatty infiltration
    (B) fatty metamorphosis
    (C) enzymatic fat necrosis
    (D) fatty change
    (E) cloudy swelling

32. Which of the following best describe granulation tissue?

    (A) collagen and giant cells
    (B) fibroblasts and macrophages
    (C) capillary buds and fibroblasts
    (D) capillary buds and lymphocytes
    (E) fibroblasts and giant cells

33. Wound healing may be impaired by all EXCEPT

    (A) infection
    (B) close approximation of the edges of the wound
    (C) ascorbic acid deficiency
    (D) corticosteroid therapy
    (E) severe vascular disease in the same area

34. Healing of a clean surgical wound by first intention involves all EXCEPT

    (A) minimal tissue loss
    (B) absent or minimal bacterial infection
    (C) moderate granulation tissue
    (D) epidermal regeneration
    (E) exuberant scar tissue

35. Hemorrhage in an acute inflammatory reaction is best explained by

    (A) fibrinolysis
    (B) release of leukocyte lysosomal enzymes
    (C) damage to blood vessels
    (D) production of lymphokines
    (E) release of chemical mediators of vascular permeability

36. The development of tensile strength in a healing wound depends primarily on

    (A) contraction of the scar
    (B) collagen content of the wound
    (C) ascorbic acid content of the scar
    (D) appearance of capillary sprouts
    (E) level of keloidogenic factor

37. Of the following events that are part of the acute inflammatory response, which would occur THIRD in correct sequence?

(A) vascular dilatation
(B) local hemoconcentration and slowing of blood flow
(C) margination of white blood cells
(D) emigration of white blood cells
(E) increased vascular permeability

38. All are true statements about tuberculosis EXCEPT

    (A) the immune response may arrest the disease
    (B) the immune response causes tissue damage
    (C) lesions resulting from past infections often differ from those produced by subsequent organisms
    (D) humoral antibody coats the organisms and destroys them
    (E) cell-mediated immunity is the most important response

39. Which of the following substances is LEAST likely to produce vasodilatation and platelet aggregation at the same time?

    (A) leukotrienes
    (B) thromboxane
    (C) prostacyclins
    (D) prostaglandins
    (E) bradykinin

Questions 40 through 42. Refer to Figure 2–5.

40. The cells are

    (A) plasma cells
    (B) peritoneal macrophages
    (C) polymorphonuclear leukocytes (PMN)
    (D) lymphocytes
    (E) malignant cells

41. The most appropriate description of the condition is

    (A) chronic peritonitis
    (B) tuberculous peritonitis
    (C) carcinomatous peritonitis
    (D) acute peritonitis
    (E) ascites

42. The most likely source of the reaction is

    (A) ovarian carcinoma
    (B) carcinoma of the stomach
    (C) tuberculosis of the intestine
    (D) ruptured appendix
    (E) heart failure

Questions 43 through 45. Refer to Figure 2–6.

43. Which type of reaction does this represent?

    (A) acute suppurative inflammation
    (B) granulomatous inflammation

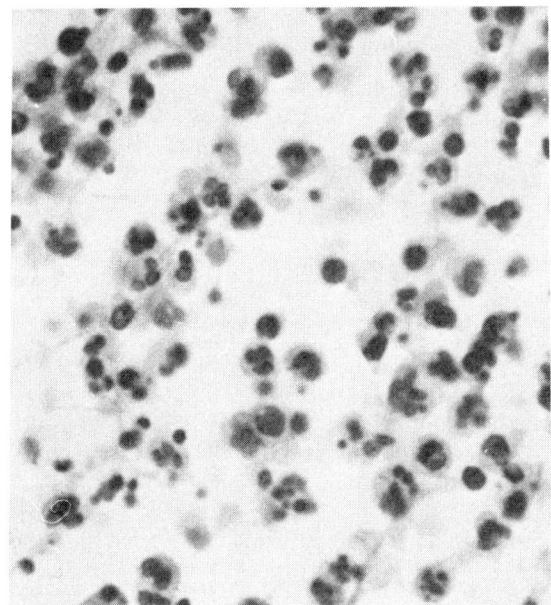

Figure 2–5. Microscopy of fluid removed from the peritoneal cavity.

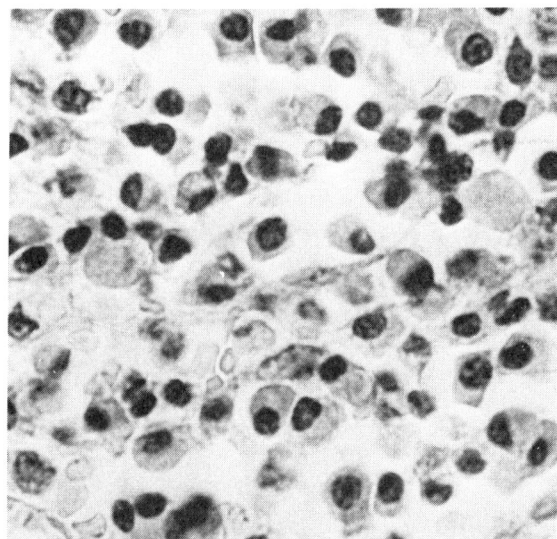

Figure 2–6. High-power photomicrograph of cells seen in a firm, painless skin nodule.

(C) subacute inflammation
(D) granulation tissue
(E) chronic inflammation

44. Which laboratory investigation is likely to be the most useful diagnostically?

    (A) gram stain
    (B) stain for acid-fast bacteria
    (C) examination of fresh tissue by darkfield illumination
    (D) stain for fungi
    (E) culture of tissue on blood agar

45. The most likely diagnosis, assuming one of the above techniques to be positive, is

(A) cat-scratch fever
(B) measles
(C) staphylococcal lymphadenitis
(D) tuberculosis lymphadenitis
(E) primary chancre of syphilis

Questions 46 through 48. Refer to Figure 2–7.

46. This most likely represents

(A) malignant lymphoma
(B) secondary carcinoma
(C) granulomatous inflammation
(D) acute inflammation
(E) healing by first intention

47. A stain for microorganisms would most likely show

(A) gram-positive cocci in clusters
(B) gram-negative bacilli
(C) Feulgen-positive inclusions for viruses
(D) acid-fast bacilli (Ziehl-Neelsen stain)
(E) malignant cells

48. What is the most likely diagnosis?

(A) tuberculosis
(B) syphilis
(C) gonorrhea
(D) *Trichinella spiralis*
(E) staphylococcal abscess

Questions 49 and 50. Refer to Figures 2–8 and 2–9.

49. The features are most consistent with

(A) acute inflammatory exudate
(B) chronic granulomatous inflammation
(C) scar tissue
(D) neoplastic transformation
(E) necrosis of tissue

50. Which is the best description of the features demonstrated?

(A) healing scar in skin
(B) tuberculosis of the skin
(C) abscess of the subcutaneous tissue
(D) foreign body granuloma of skin
(E) malignant melanoma of skin

DIRECTIONS (Questions 51 through 108): Each group of items in this section consists of lettered headings followed by a set of numbered words or phrases. For each numbered word or phrase, select the ONE lettered heading that is most closely associated with it. <u>Each lettered heading may be selected once, more than once, or not at all.</u>

Questions 51 through 56

(A) polymorphonuclear leukocytes (PMN)
(B) eosinophils
(C) basophils
(D) plasma cells
(E) monocytes

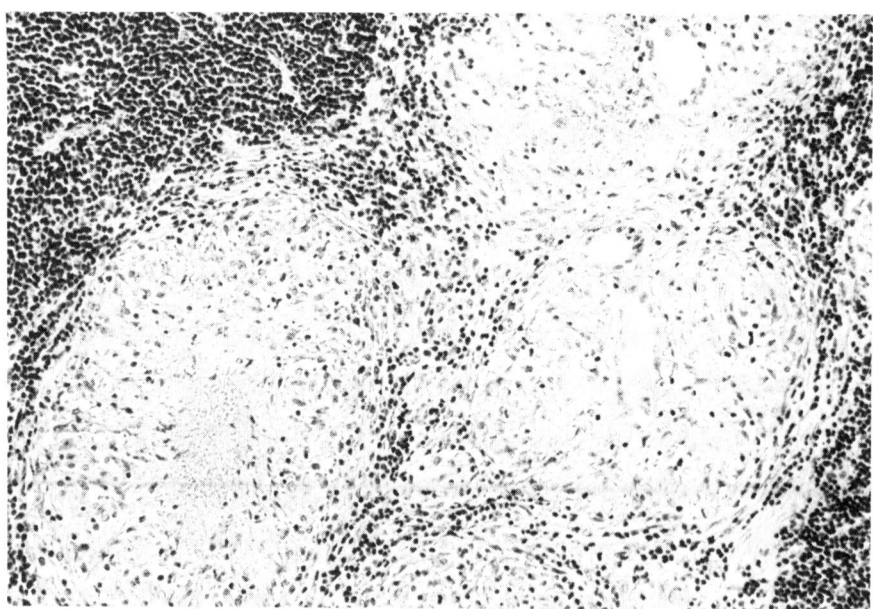

Figure 2–7. Photomicrograph of a lymph node biopsy.

Figure 2–8. Low-power magnification of skin.

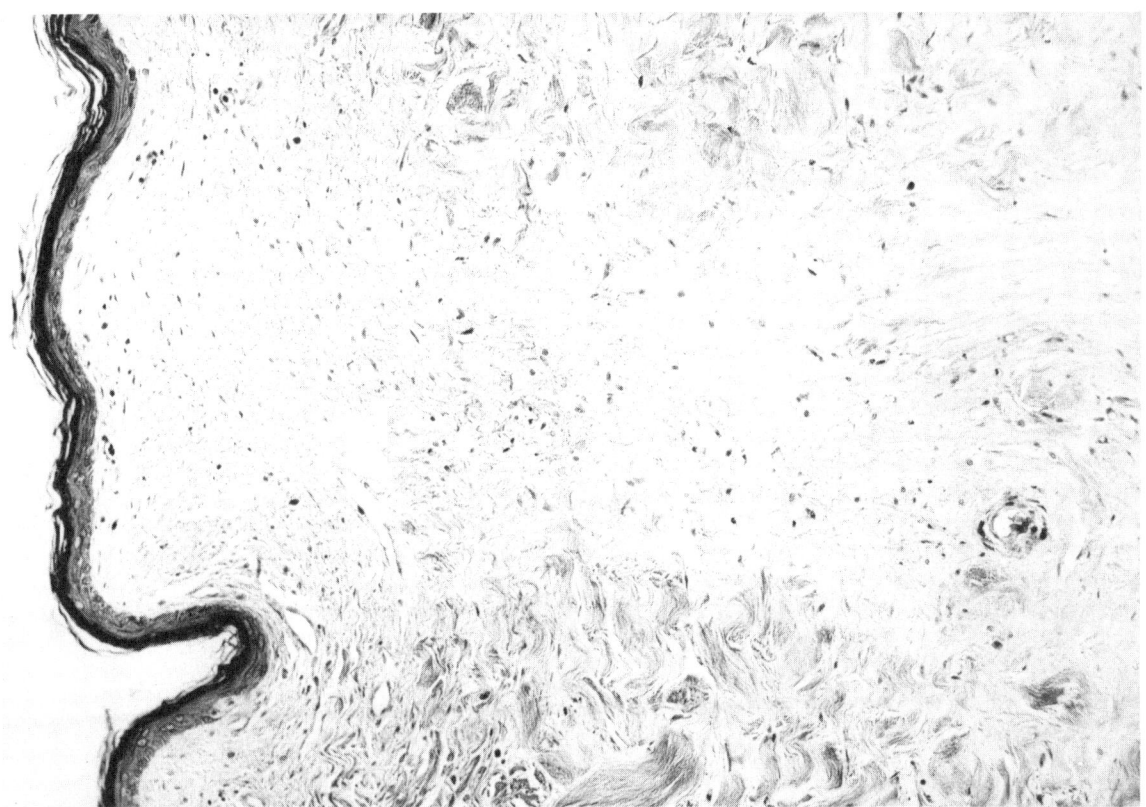

Figure 2–9. High-power magnification of skin.

51. Abscess formation

52. Immunoglobulin synthesis

53. Giant cell formation

54. Edge of recent infarct

55. Bronchial wall in asthmatic reactions

56. Response to parasites in tissue

Questions 57 and 58

(A) Hageman factor
(B) adenosine diphosphate (ADP)
(C) platelet factor III
(D) histamine
(E) bradykinin

57. Pain of acute inflammation

58. Platelet aggregation

Questions 59 through 62

(A) granulation tissue
(B) fibrous tissue
(C) fibrin
(D) amyloid
(E) fat necrosis

59. Early acute inflammation

60. Early phase of wound healing

61. Abscess

62. Chronic inflammation

Questions 63 through 67

(A) fibrin deposition on serosal surfaces
(B) fibrin and mucus on epithelial surfaces
(C) polymorphonuclear leukocytes (PMN) and localized necrosis of tissue
(D) protein-rich fluid in serous cavities
(E) diffuse PMN infiltration and fibrin throughout the tissue

63. Suppurative inflammation

64. Phlegmonous inflammation

65. Catarrhal inflammation

66. Fibrinous exudate

67. Serous exudate

Questions 68 through 71

(A) capillary buds and fibroblasts
(B) caseous necrosis and multinucleate giant cells
(C) central liquid necrotic debris mixed with neutrophils and bacteria
(D) collections of dense mature collagen
(E) coagulative necrosis and hemorrhage

68. Very early ischemic infarct

69. Abscess

70. Final stage of a healing wound

71. Response to tubercle bacilli

Questions 72 through 75

(A) fluid from pericardium with low specific gravity and no inflammatory cells
(B) fluid from pericardium with high specific gravity, many neutrophils, and bacteria
(C) fluid from pericardium with high specific gravity, multinucleate giant cells, epithelioid cells, and lymphocytes
(D) fluid from pericardium with mostly erythrocytes
(E) fluid from pericardium with high specific gravity, abundant fibrin, but only rare inflammatory cells

72. Purulent exudate following pericardial wound infection

73. Transudate of congestive heart failure

74. Exudate of tuberculous pericarditis

75. Exudate of rheumatic pericarditis

Questions 76 through 78

(A) ascorbic acid
(B) interleukin II
(C) chalones
(D) histamine
(E) fibronectin

76. Glycoprotein that is chemotactic for fibroblasts and stimulates capillary formation

77. Product of mature cells that inhibits cell division by neighboring cells

78. Vitamin that promotes proper collagen formation

Questions 79 through 82

(A) serotonin
(B) epidermal growth factor
(C) suppuration
(D) sarcoidosis
(E) eosinophilia

79. Promotes growth of surface epithelium in wounds

80. Delays proper wound healing

81. Associated with parasitic infections

82. Noncaseating granulomas

Questions 83 through 86

(A) plasminogen activator and factor VIII
(B) bradykinin
(C) aspirin
(D) myeloperoxidase
(E) leukotrienes

83. Oxidant with antimicrobial activity found in neutrophils

84. Strongly chemotactic for inflammatory cells

85. Synthesized by endothelial cells

86. Production of local pain

Questions 87 through 90

(A) C3a
(B) myofibroblasts
(C) prostacyclin
(D) plasma cells
(E) thromboxane A_2

87. Causes wound contraction

88. Anaphylatoxin

89. Inhibits platelet aggregation

90. Causes platelet aggregation

Questions 91 through 94

(A) margination of leukocytes
(B) fibrosis
(C) granulation tissue
(D) chronic foreign body inflammation
(E) histamine

91. Tissue reaction to nonabsorbable suture material

92. Early event in the acute inflammatory response

93. Chemical mediator of fluid exudation in acute inflammatory reaction

94. Fibroblasts and capillary buds

Questions 95 through 98

(A) collagen
(B) procollagenase
(C) laminin
(D) fibroblast growth factors
(E) elastin

95. Basement membrane glycoprotein

96. Major component of elastic tissue

97. Mitogenic and angiogenic

98. Crosslinking increases wound tensile strength

Questions 99 through 105

(A) hyperacute inflammation
(B) acute inflammation
(C) chronic inflammation
(D) noninflammatory fibrosis
(E) noncaseating granulomatous inflammation
(F) caseating granulomatous inflammation
(G) eosinophilic inflammation
(H) foreign body inflammation

99. A 38-year-old female is found to have bilateral hilar adenopathy on chest x-rays. She complains of a 2-month history of fever, fatigue, and increasing dyspnea. Lymphadenopathy is found on physical examination. A biopsy of one of her enlarged lymph nodes shows sarcoidosis. What pattern of inflammation did the lymph node demonstrate?

100. A 67-year-old male has been experiencing low grade fever, chest pains, cough, and bloody phlegm for about 6 weeks. A sputum sample is sent to the laboratory for examination. The sputum is found to contain numerous acid-fast bacilli. What pattern of inflammation is characteristic of this infectious disease?

101. A 45-year-old white female has noticed recent onset of symmetric swelling of the small joints of her hand, particularly in the morning. These joints are also painful and stiff. About 6 months later her knee joint also becomes swollen and painful. An arthroscopic examination of the joint finds abundant hypertrophic synovium with pannus formation. Shavings of the synovium examined pathologically display the typical histologic features of rheumatoid arthritis. What pattern of inflammation was present in the synovial tissue?

102. A 19-year-old male develops fever, right lower quadrant abdominal pain, and diarrhea. His peripheral leukocyte count is increased with many young band neutrophils and early toxic granulation. Surgery is performed to remove the appendix. At the time of surgery the appendix is tense, engorged with luminal purulent material, and has serosal fibrinous exudates. An obstructing fecalith is present at the appendiceal origin. What pattern of inflammation is the appendix most likely to display?

103. A 56-year-old female has a small 0.7 cm carcinoma of the left breast. She elects to have a lumpectomy excision followed by radiation therapy to the lumpectomy site. Five years later there is no evidence of recurrent or metastatic breast carcinoma. Her radiation site, however, is now sunken and hard. A biopsy of this tissue shows radiation damage and hypertrophic scar formation. What term best characterizes the radiation site changes?

104. A 14-year-old African boy has numerous lesions on his face. At first the skin lesions were only erythematous. But over the last 2 months he has noticed the center of these lesions to become hypopigmented and depressed. A biopsy of one of these skin lesions demonstrates tuberculoid leprosy. What pattern of inflammation was present on the biopsy?

105. At autopsy a 78-year-old male is found to have an impacted stone in his common bile duct and multiple hepatic abscesses. Pyogenic bacteria are cultured from the abscesses. What pattern of inflammation do the hepatic abscesses display?

106. A patient with a temperature of 101°F, headache, and stiff neck has the following laboratory findings: total leukocyte count of 18,000/mm³ (18 × 10⁹/L) with 70% segmented neutrophils, 18% bands, 10% lymphocytes, and 2% monocytes; cerebrospinal fluid (CSF) turbid, glucose 35 mg/dl, protein 115 mg/dl, and 500 neutrophils/mm³ (75% segmented, 25% bands); blood glucose 110 mg/dl. The most likely diagnosis is

(A) chronic lymphocytic meningitis
(B) granulomatous meningitis (tuberculous or cryptococcal)
(C) subarachnoid hemorrhage
(D) acute suppurative meningitis
(E) pituitary gland carcinoma

107. In the patient in Question 106, which is the most likely associated finding?

(A) pulmonary tuberculosis
(B) recent or current viral pneumonia
(C) middle cerebral artery aneurysm
(D) suppurative otitis media
(E) diabetes insipidus

108. In the patient in Question 106, which complication is most likely?

(A) disseminated miliary tuberculosis
(B) intracerebral hemorrhage
(C) severe viremia
(D) brain abscess
(E) hyponatremia

Answers and Explanations

1. **(E)** This question is meant to establish the well-known basic cardinal signs of acute inflammation, which should be known by all students and is a fundamental question of factual knowledge. This is based on the writings of Celsus in the first century AD: "Rubor et tumor cum calore delore"—redness, swelling, heat, and pain being the manifestations of acute inflammation. See Figure 2–1 for the sequences of events and their relationships to other aspects of inflammation. *(1:35)*

2. **(D)** The redness in the early phase of acute inflammation and in some of the later phases is basically a vascular phenomenon. In fact, acute inflammation is primarily a response of the small blood vessels to injury whatever the injury may be. (Figs 2–1, 2–10, and 2–11). Although edema of the tissue is also a manifestation of acute inflammation, it is not the cause of the redness, nor is margination of the white cells or fibrin deposition, which comes later in the event. Thrombosis of blood vessels, although it may cause a dusky discoloration of the skin, is a very late and severe complication of inflammation. *(1:35)*

3. **(D)** The outpouring of protein-rich fluid into the tissue is the main cause of the swelling associated with acute inflammation. Although swelling is related to some of the other events described, it is the actual formation of the fluid that causes the swelling. In Figure 2–4, the relationship of this particular aspect to the other events in the manifestations of acute inflammation can be seen. Although the proliferation of fibroblasts may, of course, produce some swelling, this is usually a much later complication of acute inflammation and more related to chronic inflammatory changes (Table 2–2). *(2:40–45)*

4. **(E)**

5. **(E)**

4 and 5. All of the events in Question 4 describe the hydrostatic pressure related to the production of fluid with low specific gravity that does not clot on standing because it has no fibrinogen. It is the characteristic description of a transiodate. In comparison, Question 5 describes the characteristic features of an exudate in which there is altered vascular permeability. The fluid has a high specific gravity and clots on standing because it does contain fibrinogen. Table 2–1 summarizes the main features that distinguish transudates and exudates of different degrees of severity and summarizes the main features. *(5:37)*

6. **(C)** This is another way of obtaining the information given in Questions 4 and 5; Table 2–1 summarizes the main distinguishing features, which are high protein, medium to high specific gravity, and coagulability because of the presence of fibrinogen, that characterize an exudate. Vascular changes have taken place rather than there being a transudate in which back pressure with no altered vascular permeability produces a different type of fluid. *(5:37)*

7. **(E)** The sensation of pain associated with acute inflammation is a complex phenomenon and can be produced in varying degrees by any of the mechanisms or substances mentioned. The combination of them, of course, makes the pain more severe, and the anatomic site also is of importance. For instance, a minor degree of inflammation in the subcutaneous tissue in the back of the neck will be more painful than a more extensive inflammation in the skin of the back of the hand, since the tissue tension in these two sites adds another element to the interaction. *(2:52–60)*

8. **(E)** Histamines, serotonin, the kinins, and the prostaglandins are all considered to be chemical mediators of acute inflammation. Their relative importance in different stages and their effects on different components of the inflammatory response can be seen in Figure 2–12. Some of the mediators occur early in the vascular changes of acute inflammation, and others occur both early and late and act as an amplifying system to maintain the reaction in

case the original stimulus is short-lived. Sometimes, of course, this can be a disadvantage as well as an advantage. *(1:43)*

9. **(D)** The accumulation of dead and dying polymorphs or neutrophils, dead and dying bacteria, and liquefaction necrosis of tissue is the characteristic description of suppurative inflammation. If found in a localized area, it is described as an abscess. Catarrhal inflammation may produce some of the features, including the neutrophils, and so can cellulitis, but the formation of an abscess requires all of these combined in a localized, encapsulated form. Granulomatous inflammation is considerably different and consists of a dry cellular proliferation of fibroblasts, epithelioid cells, and fibroblasts. The distinction between these two manifestations of acute and chronic inflammation can be seen in Table 2–2. *(2:69)*

10. **(B)** Although all of the events occur in acute inflammation, this particular sequence is an important distinction. It is the stasis of flow that leads to the margination of leukocytes, which leads to their emigration through the vessel wall, which results in phagocytosis. The term "lymphadenitis" is merely a description of inflammation in general in a lymph node and is in that sense an irrelevant component answer. The sequential events in acute inflammation are summarized in Figure 2–1 and outlined in the introductory pages of this chapter. *(2:40–51)*

11. **(A)** The best definition of inflammation is a reaction of the microcirculation in tissue to injury. Part of this, of course, consists of edema, chemotaxis, and some cellular changes resulting from injury. Abnormal cell growth usually is associated with neoplastic change, although some reaction may occur as a result of chronic inflammation. *(5:36)*

12. **(C)** The mediators of vascular permeability may act at different stages in the inflammatory response. They do not in and of themselves particularly increase intravascular hydrostatic pressure except by secondary events. The dissolution of the capillary basement membrane would be a very serious and irreparable injury and may occur as a complication but not as a fundamental mechanism. The binding of serum albumin into tissue is not a particularly important component. Contraction of endothelial cells, however, does open the otherwise potential spaces that have been shown to exist as gaps between endothelial cells, resulting in alterations in vascular permeability. *(3:71–73)*

13. **(D)** Histamine is a very important substance in the transient aspects of early acute inflammation but

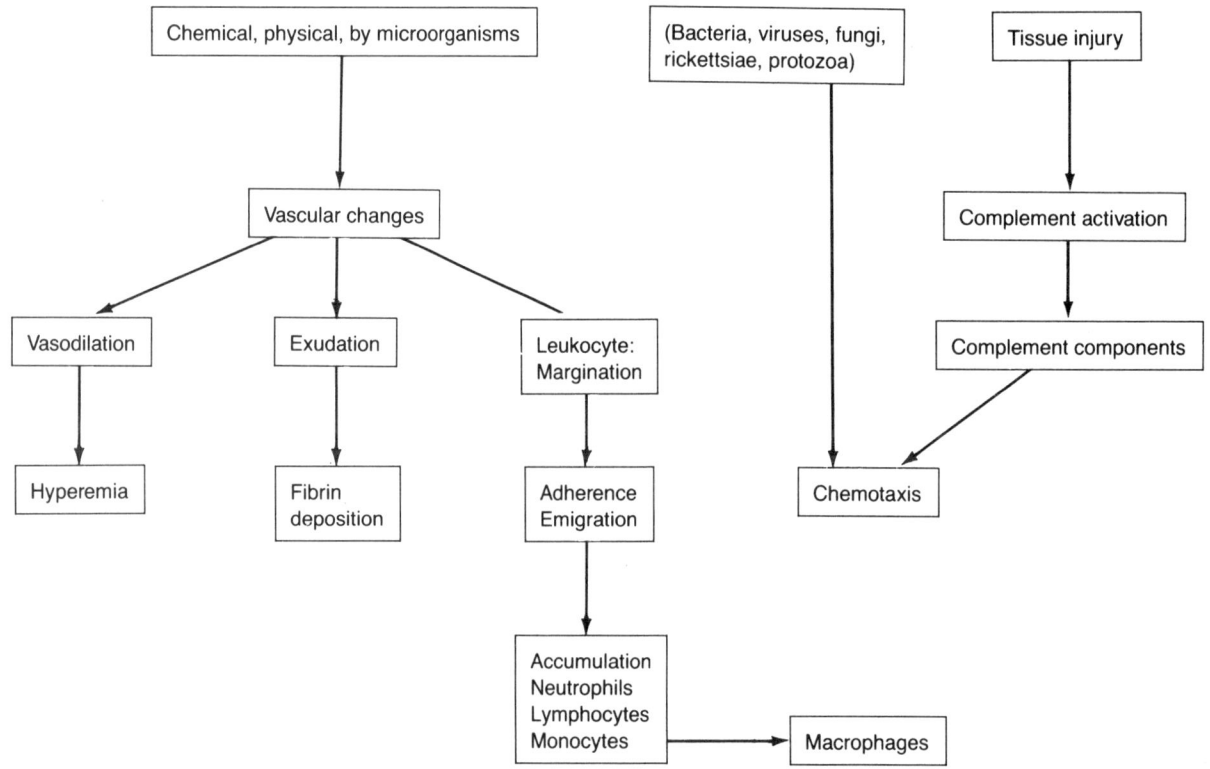

Figure 2–10. Schematic summary of events following injury.

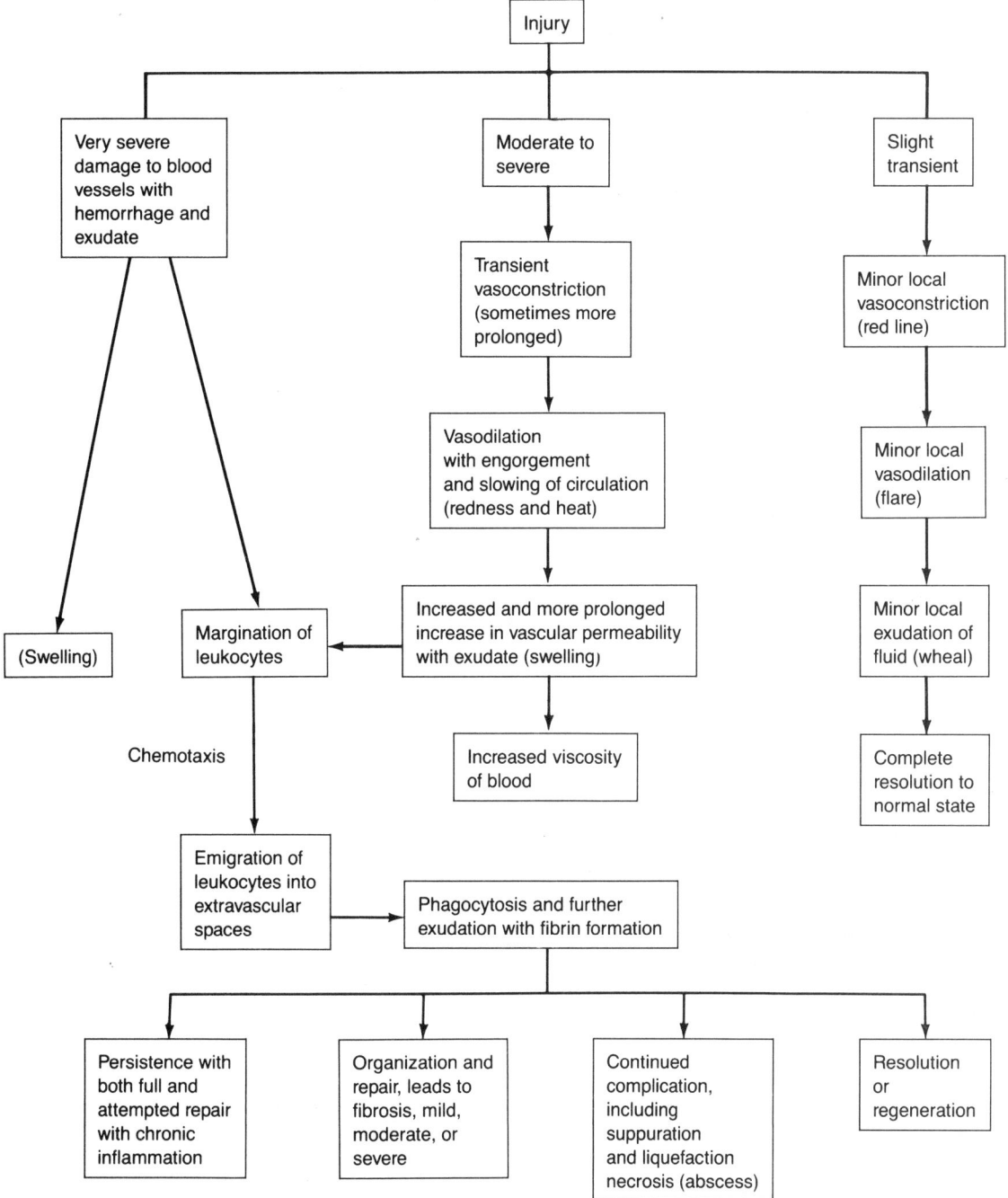

Figure 2–11. Possible sequences following tissue injury.

may act at different stages. All of the others mentioned have some effect in vascular permeability but at different stages and by different mechanisms. Histamine is by far the most important in the transient, immediate phase. This is seen also in Figures 2–12 and 2–13, which show the sequential release of chemical mediators. *(1:42)*

14. **(C)** Histamine is the most important early chemical mediator in the exudative or fluid phase of acute inflammation. The lymphokines, leukotriene B4, the prostaglandins, and interleukin I occur at different stages of the inflammatory response. Many of them act in the more cellular phases, late in chronic inflammation (Figs 2–12 and 2–13). *(1:42)*

15. **(C)** All of the other mediators mentioned are products of cell membrane phospholipid via arachidonic acid, whereas histamine is liberated from mast cells and is of a different composition and origin.

Mediators of Exudative Phase

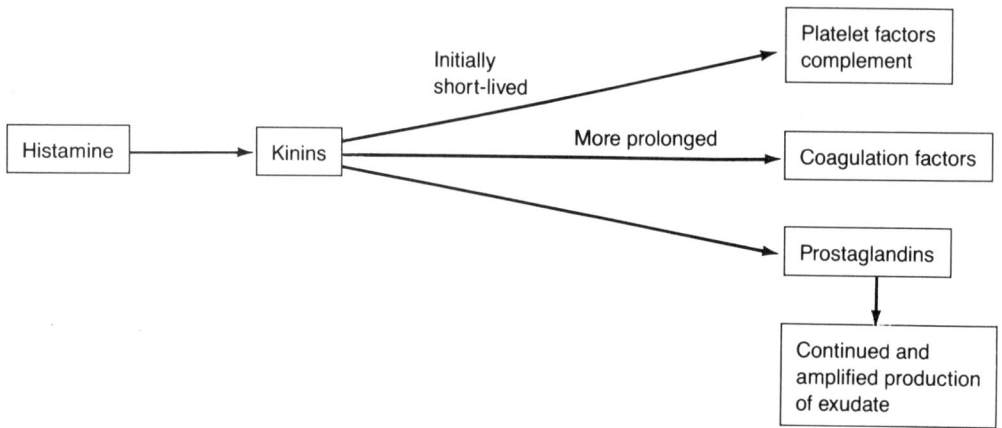

Mediators of Cellular Phase

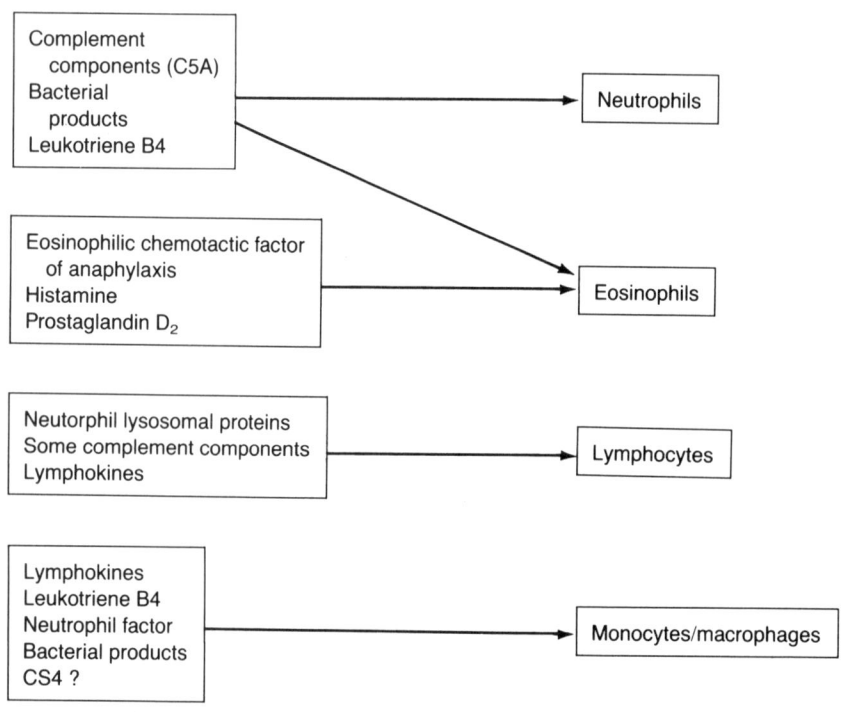

Figure 2-12. Chemical mediators of inflammation (sequential release).

Figure 2–13 is a simplified schematic of the origin of some of the substances mentioned from cell membrane phospholipids via the arachidonic acid pathway. *(2:52–60)*

16. **(D)** Aspirin is believed to have an effect via a number of complex interactions, including prostaglandins and their synthesis and action and other less well-understood pathways in acute inflammation. All of the other substances mentioned are, in fact, components of the chemical mediators of acute inflammation and, therefore, would hardly be used in the reduction of their effects. *(1:43)*

17. **(E)** The characteristic cell in acute inflammation is the polymorphonuclear leukocyte, which is seen in most forms of acute inflammation, although the amounts may be modified by either positive or negative chemotaxis later in the events. The plasma cell, foreign body giant cell, Langhans' giant cell, and lymphocytes are all characteristic of subacute and chronic inflammation (Table 2–2). *(4:9)*

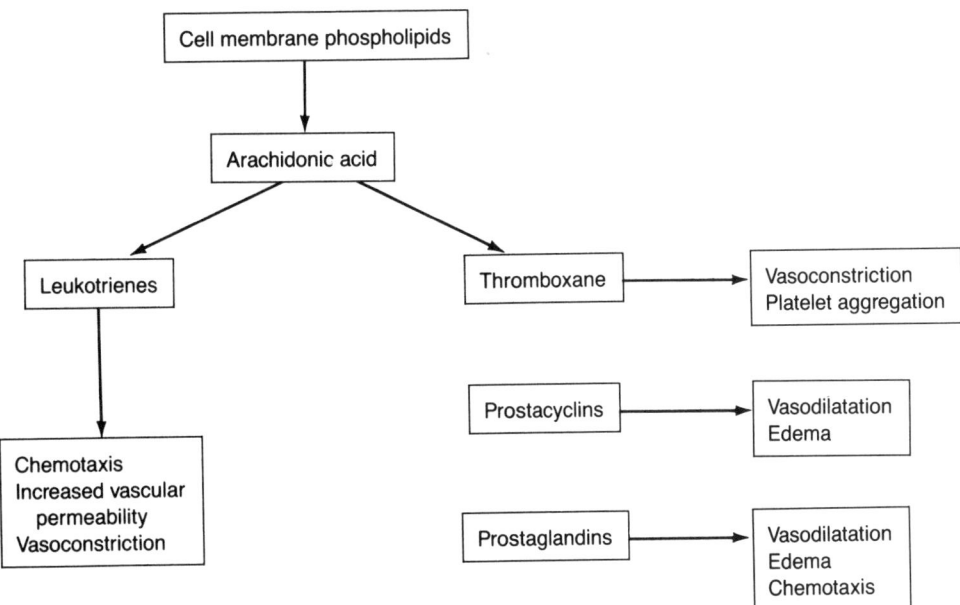

Figure 2-13. Simplified schema of role of phospholipids and their products as mediators of acute inflammation.

18. **(D)** The lymphocyte and monocyte series are the characteristic cells seen in more prolonged forms of inflammation, that is, chronic inflammation. The eosinophils and the polymorphonuclear leukocytes usually are associated with early or acute inflammatory responses. The mast cell is involved in liberating histamine in early inflammation. The platelets, although they may aggregate, are not characteristic of either. *(3:89–91)*

19. **(B)** Edema, fibrin, dilatation, and vascular engorgement are the characteristic manifestations of tissue responding to acute injury and are the underlying mechanisms for the cardinal signs of acute inflammation of redness, swelling, and heat. Chronic inflammation is a more cellular and much less vascular phenomenon (Table 2–2). Suppurative inflammation is characterized by destruction of tissue and an increase in polymorphonuclear leukocytes. Wound healing in the later stages would consist largely of a vascular connective tissue and granulation tissue. It is distinguished by its composition of newly-formed blood vessels and fibroblasts. These characteristic differences are summarized in Figure 2–2 and in the introduction to this chapter. *(4:37)*

20. **(D)** This is the reverse of Question 19. In this case, the features of monocytes, giant cells, fibroblasts, and lymphocytes are the highly cellular and relatively avascular components that occur late in response to injury and are characteristic of chronic inflammation (Table 2–2). *(4:37)*

21. **(E)** Staphylococci are pyogenic bacteria; that is, they are pus producing. To produce pus, there must be some form of chemical attraction to the characteristic cell of acute suppurative inflammation that produces pus, namely, the PMN. Characteristic examples of such infections include boils, carbuncles, and abscesses. Although lymphocytes and monocytes may play a minor role in the outer limits and in the later stages of unresolved pyogenic infections of this type, and eosinophils occasionally may accompany PMNs, it is the PMNs that are the characteristic cell in this type of inflammation and its suppurative complication. *(3:87)*

22. **(A)** Viral damage is usually at the cellular level, although in very early reactions to viral infections, an acute inflammatory response may occur. The more characteristic and prolonged viral infections usually result in a form of chronic inflammation, and since the lymphocyte is the characteristic cell of chronic inflammation, it is the one most likely to be seen. *(4:37)*

23. **(C)** Various types of protozoal proteins appear to stimulate chemotaxis of eosinophil leukocytes more than other cells. Although this is not universal, it is frequent enough to be of characteristic importance diagnostically. *(4:37)*

24. **(C)** For reasons not entirely understood, species of *Salmonella*, particularly *Salmonella typhi*, produce a negative chemotaxis toward neutrophils or polymorphonuclear leukocytes (PMN) and eosinophils.

Therefore, the predominant cell, despite acute inflammation, is the monocyte rather than the usual PMN. In many other respects, acute inflammation of typhoid is similar to that seen in other acute inflammatory situations, and only rarely do the lymphocyte and fibrosis become a characteristic response. The increase in monocytes in this form of inflammation is seen not only at the site of the lesion but also in the draining lymph nodes. *(5:359–362)*

25. **(A)** Granulation tissue is the first phase of the healing process at the end of acute inflammation. New capillaries proliferate in the tissue, with fibroblasts and the first laying down of new collagen, which eventually will become largely avascular scar tissue. It is not to be confused with granulomatous inflammation or granuloma, which is the hallmark of a form of chronic inflammation in which healing and the stimulation for damage occur concurrently. Granulation tissue is a normal response in the normal healing process (Table 2–3). *(2:73–74)*

26. **(B)** This is a corollary to Question 25. New capillaries, fibroblasts, and collagen describe granulation tissue occurring at the periphery of a hematoma or collection of blood. Although lysis of the blood clot may occur as a result, the actual formation of this response is known as organization and is an attempt to heal the area and fill the defect with collagen or scar tissue. If this occurs within a blood vessel, recanalization of the occluded lumen may take place subsequently and embolization may be an eventual complication. Infarction may be related to the formation of material in the lumen but has nothing to do with the process described. *(2:73–74)*

27. **(E)** All these complications may occur following acute inflammation. The more obvious one of suppuration is an indication of breakdown of tissue, with bacterial lysosomal enzyme release, dead and dying neutrophils, and possibly the organisms that caused the inflammation. Abscess formation may occur as a subsequent complication of such suppuration. Dense scar tissue may complicate this or less complicated forms of acute inflammation, and a scar often may be the ultimate complication of acute inflammation that does not resolve. Organization with adhesions between these epithelial surfaces is merely a local anatomic setting in which such scar tissue may occur, binding fine delicate membranes together (Table 2–3 and Fig 2–11). *(3:84–89)*

28. **(C)** Vitamin C is particularly important in the formation of procollagen in the early form of wound healing. This was known in the days when scurvy was a prevalent disease and wounds did not heal correctly or in a timely fashion. *(5:70–71)*

29. **(D)** The term "callus" describes the modified and specialized form of granulation tissue that occurs in a healing bone. It is essentially the same phenomenon as granulation tissue, with the formation of new capillaries and fibroblasts and the laying down of collagen but with the rapid conversion of the ground substance and collagen to bone by osteoblasts. The remodeling by osteoblasts makes this particular form of granulation tissue so characteristic of bone. Involucrum is dead bone that is associated with inflammation that does not lead to correct resolution and healing. Laminated bone is a description of normal bone. Fibrocartilage is as stated. Periosteal new bone, although it may form as a result of a healing fracture, is a later remodeling manifestation and is not the callus described. *(4:69)*

30. **(B)** Liver parenchymal cells are the best of the cells mentioned in regenerative capabilities. Although skeletal muscle may show some attempt at regeneration, in keeping with heart muscle and neurons, this is a very limited capacity. Neurons or the CNS have no such regenerative capacity. *(5:89–95)*

31. **(C)** The word "saponification" means the breakdown of fat, with soap formation in the tissues. Therefore, of all possible changes, the most likely one is fat necrosis. When this occurs, it inevitably produces an acute inflammatory response, and the combination of the two is best seen in enzymatic fat necrosis. A good example of this is acute pancreatitis, in which enzymes from the damaged pancreas destroy the fat in the surrounding tissue, causing saponification and resulting in an acute inflammatory response. *(4:103)*

32. **(C)** The combination of new capillary buds and fibroblasts is the hallmark of granulation tissue. The presence of collagen and giant cells is more in keeping with a prolonged response, as is seen in chronic inflammation. Similarly, fibroblasts and macrophages are seen in the later stages of chronic inflammation or in the stage before development of true healing. Capillary buds and lymphocytes would be seen when chronic inflammation was persisting and, therefore, healing was not adequate. Sometimes, this can be a mixed picture. Fibroblasts and giant cells are seen more typically in chronic granulomatous inflammation (Table 2–2 and Fig 2–12). *(2:73–76)*

33. **(B)** Close approximation of the edges of a wound is clearly the best way in which to insure that healing will occur by the minimum amount of replacement of tissue with granulation tissue and fibrosis. This

is sometimes referred to as "healing by first intention." Infection, ascorbic acid deficiency, corticosteroid therapy, and vascular disease in the same area are characteristic complications that would not allow the healing process to occur smoothly and swiftly. *(2:82–84)*

34. **(E)** This is related to Question 33. Exuberant scar tissue is not characteristic of healing by first intention, in which an approximated wound produces the minimum amount of collagen necessary to hold the wound together. It is seen typically in more advanced wounds by second intention and healing by granulation, since much more fibrous tissue is produced. All of the other events listed are factors that are seen characteristically in an uncomplicated wound healing by first intention. *(2:82–84)*

35. **(C)** Hemorrhagic inflammatory response usually results in a severe and more violent form of inflammation in which the small blood vessels are damaged in the inflammatory response (Figs 2–1 and 2–11). *(3:70–71)*

36. **(B)** It is the amount of collagen in a wound that determines the tensile strength. The contractility of the wound should not be confused with this since it can occur at several stages and is not entirely dependent on collagen but on other factors. The ascorbic acid content of the scar does not appear to be significant, since ascorbic acid availability in the body in general is adequate. The appearance of capillary sprouts merely indicates the early stages of the production of such a scar, and the level of substance that may produce keloid is not known and does not appear to have anything to do with the tensile strength of the developing scar tissue. *(5:69–73)*

37. **(B)** The correct order of the events in acute inflammation are vascular dilatation, increased vascular permeability, local hemoconcentration and slowing of blood, margination of white cells, and emigration of white cells (Figs 2–1 and 2–11). *(1:45)*

38. **(D)** The humoral immune response in the body's reaction to the tubercle bacillus is characteristically that of a chronic cellular granulomatous reaction, and, therefore, humoral or serum antibody is very unlikely to be seen. In fact, it plays a minor role in tuberculosis except in the very early stages. All of the other events or considerations are correct and typify this type of reaction. *(2:373–380)*

39. **(B)** Thromboxane is a by-product of arachidonic acid, which is a potent vasoconstrictor as well as a platelet aggregator and would, therefore, not produce vasodilatation. The leukotrienes produce vasoconstriction but not platelet aggregation. Prostacyclins cause vasodilatation, and most of the prostaglandins cause vasodilatation with edema and chemotaxis. Bradykinin is also a vasodilator. Some of the mechanisms and effects of these substances are summarized in Figures 2–12, 2–13, and 2–14. *(1:43)*

40. **(C)** The cells have the multilobe structure and size of a PMN. This is the typical cell seen in acute inflammation. *(4:17)*

41. **(D)** The presence of polymorphonuclear leukocytes (PMN) in peritoneal fluid is typical of an acute inflammatory response of the suppurative type, as seen in acute peritonitis. In ascites, although PMNs may be present, they are not necessarily characteristic. In chronic peritonitis, the lymphocytes are the predominant cell, with perhaps some monocytes. In tuberculous peritonitis, lymphocytes and monocytes are seen. In carcinomatous peritonitis, in some instances, PMNs may be present, but again, peritoneal macrophages also would be very strongly represented. *(4:37)*

42. **(D)** If one assumes that this is acute peritonitis and that these are polymorphonuclear leukocytes (PMN), rupture of the appendix would be by far the most common form of acute inflammation with suppuration occurring in the peritoneal cavity. *(4:10–19)*

43. **(C)** The cells have eccentric nuclei of a cartwheel variety, and their shape and size are characteristic of plasma cells. The plasma cell is seen most frequently in subacute or in some early chronic inflammation but is not characteristic of acute suppurative inflammation. *(4:37–43)*

44. **(C)** A firm painless skin nodule consisting entirely of plasma cells is a highly characteristic response to a very few types of organisms, and the primary chancre of syphilis is the most common. Darkfield illumination for the presence of live spirochetes is more valuable than are gram stains, acid-fast stains, or stains for fungi or malignant cells. *(4:37–43)*

45. **(E)** The only reasonable positive finding by darkfield illumination in a painless skin nodule containing plasma cells is spirochetes of syphilis and, therefore, the alternative are much less likely. *(4:37–43)*

46. **(C)** Figure 2–7 shows a collection of cells in a background of lymphocytes. The cells form tubercles or granulomas in which giant cells can be seen. This is typical of a granulomatous form of chronic inflammation. *(2:373–374)*

47. **(D)** Of the alternatives presented, a giant cell granulomatous lesion in a lymph node is not typical of a

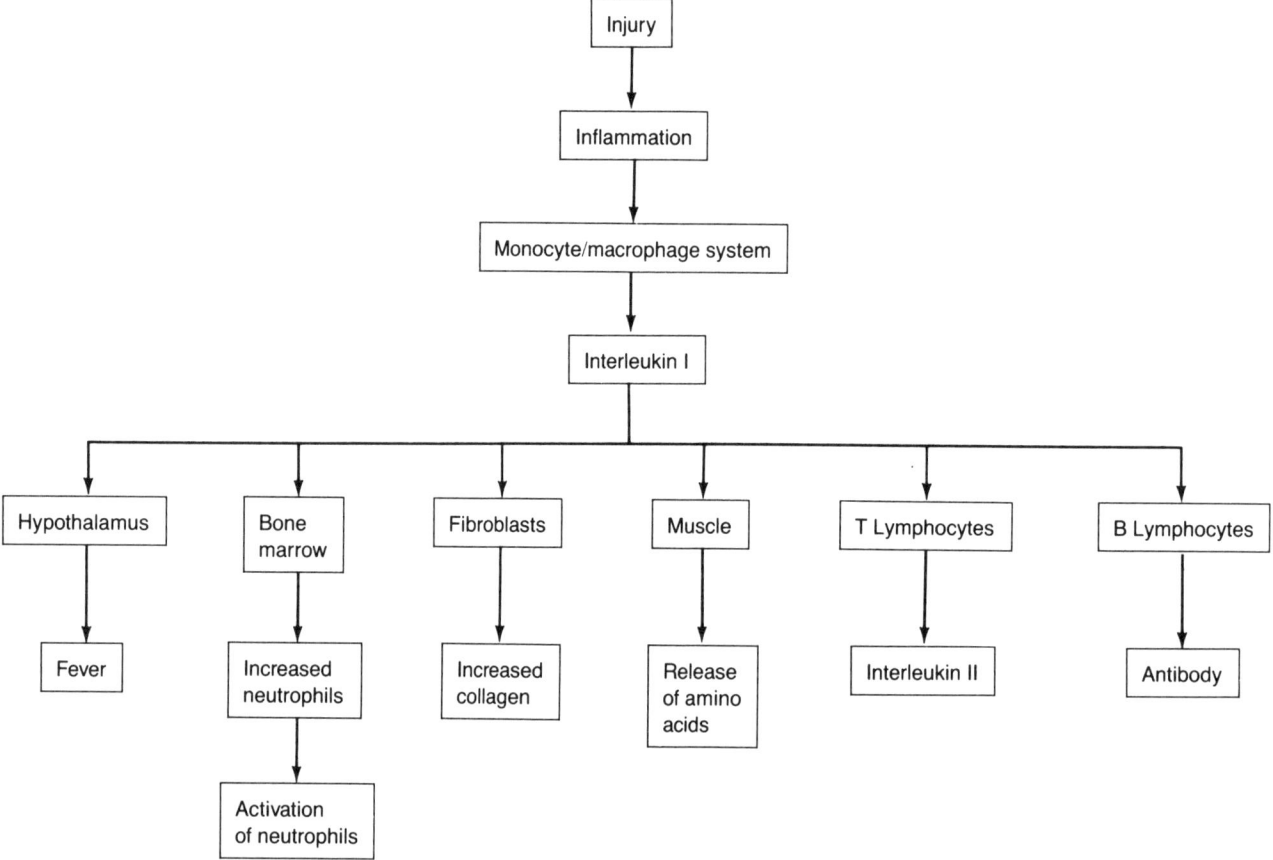

Figure 2-14. Diverse actions of interleukin I activation.

pyogenic infection produced by gram-positive cocci or gram-negative bacilli. *(3:89–94)*

48. **(A)** Since the organisms are acid-fast bacilli, the only reasonable diagnosis is tuberculosis. *Trichinella spiralis* and the organisms causing syphilis, gonorrhea, and staphylococcal abscesses are not acid-fast bacilli. *(4:58–59)*

49. **(C)**

50. **(A)**

49 and 50. Figures 2–8 and 2–9 depict sections through skin and subcutaneous tissue. **A** is epidermis, **B** is normal collagen bundles of the dermis, **C** is scar tissue that extends vertically from the surface into the dermis and is more amorphous in appearance than the surrounding epidermis. There is no evidence of acute or chronic inflammation cells or exudate and no evidence of necrosis or tumor. The appearance of bland, almost structureless collagen in this linear fashion is characteristic of scar tissue and is the end result of healing. *(4:69–73)*

51. **(A)**

52. **(D)**

53. **(E)**

54. **(A)**

55. **(B)**

56. **(B)**

51 through 56. The PMN is the characteristic cell of acute inflammation (Table 2–2) and, therefore, would be expected in an abscess, which is a focal collection of such white cells in response to a number of stimuli in the presence of liquefaction necrosis. The PMNs also would be seen at the edge of a recent infarct, since the tissue damage elicits chemotaxis of PMNs early in the evolution of the process. Eosinophils are attracted to tissue by chemotactic substances in the walls of many protozoal and other forms of parasites. They would be seen in this condition and are seen classically in the bronchial wall in asthmatic reactions. Eosinophils are involved also in attraction to tissue in which certain types of allergic reactions have taken place presumably because of immune complexes and some complement pathways. They are seen in bronchial asthma in increased numbers both in the peripheral blood and in the tissue concerned.

Plasma cells are the main end production cells of the B lymphocyte series and produce immunoglobulins. The monocyte is the cell of origin of many of the cells of chronic inflammation, including the epithelioid cells of granulomas and the fused monocytes and epithelioid cells that produce the Langhans' giant cells in certain types of granulomatous inflammation and foreign body giant cells. *(4:37)*

57. **(E)**

58. **(B)**

57 and 58. Although there are many factors that can be responsible for the pain of acute inflammation, the kinin group of chemical mediators is particularly known to be pain producing. Platelet aggregation can occur through a number of chemical mediators, some of which are summarized in Figures 2–12 and 2–13. However, ADP is both liberated by platelets and can cause further platelet aggregation and is, therefore, particularly important in this respect. *(2:52–60)*

59. **(B)**

60. **(A)**

61. **(E)**

62. **(B)**

59 through 62. Early acute inflammation produces an exudation of fluid rich in fibrinogen, and fibrin is precipitated on the surfaces of tissues. In the early phase of wound healing, granulation tissue is present, which eventually becomes fibrous tissue. Therefore, the early phase is associated with the production of granulation tissue. Chronic inflammation occurs after the early phase and is characterized by a number of events. Fibrous tissue is the hallmark, although it also could be the end result of a successful healing process (Figs 2–5 and 2–6). An abscess clearly is associated with pus and the presence of liquefaction necrosis and polymorphonuclear lymphocytes. *(2:39–84)*

63. **(C)**

64. **(E)**

65. **(B)**

66. **(A)**

67. **(D)**

63 through 67. These descriptions of the various manifestations of acute inflammation still are used extensively, although some of them are somewhat archaic. The deposition of fibrin on mucosal surfaces (fibrous exudate) is characteristic of the exudative phase of acute inflammation. Suppurative inflammation is characterized by the breakdown of tissue, with the presence of large numbers of leukocytes. In catarrhal inflammation, there is a mixture of fibrin on the surface of epithelium and mucus. A serous exudate is one in which fluid of high protein content accumulates in body cavities as a result of the inflammatory response. *(3:84–94)*

68. **(E)**

69. **(C)**

70. **(D)**

71. **(E)**

68 through 71. A very early ischemic infarct, such as a myocardial infarct due to coronary atherosclerosis, is characterized by coagulative necrosis and hemorrhage. Later there is neutrophilic and phagocytic resolution of the dead tissue. Granulation tissue ingrowth then occurs. The final stages of wound maturation are typified by collections of dense mature avascular collagen. Tissue reactions to pyogenic bacteria, such as staphylococci or streptococci, are typified by suppuration and abscess formation. The histology of an abscess includes liquid debris, neutrophils, and bacterial organisms. Tissue reactions to infections due to tubercle bacilli include granuloma formation, fibrosis, and lymphoplasmacytic inflammatory infiltrates. Capillary buds and fibroblasts are seen in the early healing stages of all wounds, regardless of etiology. *(2:65–70,73–74)*

72. **(B)**

73. **(A)**

74. **(C)**

75. **(E)**

72 through 75. Most abnormal collections of fluid (effusions) in a body cavity, such as a pericardial effusion, can be classified as either a transudate or as an exudate. Transudative fluid has a low specific gravity below 1.012, a total protein below 2 gm/dl, and is essentially devoid of inflammatory cells. Transudates are an ultrafiltrate of blood and are usually caused by elevated hydrostatic pressure, such as during congestive heart failure. Exudates have a high specific gravity of 1.020 or more, a total protein of 2 gm/dl or higher, and many inflammatory cells. Exudates usually occur with infectious or inflammatory processes. The type of inflammatory cell present in the exudate is determined by the etiology of the effusion. For example, tubercle bacilli characteristically evoke a mixture of multinucleate giant cells, lymphocytes, epithelioid histiocytes, and fibroblasts. Pyogenic bacteria in an exudative effusion usually result in an abscess formation composed of many neutrophils and necrotic debris. Some immunologic disorders, such as rheumatic pericarditis, produce an exudate rich in fibrin with only a few lymphocytes. *(2:40–41)*

76. **(E)**

77. **(C)**

78. **(A)**

76 through 78. A large number of chemical mediators are active in wound healing and repair. Growth-stimulating factors include fibronectin, platelet-derived growth factor, lymphokines, macrophage-derived growth factor, and fibrin. Fibronectin is a glycoprotein synthesized by fibroblasts that stimulates capillary formation and is chemotactic for fibroblasts. Platelet-derived growth factor is produced by platelets and stimulates capillary and fibroblast proliferation. Interleukin II is a lymphokine synthesized by T cell lymphocytes. Interleukin II stimulates T cell production. Macrophage-derived growth factor is mitogenic for fibroblasts. Chalones are growth-inhibiting chemical factors secreted by leukocytes and epidermal cells. Chalones inhibit cell division of neighboring cells (contact inhibition). Vitamin C, ascorbic acid, promotes proper collagen and matrix formation through hydroxylation of proline and lysine, and through the aggregation of tropocollagen fibrils. Histamine is present in mast cells and acts as a mediator of the acute inflammatory response through increasing vascular permeability. *(1:58,87,160–161)*

79. **(B)** A healing wound goes through several stages. The initial wound trauma engenders an acute inflammatory response with attendant leakage of plasma proteins, fibrin clot formation, and diapedesis of inflammatory cells. Next, granulation tissue composed of young collagen and capillary buds fill the wound defect. The surrounding epithelium and fibroblasts are stimulated by epidermal growth factor, a mitogenic polypeptide of about 6000 daltons. Epidermal growth factor stimulates cell division by binding to specific fibroblastic and epithelial tyrosine kinase receptors which trigger subsequent RNA synthesis, DNA synthesis, and mitosis. The final stages of wound healing are characterized by collagen deposition, collagen maturation, decreasing vascularity, and wound contraction. *(2:76–77; 3:94–104)*

80. **(C)** A number of detrimental factors impede proper wound healing. Suppuration or pus formation is toxic to many cell types and delays the ingrowth of granulation tissue into a wound. If the suppurative process is unable to drain spontaneously, an abscess can develop further complicating the resolution phase of wound healing. Abscesses may resolve spontaneously (pointing of an abscess) or through surgical drainage. Another adverse factor in wound healing is the presence of foreign material in the wound. Glass, wood splinters, and dirt in traumatic wounds mechanically obstruct orderly healing and provide a nidus for infection and suppuration. Additional factors that delay wound healing include vascular insufficiency, gapping wound defects, and a lack of collagen strengthening cofactors, such as ascorbic acid. Glucocorticoid therapy and diabetes also delay proper wound healing. *(1:90–91)*

81. **(E)** Eosinophils usually comprise less than 5% of peripheral blood leukocytes. A wide range of inflammatory, infectious, allergic, and neoplastic disorders produce increased circulating eosinophils (eosinophilia). Eosinophilia is a common manifestation of parasitic infections, especially with metazoan infestations. Allergic disorders that produce eosinophilia include allergic rhinitis, asthma, urticaria, drug allergies, and eczema. Immunologic diseases in which eosinophilia may occur include polyarteritis nodosa, pemphigus vulgaris, Loffler's syndrome, and eosinophilic gastroenteritis. Neoplasms associated with eosinophilia include Hodgkin's disease, mycosis fungoides, and eosinophilic leukemia. *(1:410)*

82. **(D)** Sarcoidosis is a disease of unknown etiology characterized by noncaseating granulomas in multiple sites throughout the body. The presence of these distinctive granulomas suggests an immunologic or hypersensitivity reaction to an infectious agent. Clinically there may be peripheral lymphadenopathy, splenomegaly, hepatomegaly, fever, fatigue, cutaneous lesions, or eye involvement. Laboratory findings may identify hypercalcemia, elevated angiotension-converting enzyme levels, and hyperglobulinemia. Radiographic studies usually demonstrate bilateral hilar adenopathy and lytic lesions of the phalangeal bones. There is no specific therapy, although some success is achieved with immunosuppression. The clinical course of the disorder is variable. Over half of affected individuals recover with minimal or no sequela. About 20% have permanent moderate pulmonary impairment.

About 10% have progressive disease with terminal cor pulmonale, cerebral dysfunction, or cardiac insufficiency. *(2:427–429)*

83. **(D)** Myeloperoxidase is an enzyme present in the azurophilic granules of neutrophilic leukocytes. This enzyme actively converts peroxidase into a potent oxidative-free radical form which is bactericidal. The conversion reaction requires a halide cofactor, such as a chloride ion. The infrequent individuals who are born without normal myeloperoxidase activity suffer from a disorder termed "chronic granulomatous disease." With this genetic disease there is normal phagocytosis of bacteria. But the ingested organisms cannot be killed due to the hereditary impairment of myeloperoxidase. Thus, the organisms continue to multiply intracellularly. Histologically this sequence of events is observed as multifocal granulomas and microabscesses. The disease is usually inherited in an X-linked recessive mode, although a few individuals inherit the disorder in an autosomal recessive fashion. *(2:50–51,5:1049–1050)*

84. **(E)** Arachidonic acid is found in the cell membranes of many inflammatory cells, such as neutrophils, macrophages, and mast cells. The enzymatic release of this twenty carbon unsaturated fatty acid by stimulated phospholipases initiates a subsequent cascade of metabolites, including leukotrienes and prostaglandins, which serve as chemical mediators of the acute inflammatory response. Leukotrienes are strongly chemotactic for inflammatory cells. Additionally, leukotrienes increase vascular permeability. The prostaglandins cause vasodilation, increase vascular permeability, and are chemotactic. Inhibitors of the acute inflammatory response act by either blocking the phospholipase release of free arachidonic acid (corticosteroids) or by blocking the cyclooxygenase pathway (aspirin). *(1:42–45)*

85. **(A)** Endothelial cells line the interior wall of blood and lymphatic vessels providing a smooth nonclotting surface. Between the individual endothelial cells are small pores through which water and small molecules exchange with the interstitium. The widening of these pores by histamine results in edema formation during the acute phase of the inflammatory response. Endothelial cells, in addition, synthesize a diverse group of substances, including factor VIII, plasminogen activator, and prostaglandins. *(1:317)*

86. **(B)** Bradykinin is painful when injected into the skin. It also causes contraction of smooth muscles and dilation of blood vessels. Bradykinin is the end product of the kinin system. The kinin system is a series of plasma proteases that begins with activation of factor XII (Hageman factor) and ends with bradykinin production. Initial contact with collagen, basement membrane material, bacterial endotoxin, or other surface agents converts factor XII into factor XIIA (prekallikrein activator). The next step in the kinin system is the conversion of prekallikrein into kallikrein by factor XIIA. The kallikrein produced then cleaves high-molecular weight kininogen to produce bradykinin. The kinin system is only one of three plasma proteases whose components are useful in the acute inflammatory response. The other plasma proteases are the complement system and the blood clotting system. *(2:54)*

87. **(B)** Myofibroblasts are mesenchymal-derived cells with features of both smooth muscle cells and fibroblasts. Like smooth muscle cells, the myofibroblasts contain the contractile protein bundles of actin and myosin. However, the myofibroblasts still retain the fibroblastic quality of collagen production. When a wound develops the myofibroblasts enter the defect on the second or third day concomitant with the ingrowth of granulation tissue. The contractile properties of the myofibroblast provide a mechanical reduction in the size of the wound defect to be repaired. In general, the smaller the defect to be repaired the more rapid the closure is completed. *(5:77)*

88. **(A)** Complement is a cascade of plasma proteases whose final goal is the lysis of cell membranes. In the classic pathway, complement is bound to the Fc portion of an antibody-antigen complex. In the alternative pathway, properdin initiates complement activation independent of an antibody-antigen complex. After initiation the complement cascade generates a wide number of fractions with diverse biologic activities. The C3a and C3b fractions are anaphylatoxic and opsonic, respectively. The C5a fraction is anaphylatoxic and chemotactic. The C1 and C5b67 fractions are chemotactic. These active products can modify the inflammatory response through the recruitment of additional inflammatory cells (chemotaxis) or through increasing vascular permeability (anaphylaxis). *(3:510–511)*

89. **(C)** Prostacyclin (prostaglandin PGI_2) is a potent inhibitor of platelet aggregation and is secreted principally by endothelial cells and macrophages. Prostacyclin is synthesized from free arachidonic acid via the cyclooxygenase pathway. A number of unstable prostaglandins (PGH_2 and PGG_2) are synthesized as intermediates prior to final synthesis of stable prostacyclin. Prostacyclin is a modifier of the inflammatory response through its vasodilatory action. The vasodilation increases the blood flow to an inflamed area, potentially increasing the plasma proteins and inflammatory cells available to mount an inflammatory response. Prostacyclin also reduces the functional activity of platelets and neutrophils by increasing their intracellular cyclic

adenosine monophosphate levels. Prostacyclin synthesis, like most of the other prostaglandins, is reduced by aspirin, indomethacin, and corticosteroids. *(1:43–45,5:47–54)*

90. **(E)** Thromboxane A_2 is a potent mediator of platelet aggregation. Thromboxane A_2 is synthesized from free arachidonic acid via the cyclooxygenase pathway. It is present in high concentrations within platelet granules. Its release plays a major role in the "second wave" of platelet aggregation. Thromboxane A_2 is also an active vasoconstrictor. Its dual ability to recruit platelets and constrict blood vessels is particularly useful in states of vascular disruption. *(5:47–48)*

91. **(D)** Foreign body inflammation displays a constellation of histologic features: multinucleate giant cells, lymphocytes, nonepithelioid histiocytes, and fibrosis. The multinucleate giant cells seen in foreign body reactions demonstrate multiple nuclei randomly arranged throughout the cytoplasm, including nuclei present in the center of the cell. This is in contradistinction to the Langhans' giant cell seen with granulomatous inflammation. The Langhans' cells has its multiple nuclei arranged at the periphery of the cytoplasm, usually without any nuclei in the center of the cell. The mononuclear epithelioid histiocytes from which the Langhans' cell is derived are also seen in granulomatous inflammation. With foreign body inflammation only normal, nonepithelioid histiocytes are usually seen. Fibrosis may be a very prominent feature of foreign body inflammation, such as that seen with inhaled silicon particles (silicosis). Fibrosis plays only a minor role in granulomatous inflammation until the final healing stages. Nonabsorbable sutures, such as those made of silk or plastic, would evoke a foreign body inflammatory response. The use of adsorbable suture material, such as chromic-treated cat gut, would evoke a foreign body response until the suture material was completely metabolized. *(5:58–63)*

92. **(A)** In the acute inflammatory response, there is immediate transient vasoconstriction (blanch), followed by vasodilation (flare), and fluid exudation (wheal). Margination of leukocytes occurs early in the acute inflammatory response. A number of chemical mediators, including epinephrine, are able to marginate leukocytes. The presence of leukocytes on the inner wall of blood vessels insures that sufficient leukocytes will be available for recruitment into the adjacent damaged tissue. As the inflammatory process progresses, the marginated leukocytes will exit through the newly expanded holes in the blood vessel walls (diapedsis) in response to chemotactic products liberated by tissue damage. *(3:76–78)*

93. **(E)** Histamine is a chemical mediator of fluid exudation in the acute inflammatory response through its ability to produce endothelial cell contraction. Histamine is found mainly in mast cells and basophils, and to a lesser extent in platelets. Histamine acts on the vasculature by binding to specific H_1-receptor sites on endothelial cells. Once bound, histamine initiates a reversible contraction of the endothelial cell cytoplasm. This cytoplasmic contraction widens the miniscule gaps already present between endothelial cell membranes and allows the exudation of fluid and larger molecules out into the interstitium. *(5:40–42)*.

94. **(C)** Granulation tissue is composed of fibroblasts and capillary buds. Histologically, there is usually accompanying mild edema, a few inflammatory cells, and a rare extravisated erythrocyte. In a clean, nonsuppurative wound granulation tissue appears during the second through fifth day. Beginning at the periphery of the defect it advances centrally. As the wound matures the granulation tissue becomes less vascularized and more collagenized. There is contraction of the wound site from myofibroblasts and the crosslinking of the young collagen imparts increased tensile strength to the healing tissue. The final stages of a healed wound result in fibrosis. *(5:66–83)*

95. **(C)** Basement membranes separate the epithelial and mesenchymal compartments. The basement membrane is composed of type IV collagen, laminin, and heparin sulfate proteoglycan. The glycoprotein laminin is the major component of the basement membrane and serves a glue-like function simultaneously attaching to collagen, epithelial cells, and proteoglycans. The large laminin molecule has three short arms, a central core, and a single long arm. Type IV collagen can bind to each of the laminin molecule's three short arms. The central core of the laminin molecule attaches to specific receptors present on the external surface of epithelial cells. The long arm of laminin binds to heparin. The laminin molecule is an important structural barrier that malignant cells must overcome before they can invade into the interstitium. *(2:257–259)*

96. **(E)** Elastic connective tissue is found at many sites throughout the body such as the ears, the spinal column, skin, lungs, the epiglottis, and in blood vessels. The major component fiber of elastic connective tissue is elastin. The precursor fiber, tropoelastin, measures about 70,000 daltons and matures into elastin by covalent desmosine and isodesmosine crosslinkages. The half-life of elastin is longer than the normal human life span. However, actinic damage, trauma, and certain bacterial elastases can all retard the longevity of elastin. *(2:81)*

97. **(D)** In the repair phase of a healing wound, a number of growth factors are active. These growth factors include fibroblast growth factor, epidermal growth factor, transforming growth factors, interleukin I, and tissue necrosis factor. The fibroblast growth factor is synthesized by a wide variety of epithelial and mesenchymal tissues. It is mitogenic for fibroblasts. In addition, it has the ability to stimulate the production and growth of new blood vessels (angiogenesis). *(2:77)*

98. **(A)** Collagen crosslinking increases wound tensile strength. This crosslinkage takes place between tropocollagen fibers at the site of previously oxidized lysine and hydroxylated proline residues. The oxidation and hydroxylation steps require the presence of ascorbic acid (vitamin C) and specific enzymes. *(1:85)*

99. **(E)** Sarcoidosis produces a noncaseating pattern of granulomatous inflammation. Although the exact cause is unknown, an infectious or disordered immune etiology is suspected. Sarcoidosis occurs more frequently in North American blacks than in whites, and is common in Scandinavia. The clinical symptoms include fever, fatigue, malaise, weight loss, dyspnea, skin lesions, splenomegaly, eye lesions, and lymphadenopathy. Affected sites demonstrate the characteristic noncaseating granulomas on histologic examination. The majority of individuals with sarcoidosis recover uneventfully or suffer only minor pulmonary impairment. Only about 10% of patients suffer end-stage lung disease or succumb to cardiac complications. *(5:607–698)*

100. **(F)** Tuberculosis produces a caseating pattern of granulomatous inflammation. Tuberculosis is divided into primary and secondary forms. An individual's first infection with tubercle bacilli is termed "primary tuberculosis." The inhaled bacilli lodge in the distal airways of the lung where they multiply freely until cell-mediated immunity develops. The typical caseating granulomatous pattern of inflammation coincides with the development of cellular immunity. Secondary tuberculosis occurs with reinfection of an individual from a dormant primary focus. If there is adequate cellular immunity, a caseating granulomatous reaction occurs. Histologically, there is central cheesy necrosis and a peripheral wall formed by lymphocytes, epithelioid histiocytes, Langhans' giant cells, and early fibrous tissue. The waxy cell walls of the tubercle bacilli retain carbolfuchsin dyes after acid rinsing. This "acid-fast" property is useful in the laboratory identification of mycobacterial infections. *(5:394–397)*

101. **(C)** The pattern of inflammation seen in rheumatoid arthritis is chronic inflammation. The synovium displays villiform hypertrophy, a mixed lymphocytic and plasmacytic infiltrate, germinal follicle formation, and fibrin deposition. Most affected individuals possess a rheumatoid factor in their serum which can be detected by laboratory testing. This factor is an IgM molecule that reacts against IgG. The disease is most commonly observed to occur in middle-aged females. Symmetric swelling of the small joints of the hands is the usual presenting feature. *(3:2077–2086)*

102. **(B)** The basic fact that the narrow lumen of the appendix is continuous with that of the bowel predisposes to its obstruction by an impacted fecalith. Continued secretion of mucinous fluid distal to the obstruction causes increased intraluminal pressure, which impedes venous drainage and causes ischemic damage and transudation of fluid into the wall, and possibly venous thrombosis, as well. The mucosa, especially if eschemically injured, is subject to damage by the fecalith, leading to invasion by the normal mixed bacterial flora of the bowel, with consequent exudation of fluid and neutrophils into the wall and onto the serosa. The vicious cycle of ischemia, bacterial infection, and swelling due to acute inflammation often increases tension in the tissue enough to impede blood flow, causing more ischemia and even gangrene, with rupture and peritonitis. This sequence of events is a particular problem in this location because the venous return and end-arterial supply are easily compromised, and adequate collateral circulation is not present. Thus, resolution is not likely to follow significant acute inflammation in this anatomic site. The appendix may also be occluded by calculus, tumor, *Enterobius vermicularis* infestation, and possibly lymphoid hyperplasia associated with viral or bacterial infection. Some cases of acute appendicitis apparently are not associated with luminal obstruction and may result from sharp angulation of the appendix caused by adhesions, fibrous bands, or retrocecal location. The pathogenesis of similar situations can be predicted, such as a loop of bowel incarcerated within a hernia and possibly strangulated, twisted around its mesentery (volvulus), or telescoped into itself (intussusception), or a colonic diverticulum can become obstructed and inflamed. *(4:10–19)*

103. **(D)** Noninflammatory fibrosis commonly follows in sites of radiation therapy. Chronic radiodermatitis is characterized by loss of adnexal structures, poor vascularity with perivascular fibrosis, increased collagen deposition in the dermis, and a thinning of the epidermis. These histologic changes are accompanied by the clinical observations of a shrunken, hard, thin-skinned surface that heals poorly, or not at all, if injured. *(3:273–274)*

104. **(F)** Tuberculoid leprosy displays a caseating granulomatous pattern of inflammation. In tuberculoid

leprosy there is a type IV delayed hypersensitivity reaction to leprosy bacilli antigens producing caseating granulomas. Clinically, these lesions are hypopigmented and are depressed centrally. Leprosy bacilli characteristically involve nerves producing the additional later clinical findings of wristdrop, footdrop, and other palsies. Leprosy is seen in tropical countries, including portions of the southern United States, California, and Hawaii. *(1:882–883)*

105. **(B)** Hepatic abscesses have an acute inflammatory reaction pattern. Bacterial hepatic abscesses usually result from either biliary obstruction or septicemia. The pyogenic and coliform bacteria are the most frequent pathogens. The mortality rate for hepatic abscesses is about 60%. Histologically, there is central necrotic debris, fibrin precipitates, abundant neutrophils, and scattered bacteria. *(1:645–646)*

106. **(D)**

107. **(D)**

108. **(D)**

106 through 108. The presence of fever, headache, and stiff neck may be seen in all of the conditions and simply results from irritation of the meninges. However, the blood and CSF neutrophilic leukocytosis with an increased proportion of immature forms (left shift) is strong evidence of acute suppurative inflammation, most probably due to bacterial infection most likely associated with bacterial otitis media. Chronic lymphocytic meningitis, tuberculous and fungal meningitis, and allergic encephalomyelitis classically produce a lymphocytic or monocytic cellular response. The most likely complication is brain abscess. *(2:1392–1393)*

REFERENCES

1. Chandrasoma P, Taylor CR: Concise Pathology, Norwalk, Appleton and Lange, 1991
2. Cotran RS, Kumar V, Robbins SL: Robbins Pathologic Basis of Disease, 4th edition, Philadelphia, Saunders, 1989
3. Kissane JM (ed): Anderson's Pathology, 9th edition, St. Louis, Mosby, 1990
4. Lewis MG, Rowden G: Histopathology: A Step by Step Approach, Boston, Little, Brown, 1987
5. Rubin E, Farber JL: Pathology, Philadelphia, Lippincott, 1988

CHAPTER 3

Alterations of Fluid Balance, Hemodynamics, Coagulation, and Acid-Base

The constant cellular demand for oxygen, metabolites, electrolytes, and waste removal requires precisely tuned homeostatic mechanisms for fluid balance and hemodynamics. Perturbations in fluid balance, acid-base, hemodynamics, and coagulation are commonly encountered in medicine and can result in a wide range of pathologic entities such as dehydration, edema, shock, thrombosis, embolization, infarction, and hemorrhage.

BASIC FACTS AND CONCEPTS

The human body is mostly (60%) water, and total body water is divided between intracellular and extracellular compartments. The relative volume of intracellular water is about twice that of extracellular water. In the normal physiologic state, the interstitium is free of excess water (nonedematous) because of the draining action of terminal lymphatics.

CAPILLARY	DIRECTION OF FLUID FLOW (MM HG)		INTERSTITIUM
Oncotic pressure	← (28)	→ (5)	Oncotic pressure
Hydrostatic pressure	→ (17)	→ (−6.5)	Hydrostatic pressure
	net 0.5 → drawn off by lymphatics		

When the ability of the terminal lymphatics to absorb excess fluid is impaired or the quantity of fluid is excessive, edema can occur. Depending on the site and disease process considered, the resultant edema may be either localized (eg, urticaria) or diffuse (eg, anasarca). The usual pathologic mechanisms of edema formation are:

1. Decreased plasma oncotic pressure: Hypoalbuminemia secondary to cirrhosis, severe starvation, or nephrotic syndrome.
2. Increased hydrostatic capillary pressure: Congestive heart failure.
3. Lymphatic obstruction: Filariasis or metastatic cancer.
4. Increased endothelial permeability: Urticaria or thermal burns.
5. Increased sodium retention: Excessive salt intake.

Decreased total fluid volume is termed "dehydration" and may be seen with insufficient fluid intake and/or with excessive loss of bodily fluids. Excessive loss of selective bodily fluids, such as loss of gastric acid by repeated vomiting, may result not only in dehydration, but may additionally cause abnormalities in electrolyte and acid-base balance.

Decreased vascular perfusion of tissues is termed "shock" and may be due to:

1. Hypovolemic shock: Hemorrhage, dehydration, or diarrhea.
2. Vasodilatory shock: Sepsis or anaphylaxis.
3. Cardiogenic shock: Myocardial infarct, myocarditis, or tamponade.

Normal hemodynamics is defined as nonturbulent laminar flow of liquified blood within blood vessels. Abnormal hemodynamics usually occurs with damaged endothelium, vascular stasis, or increased blood coagulability. Pathologic hemodynamics predisposes to intravascular clotting and thrombogenesis which may further engender embolization, hemorrhage, and infarction. Occlusive thrombi or emboli in distal-end arteries of the heart, spleen, or kidney produce wedge-shaped pale infarcts with coagulative necrosis. Thromboses in a dual blood supply organ, such as lung and intestine, characteristically produce a hemorrhagic infarct. Brain infarcts display a unique pattern of liquefaction necrosis.

Bleeding, coagulation, and hemorrhage are intimately related to abnormal hemodynamics, usually as a contributor to the disordered process, a result of the process, or both. The normal coagulation system is a complex cascade of interactive proteins with varying activator, inhibitor, and modifying properties. The task of the coagulation system alternates between the maintenance of blood in the native liquid state and the prompt formation of a stable fibrin clot when activated. The two initiating arms of the coagulation system are divided into the extrinsic and intrinsic systems. The intrinsic system is usually activated by intravascular damage, such as collagen exposed at an ulcerated atheromatous plaque. The extrinsic system is activated by tissue damage, such as a surgeon's incision with liberation of lipoprotein tissue factors. In many instances the dual systems are coactive. Both pathways share a terminal goal of thrombin-fibrin production. "Fibrinolysis" is the term used to describe the physiologic dissolution of the fibrin clot. Hyperactive fibrinolysis is operative in a number of disease states, such as disseminated intravascular coagulation, carcinomatosis, and multiple recurrent deep vein thromboses.

Alterations of pH deleteriously affect a myriad of intracellular enzymatic processes that sustain life. Disturbances of acid-base in their pure form are pathologically sorted into four categories: respiratory acidosis, respiratory alkalosis, metabolic acidosis, and metabolic alkalosis.

FORM	pH	P_{CO_2}	HCO_3	EXAMPLE
Respiratory acidosis	↓	↑	↑	Hypoventilation
Respiratory alkalosis	↑	↓	↓	Hyperventilation
Metabolic acidosis	↓	Normal	↓	Diabetic ketoacidosis
Metabolic alkalosis	↑	Normal	↑	Gastric suction

Questions

DIRECTIONS (Questions 1 through 49): Each of the numbered items or incomplete statements in this section is followed by answers or by completions of the statement. Selection the ONE lettered answer or completion that is BEST in each case.

1. The single largest constituent of the body by weight is

    (A) lysosomes
    (B) ribosomes
    (C) nucleic acid
    (D) water
    (E) blood

2. The tissue that has the lowest percentage of water is

    (A) spleen
    (B) heart
    (C) liver
    (D) adipose tissue
    (E) skeletal muscle

3. Identify the incorrect statement

    (A) about 35% of lean body weight is water
    (B) the body has twice as much intracellular as extracellular water
    (C) plasma is approximately 5% of lean body weight
    (D) there is about three times as much interstitial fluid as plasma
    (E) plasma and interstitial fluid are separated by a semipermeable endothelial barrier

4. Which pressure is highest (in mm Hg)?

    (A) capillary hydrostatic pressure
    (B) interstitial hydrostatic pressure
    (C) interstitial oncotic pressure
    (D) capillary oncotic pressure
    (E) terminal lymphatic pressure

5. The purpose of the lymphatic valves is

    (A) to allow lymph flow in only one direction
    (B) nonexistent, since lymphatics do not have valves
    (C) to reduce lymphatic oncotic pressure
    (D) to reduce lymphatic hydrostatic pressure
    (E) to increase lymphatic oncotic pressure

6. Predisposing conditions for vascular thrombosis include all of the following EXCEPT

    (A) turbulent blood flow
    (B) increased blood viscosity
    (C) thrombocytopenia
    (D) injury to the endothelial barrier
    (E) stasis of blood

7. Which statement concerning edema is true?
    (A) edema is an accumulation of excess fluid in the interstitial tissue spaces or body cavities
    (B) edema always is a systemic process and rarely is localized
    (C) ascites is generalized edema particularly noticeable in the subcutaneous tissue
    (D) collection of edema fluid in the peritoneal cavity is termed "hydropericardium"
    (E) noninflammatory protein-poor edema is an exudate

8. Hypostatic pneumonia is

    (A) usually caused by a virus
    (B) secondary infection of chronic pulmonary edema
    (C) associated with low blood pressure
    (D) associated with low electrical charges
    (E) infections of the legs with pulmonary complications

9. These are likely causes of edema EXCEPT

    (A) increased vascular hydrostatic pressure
    (B) lymphatic obstruction
    (C) increased vascular oncotic pressure
    (D) increased vascular permeability
    (E) increased interstitial oncotic pressure

10. Clinical states associated with generalized edema may include all EXCEPT

    (A) congestive heart failure
    (B) nephrotic syndrome
    (C) protein malnutrition
    (D) cirrhosis
    (E) multiple myeloma

11. Identify the incorrect statement about hydropericardium

    (A) always less than 50 ml
    (B) can produce cardiac tamponade
    (C) seen with congestive heart failure (CHF)
    (D) usually a transudate
    (E) associated with myxedema

12. When viewed under the microscope with routine hematoxylin and eosin (H & E) stains, edema fluid appears as

    (A) pink acellular precipitates
    (B) blue nuclei, pink cytoplasm
    (C) depends on cell type
    (D) bile-stained gelatinous plugs
    (E) lines of Zahn

13. Chronic passive congestion of the lung might include all the following EXCEPT

    (A) brown induration
    (B) hemosiderin macrophages
    (C) erythema
    (D) pulmonary edema
    (E) congested alveolar capillaries

14. Which statement is INCORRECT?

    (A) cations carry positive electrical charges
    (B) proteins contribute osmotic pressure to the vascular compartment
    (C) venous congestion may lead to edema
    (D) sodium is the major intracellular cation
    (E) the major osmoles in blood are Na, Cl, HCO_3

15. Hydrogen ion concentration is expressed as

    (A) mg/dl
    (B) mg%
    (C) pH
    (D) Pco_2
    (E) mEq/L

16. An anxious man is brought to the emergency department feeling light-headed. His arterial blood gas is pH 7.52, HCO_3 is 21 mmol/L, and Pco_2 is 20 mm Hg. The most likely diagnosis is

    (A) metabolic acidosis
    (B) respiratory alkalosis
    (C) inappropriate anion gap
    (D) respiratory acidosis
    (E) metabolic alkalosis

17. A 63-year-old female has been vomiting for several hours. Her blood gases are pH 7.51, HCO_3 32 mmol/L and Pco_2 40 mm Hg. The most likely diagnosis is

    (A) anion gap metabolic acidosis
    (B) nonanion gap metabolic acidosis
    (C) metabolic alkalosis
    (D) respiratory acidosis
    (E) respiratory alkalosis

18. Which would be an UNEXPECTED finding with an elevated serum hydrogen ion concentration?

    (A) acidosis
    (B) renal compensation by increased urinary H^+
    (C) pulmonary compensation by hypoventilation
    (D) pH 7.20
    (E) elevated serum K^+

19. Which item is the LEAST important in determining if a vascular occlusion will cause infarction

    (A) rate at which the occlusion develops
    (B) anatomic pattern of blood supply
    (C) vulnerability of the tissue to ischemia
    (D) presence of a collateral blood supply
    (E) serum osmolality

20. Hyperkalemia may be caused by all of the following EXCEPT

    (A) triamterene
    (B) acidosis
    (C) juvenile diabetes mellitus
    (D) adrenal insufficiency
    (E) aldosterone-secreting tumor

21. Identify the INCORRECT statement concerning buffers

    (A) bicarbonate is the most important extracellular buffer
    (B) a buffer is a weak acid and its salt
    (C) buffers tend to exaggerate changes of hydrogen ion concentration
    (D) intracellular buffers include proteins and phosphates
    (E) buffers help to maintain pH near 7.4 in healthy people

22. Important intracellular buffers include all of the following EXCEPT

    (A) inorganic phosphates
    (B) hemoglobin
    (C) organic phosphates
    (D) sodium
    (E) proteins

23. The enzyme responsible for the conversion of bicarbonate and carbon dioxide into carbonic acid is

    (A) adenosine triphosphatase (ATPase) sodium pump
    (B) chloride anhydrase
    (C) carbonic acid transferase
    (D) carbonic anhydrase
    (E) acetazolamide

24. Normal serum osmolality is about

    (A) 210 mmol/kg
    (B) 250 mmol/kg
    (C) 290 mmol/kg
    (D) 325 mmol/kg
    (E) 350 mmol/kg

25. Which statement about anion gap is false?

    (A) elevated in lactic acidosis
    (B) Na − (HCO$_3$ + Cl)
    (C) usually 10–14 mEq/L
    (D) represents anions, such as protein, phosphates, and sulfates
    (E) total body positive charges minus negative charges

26. The development of new blood channels through an occlusive thrombus is called

    (A) infarction
    (B) fibrinolysis
    (C) recanalization
    (D) propagation
    (E) embolization

27. Chronic passive congestion of the spleen would be expected to include all of the following EXCEPT

    (A) increase in splenic weight
    (B) shrunken capsule
    (C) cyanosis
    (D) hemosiderin deposition
    (E) sinusoids filled with erythrocytes

28. All of the following describe forms of hemorrhage EXCEPT

    (A) hemopericardium
    (B) hemothorax
    (C) hemostasis
    (D) petechiae
    (E) purpura

29. All of the following would be expected in hepatic passive congestion EXCEPT

    (A) increase in weight
    (B) nutmeg pattern
    (C) centrilobular regions distended by blood
    (D) increase in size
    (E) pyramid-shaped infarcts

30. Identify the solution with the highest osmolality

    (A) 2 mol of NaCl dissolved in 1 L of H$_2$O
    (B) 1 mol of MgSO$_4$ dissolved in 1 L of H$_2$O
    (C) 1 mol of KCl dissolved in 1 L of H$_2$O
    (D) 1 mol of KCl dissolved in 2 L of H$_2$O
    (E) 1 mol of NaCl dissolved in 2 L of H$_2$O

31. Which tissue undergoes liquefaction when infarcted?

    (A) kidney
    (B) small bowel
    (C) heart
    (D) spleen
    (E) brain

32. Which statement about platelets is true?

    (A) nucleus is about 5 μm in diameter
    (B) contain alpha granules rich in adenosine diphosphate (ADP)
    (C) precursors are monocytes
    (D) contain dense bodies rich in fibrinogen
    (E) contain ectomyosin, microfilaments, and microtubules

33. Which statement concerning arterial emboli is false?

    (A) arterial emboli rarely embolize to the lower extremities
    (B) most arterial emboli arise from cardiac thrombi
    (C) most arterial emboli cause infarction
    (D) emboli from infective endocarditis can cause septic infarcts
    (E) embolization to the middle cerebral artery can be fatal

34. The single necessary criterion to define shock is

    (A) rapid bleeding
    (B) inadequate tissue perfusion
    (C) loss of plasma proteins
    (D) severe burns
    (E) massive internal injuries

35. Which statement about the coagulation system is false?

    (A) amplification at each step produces cascade effect
    (B) factors are lipids
    (C) end product is fibrin
    (D) factors may be genetically deficient
    (E) calcium and platelets are necessary cofactors

36. The earliest step in arterial thrombosis is

    (A) activation of common pathway
    (B) adherence of platelets to vessel walls
    (C) activation of intrinsic pathway
    (D) activation of plasminogen
    (E) activation of Hageman factor

37. The factor least likely to cause thrombosis is

    (A) damaged vascular wall
    (B) turbulent blood flow
    (C) decreased factor VIII
    (D) venous stasis
    (E) increased platelet count

38. Which cell secretes von Willebrand factor?

    (A) hepatocyte
    (B) neutrophil
    (C) lymphocyte
    (D) endothelial cell
    (E) platelet

39. A mural thrombus is most likely found in the

    (A) heart
    (B) coronary artery
    (C) right middle cerebral artery
    (D) right anterior cerebral artery
    (E) spleen

40. The evolution of a thrombus may include all of the following EXCEPT

    (A) lysis
    (B) organization
    (C) recanalization
    (D) retrostasis
    (E) propagation

41. Which would be an unexpected finding in occlusive coronary thrombosis?

    (A) thrombus at site of abnormal blood vessel wall
    (B) ischemic necrosis
    (C) myocardial infarct
    (D) coronary atherosclerosis
    (E) thrombocytopenia

42. Which statement concerning thromboxane A_2 (TxA_2) is false?

    (A) TxA_2 is a platelet-aggregating substance
    (B) TxA_2 may act through cyclic adenosine monophosphate (cAMP) mediation
    (C) TxA_2 is a vasoconstriction agent
    (D) TxA_2 is synthesized by platelets
    (E) Prostacyclin accelerates TxA_2 actions

43. Which factor is not part of the intrinsic clotting system?

    (A) factor VII
    (B) factor XII
    (C) factor XI
    (D) factor IX
    (E) factor VIII

44. Thrombi would not be likely to form with

    (A) deficiency of antithrombin III (AT III)
    (B) venous stasis
    (C) endothelial damage
    (D) turbulent blood flow
    (E) decreased clotting factors

45. A hemorrhagic infarct is most likely in which site?

    (A) spleen
    (B) kidney
    (C) anterior left cardiac ventricle
    (D) posterior left cardiac ventricle
    (E) lung

46. Which statement is false concerning occlusive arterial thrombi?

    (A) encountered frequently in coronary arteries
    (B) may be associated with atherosclerotic lesion
    (C) arteritis may be the initiating event
    (D) may be seen in arterial trauma
    (E) commonly embolize to the lungs

47. The term "paradoxical embolism" is best defined as

    (A) death in a healthy person from a saddle-type pulmonary embolism
    (B) an embolism that does not cause an infarct
    (C) an organized embolus
    (D) a venous embolus that gains access to the arterial side through a heart wall defect
    (E) emboli from deep venous thrombosis

48. Gas embolism can be seen in all of the following EXCEPT

    (A) uterine delivery or abortion
    (B) caisson disease
    (C) traumatic injury to chest wall or lung
    (D) decompression sickness
    (E) hypertension

49. Shock can be seen commonly in all of the following EXCEPT

    (A) massive hemorrhage
    (B) congestive heart failure
    (C) myocardial infarct
    (D) anaphylaxis
    (E) disseminated intravascular coagulation

DIRECTIONS (Questions 50 through 96): Each group of items in this section consists of lettered headings followed by a set of numbered words or phrases. For each numbered word or phrase, select the ONE lettered heading that is most closely associated with it. **Each lettered heading may be selected once, more than once, or not at all.**

Questions 50 through 53

(A) alpha-1 antitrypsin
(B) streptokinase
(C) Stuart-Prower factor
(D) adenosine diphosphate (ADP)
(E) thrombin

50. Exogenous plasmin B

51. Common name for factor II E

52. Plasmin inhibitor A

53. Platelet adherence factor D

Questions 54 through 57

(A) aldosterone
(B) lactic acid
(C) methotrexate
(D) acetazolamide
(E) bicarbonate

54. Important extracellular buffer E

55. Markedly elevated with tissue anoxia B

56. Hormone involved in sodium regulation A

57. Carbonic anhydrase inhibitor D

Questions 58 through 61

(A) total body water
(B) intracellular water
(C) extracellular water
(D) plasma
(E) fibrin

58. 40% of lean body weight B

59. 60% of lean body weight A

60. 5% of lean body weight D

61. 20% of lean body weight C

Questions 62 through 65

(A) hydropericardium
(B) hydroperitoneum
(C) hydrosalpinx
(D) hemothorax
(E) pyarthrosis

62. Collection of blood in a pleural cavity D

63. Collection of pus in a joint space E

64. Collection of fluid in the peritoneal cavity B

65. Collection of fluid in a fallopian tube C

Questions 66 through 69

(A) bleeding time
(B) prothrombin time
(C) partial thromboplastin time
(D) clot retraction test
(E) clot lysis test

66. In vitro test that evaluates the extrinsic clotting system B

67. In vitro test that evaluates the intrinsic clotting system C

68. In vivo test that evaluates platelet and capillary function A

69. In vitro test that evaluates platelet actomyosin contraction D

Questions 70 through 73

(A) filariasis
(B) urticaria
(C) psoriasis
(D) congestive heart failure
(E) hypoalbuminemia

70. Edema due to decreased vascular oncotic pressure E

71. Edema due to increased endothelial permeability B

72. Edema due to lymphatic obstruction A

73. Edema due to increased capillary hydrostatic pressure D

Questions 74 through 77

(A) air embolism
(B) fat embolism
(C) amniotic fluid embolism
(D) nitrogen embolism
(E) serosal embolism

74. Usually associated with DIC and caused by childbirth C

75. Usually seen with multiple fractures of large bones B

76. Usually seen as decompression sickness in scuba divers

77. Usually seen with thoracic puncture wounds and pneumothorax

Questions 78 through 81

(A) renal infarct
(B) angina pectoris
(C) intermittent claudication
(D) stroke
(E) amaurosis fugax

78. Emboli to ophthalmic artery

79. Emboli to middle cerebral artery

80. Thrombosis of a coronary artery

81. Emboli to branches of the renal artery

Questions 82 through 85

(A) calcium
(B) chloride
(C) potassium
(D) bicarbonate
(E) sodium

82. Major intracellular cation

83. Major extracellular cation

84. Anionic form of a major body buffer

85. Cation active in coagulation and muscle contraction

Questions 86 through 88

(A) acute metabolic acidosis
(B) acute metabolic alkalosis
(C) acute respiratory acidosis
(D) acute respiratory alkalosis
(E) chronic metabolic acidosis
(F) chronic metabolic alkalosis
(G) chronic respiratory acidosis
(H) chronic respiratory alkalosis

86. A medical student is taking part in an experiment and volunteers to breathe air to which 10% carbon dioxide has been added. After 10 minutes the student's blood gases are pH 7.28, P_{CO_2} 51 mm Hg, and HCO_3 32 mmol/L.

87. A young child is about to have an arterial blood gas study and begins hyperventilating. The laboratory reports the blood gases as pH 7.51, P_{CO_2} 26 mm Hg, and HCO_3 18 mmol/L.

88. A depressed man drinks ethylene glycol in an attempted suicide. In the emergency department his blood gases are pH 7.19, P_{CO_2} 40 mm Hg, HCO_3 19 mmol/L.

Questions 89 through 91

(A) air emboli
(B) amniotic fluid emboli
(C) fat emboli
(D) nitrogen emboli
(E) mesenteric venous thromboses
(F) candidiasis
(G) hydropericardium
(H) hemopericardium

89. A 32-year-old female with a family history of antithrombin III deficiency dies suddenly after complaining of abdominal pain for 7 days. At autopsy there is a segment of gangrenous bowel which anatomically is drained by the superior mesenteric vein. What is most likely to be found in this vein?

90. A 21-year-old pregnant female is having a very difficult and prolonged labor. She begins to develop disseminated intravascular coagulation. What is likely to be found in her lungs?

91. A 47-year-old man with Marfan's syndrome complains of chest pain and dies suddenly. At autopsy there is a dissecting aneurysm of the thoracic aorta due to cystic medial necrosis. Proximally the dissection extends through the root of the aorta into the pericardial sac. What is likely to be found in the pericardial space?

Questions 92 through 96

(A) fat embolism
(B) pulmonary embolism
(C) nitrogen embolism
(D) amniotic fluid embolism
(E) anasarca
(F) hydrosalpinx
(G) exudate
(H) transudate

92. An inexperienced scuba diver ascends from a depth of 60 meters to the surface in about 4 minutes. Shortly after surfacing the diver complains of severe muscle contractions and intense abdominal pain.

93. A 26-year-old male fractures his pelvis and femur in a motor vehicle accident. On the third hospital day he dies after developing a hemorrhagic rash, respiratory distress, and cerebral dysfunction. At autopsy fat globules are found scattered in the cerebral cortex, kidney, and lung.

94. A 43-year-old obese female is admitted to the hospital for treatment of deep vein thromboses. On the night of admission she suddenly dies. At autopsy a large plug of laminated blood clot is found to occlude the main pulmonary artery.

95. A 63-year-old man in congestive heart failure has a fluid accumulation withdrawn from his right pleural space. The laboratory analysis of the fluid is: specific gravity 1.008, albumin 0.2 gm/dL, white blood cells 2/uL, and red blood cells 0/uL.

96. A 59-year-old female with widely metastatic breast carcinoma has a fluid accumulation withdrawn from her left pleural space. The laboratory analysis of the fluid is: specific gravity 1.028, albumin 3.1 gm/dL, white blood cells 32,200/uL, and red blood cells 2900/uL.

Answers and Explanations

1. **(D)** The body is about 60% water. All the other listed constituents comprise only a small percentage (5 to 0.2%) of the body by weight. *(2:87–88)*

2. **(D)** Adipose tissue is 10% water. The other tissues are about 60% water. Because adipose tissue contributes 100% of its mass to total body weight but only 10% of its mass to total body water, all discussions of total body water use an idealized lean body, without any significant adipose tissue. In this way, water compartments can be discussed regardless of the body's nutritional status or habitus. *(2:87–88)*

3. **(A)** Water is the single largest constituent of the body, making up 60% of its lean mass. Water is distributed two thirds as intracellular water and one third as extracellular water. The extracellular compartment is divided into one-fourth plasma and three-fourths interstitial fluid by a semipermeable endothelial barrier. *(2:87–88)*

4. **(D)** Capillary oncotic pressure is about 28 mm Hg. The next highest, capillary hydrostatic pressure, is about 17 mm Hg. Interstitial oncotic and hydrostatic pressure are 5 mm Hg and −6.5 mm Hg, respectively. Terminal lymphatic pressure is negative. *(3:178–180)*

5. **(A)** The lymphatic valves are important in maintaining unidirectional flow. Both lymphatics and capillaries possess valves. The oncotic pressure is a function of the number of particles in solution, and valves do not affect it. Lymph trying to flow backwards tends to build up next to valves, raising the lymphatic hydrostatic pressure, not lowering it. *(5:791–792)*

6. **(C)** Vascular thrombosis is usually seen in association with alterations in blood flow, damage to the endothelial barrier, and in hypercoagulable states. Normal blood flow is laminar and nonturbulent. Abnormalities of blood flow that predispose to thrombus formation include sluggish flow, stasis, increased viscosity, and turbulence. Damage to the endothelial barrier may expose collagen or lipid fractions that are potent initiators of thrombogenesis. Hypercoagulable blood has an increased potential for thrombosis. Hypercoagulable states include those with increased platelets (thrombocytosis), acquired or hereditary absence of coagulation cascade inhibitors (antithrombin III deficiency), and premature activation of protein clotting factors (disseminated intravascular coagulation). A deficiency of circulating platelets, thrombocytopenia, would be an antagonist of thrombogenesis. *(1:137–138)*

7. **(A)** Edema is an accumulation of excess fluid in the interstitium or body cavities. It may be a localized or generalized process. Anasarca, not ascites, defines prominent systemic subcutaneous edema, and ascites is peritoneal cavity collections. Hydropericardium is a collection of fluid in the pericardial sac. Exudates are associated with inflammation and are protein rich. A transudate would be noninflammatory and protein-poor edema. *(6:258–265)*

8. **(B)** Secondary infection of chronic pulmonary edema is termed "hypostatic pneumonia." It is almost always a bacterial not a viral infection. It has no specific relationship to low blood pressure, low electrical charges, or leg infections. *(2:90)*

9. **(C)** Edema, the fluid expansion of the interstitial space, has numerous causes, including increased vascular hydrostatic pressure (congestive heart failure), decreased vascular oncotic pressure (hypoalbuminemia), lymphatic obstruction (lymphedema), increased capillary permeability (burns), and increased interstitial osmotic pressure (poor renal perfusion). Increased vascular oncotic pressure would tend to pull fluid out of the interstitium into the blood vessels, making edema less likely. *(2:87–90)*

10. **(E)** Only multiple myeloma (with increased plasma oncotic pressure) acts to counter edema. Congestive heart failure increases the venous hydrostatic pressure, favoring edema formation. Protein malnutrition and nephrotic syndrome both lower vascular oncotic pressure, and cirrhosis increases venous hy-

drostatic pressure and, by hypoalbuminemia, lowers vascular oncotic pressure. Both of these factors promote edema. *(2:87–90)*

11. **(A)** The normal pericardial sac contains about 5 to 50 ml of fluid. Accumulation of 100 ml or more of transudative fluid is a hydropericardium. The term "hydropericardium" is not applied to exudative expansions of the pericardium, as seen in pericarditis. Hydropericardium can occur in most edematous states, including CHF and myxedema. A rapid accumulation of fluid can cause cardiac tamponade. Slow accumulation of fluid can distend the pericardial sac to as great as 1000 ml if there is no adherent pericardial disease offering resistance to gradual expansion. *(2:648)*

12. **(A)** Edema fluid is acellular proteinaceous material that appears as a pink precipitate with H & E stain. Since edema fluid is acellular, it is not dependent on cell type, nor does it have nuclei or cytoplasm. Lines of Zahn describe alternating strata of fibrin and red blood cells in thrombi. Bile-stained gelatinous plugs bear no relationship to the microscopic appearance of edema fluid. *(2:87–90)*

13. **(C)** Chronic passive congestion must, by definition, have congested alveolar capillaries. In more severe or long-standing cases, fluid and red blood cells leak out into the alveolar spaces. This transudate fluid in the alveolar space is termed "pulmonary edema." The red blood cells are broken down to form hemosiderin (brown pigment) inside macrophages. Occasionally, a fibrotic process will occur grossly that is called "brown induration." Erythema, a reddish hue, is seen in states of active hypermia not the passive hyperemia of pulmonary passive congestion. The lungs of passive congestion are bluish (cyanosis) not reddish (erythema). *(6:254)*

14. **(D)** Cations are positively charged ions, such as potassium, calcium, and sodium. The major intracellular cation is potassium, at about 160 mEq/L. Sodium is the major extracellular, not intracellular, cation; intracellular sodium measures only 10 mEq/L. Major osmolytes in blood include Na, Cl, and HCO_3. Together they comprise about 90% of the blood's osmolality. Proteins are important osmotic forces in blood. Venous congestion is one of the major factors in edema formation. *(3:276–278)*

15. **(C)** Hydrogen ion concentration is expressed as pH units, representing the antilog of hydrogen ion concentration. This logrithmic expression is useful to cover the wide range of hydrogen ion concentration found in nature. *(4:134–135)*

16. **(B)** When evaluating acid-base problems, look first at the pH and Pco_2. The man's pH is more than 7.4, so he is alkalotic (acidotic choices then cannot be correct). The Pco_2 is not 40 mm Hg, so there is a respiratory component. Changes in Pco_2 are only respiratory, not metabolic. With these two data points, only one choice remains, respiratory alkalosis. The presentation, one of nervous hyperventilation, is the classic example. The anion gap is useful in separating forms of metabolic acidosis but provides no useful information in this instance. *(3:340–342)*

17. **(C)** The pH is elevated (alkalotic), so there is no acidosis. The Pco_2 is normal at 40 mm Hg, indicating that there is no respiratory component. This clinical presentation is classic for metabolic alkalosis. Prolonged vomiting loses HCl from the stomach and allows a metabolic alkalosis to develop. In a real clinical setting, there usually would be compensatory hypoventilation (respiratory acidosis) to attempt to correct the pH to 7.4. *(3:340–342)*

18. **(C)** An increased serum hydrogen ion concentration is an acidotic state with a pH less than 7.4. Common bodily compensatory mechanisms include movement of K^+ out of cells into the serum in exchange for H^+, increased renal secretion of H^+, and hyperventilation. Hypoventilation would exacerbate the acidosis by alveolar retention of Pco_2. *(3:330–342)*

19. **(E)** Every occlusive vascular thrombosis does not produce subsequent infarction of the involved tissues. For each occlusion there is a complex interplay of factors which determine if an infarct will result. These factors include the rate at which the occlusion develops, the anatomic pattern of blood supply, the presence of a collateral blood supply, the susceptibility of the tissues to ischemia, the oxygen saturation of the blood, the overall hemodynamic status of the individual, the rate of thrombolysis, and the rate of recanalization. In general, infarction is usually seen with sudden, complete arterial occlusions of highly active metabolic tissues in patients with poor cardiovascular status. A common example is occlusion of a dominant coronary artery followed by a myocardial infarct. The serum osmolality is not directly related to vascular occlusion or the development of an infarct. *(2:102)*

20. **(E)** Hyperkalemia is an increase in blood potassium concentration. Increases are associated with acidosis, such as in diabetes, with K^+ moving out of the cell into plasma in exchange for H^+. Triamterene is a potassium-sparing diuretic and, unlike most of the other diuretics, can cause hyperkalemia by renal potassium retention. Aldosterone saves renal sodium at the expense of K^+. In states of low aldosterone (such as adrenal insufficiency), there is hyperkalemia. In states of high aldosterone (such as aldosterone-secreting tumors), there is hypernatremia with hypokalemia. *(4:130–131)*

21. **(C)** Buffers are weak acids and their salts, such as carbonic acid (H_2CO_3, pK 6.8) and bicarbonate (HCO_3). Bicarbonate is the most important extracellular buffer, and proteins and phosphates are important intracellular buffers. The buffers tend to minimize, not exaggerate, changes of hydrogen ion concentration. pH is the logrithmic reciprocal of hydrogen ion concentration and, with the help of buffers, is maintained near 7.4 in healthy people. *(3:331–334)*

22. **(D)** A buffer is a weak acid and its salt. Of the listed choices, only sodium is not a buffer. The others help stabilize intracellular pH in the 7.4 range despite addition or subtraction of hydrogen ions. *(3:331–334)*

23. **(D)** The enzyme responsible for the conversion of carbon dioxide and bicarbonate into carbonic acid is carbonic anhydrase. Acetazolamide is a potent inhibitor of carbonic anhydrase and a diuretic. *(3:331–334)*

24. **(C)** Normal serum osmolality is about 290 mmol/L. A quick approximation is given by the formula

    osmolality = 2(sodium) + (glucose/20) + (BUN/3)

    where osmolality is calculated as mmol/L, the sodium is in mmol/L, the glucose is in mg/dL, and the BUN (blood urea nitrogen) is in mg/dL. The factors of 20 and 3 convert the mg/dL units of glucose and BUN, respectively, into mmol/L. Serum osmolality is controlled principally by antidiuretic hormone (ADH) which is synthesized by the hypothalamus and then stored in the posterior pituitary. States of high serum osmolality (dehydration) result in increased ADH release. Circulating ADH acts on the kidney to elevate urinary osmolality. The free water generated in the kidney is used to dilute the blood back to its normal osmolality of about 290 mmol/L. *(4:125–126)*

25. **(E)** The anion gap is a clinically useful measurement defined by Na − (Cl + HCO_3). It is normally 10–14 mEq/L and represents unmeasured anions, such as protein, phosphates, and sulfates. It is elevated in lactic acidosis because the lactic acid anion is increased. The difference in the body's positive and negative charges is zero, since the body is electrically neutral. *(4:133–134)*

26. **(C)** Recanalization is the development of new channels in an occlusive thrombus. Infarction is tissue death from inadequate blood supply, a common result of arterial occlusive thrombi. Fibrinolysis is the dissolving of thrombus clot by plasma proteins, particularly plasmin. Propagation is the continued enlargement of a thrombus and predisposes to embolization, which is the breaking off of parts of a thrombus that are then carried in the bloodstream to a different site. *(1:141–143)*

27. **(B)** Passive splenic congestion produces a heavy, cyanotic spleen. The cut surface freely exudes blood. The sinusoids are dilated and filled by erythrocytes. The splenic capsule is expanded and tense, not shrunken and contracted. *(2:750–751)*

28. **(C)** Hemopericardium and hemothorax are hemorrhages into the pericardial sac and pleural cavity, respectively. Petechiae and purpura are hemorrhages in skin or serosal surfaces and differ only in size. Petechiae are minute, whereas purpura can be up to about 1.0 cm in diameter. Hemostasis is the process of clotting, the opposite of hemorrhage. *(2:93)*

29. **(E)** Passive congestion of the liver is a form of passive hyperemia caused by impaired venous drainage. The increased hepatic blood volume increases the weight and size of the liver. The pattern of blood distribution is skewed into the centrilobular (venous) areas and appears grossly as a nutmeg pattern. Pyramid-shaped infarcts do not occur in hepatic passive congestion; they are characteristic of arterial thromboemboli of end-artery type. The liver has a dual blood supply, not an end-artery blood supply, and would not be expected to have pyramid-shaped infarcts. *(6:786–787)*

30. **(A)** Osmolality depends on the number of particles per unit volume, irrespective of charge. The term used to describe electrical charges per unit volume is "equivalents." In the choices listed, each chemical rapidly separates into ions in H_2O. To find the choice with the highest osmolality, find the one with the most particles per unit volume.

    RELATIVE OSMOLALITY
    A 2
    B 1
    C 1
    D ½
    E ½

    To find the solution with the highest equivalence, find the one with the most electrical charges per concentration. *(4:42–43,125–126)*

31. **(E)** Infarcts cause coagulative necrosis in most organs (including kidney, small bowel, heart, and spleen) whether caused by a white or a red infarct. Coagulative necrosis microscopically appears as an acellular, nuclei-depleted ghost image of the normal tissue architecture. The brain is an exception and undergoes liquefaction with infarcts. The in-

farcted brain tissue is rapidly liquefied, losing its usual architecture, and phagocytized by microglia. *(2:111–114)*

32. **(E)** Platelets measure about 2 mm in diameter and contain no nuclei. Their precursors are megakaryocytes, not monocytes. There are two kinds of granules in platelets, alpha and dense. The alpha contains fibrinogen, fibronectin, and beta-thromboglobin, but not ADP. The dense granules contain ADP, calcium, and histamine, but not fibrinogen. Platelets contain actomyosin, microfilaments, and tubules that are important in pseudopod formations. *(4:717–721)*

33. **(A)** Most arterial emboli arise from thrombi in the heart. Of those, about 65% arise in the left ventricle and about 20% in the left atrium. Less common sources of arterial emboli are thrombi in ulcerated aortic plaques, aortic aneurysms, and abnormal cardial valves. Arterial emboli follow varied paths, but the majority (70%) lodge in the lower extremities. Those that embolize in the brain via the middle cerebral artery may be rapidly fatal. Most arterial emboli are bland (nonseptic). Septic emboli, usually arising from infective endocarditis, are likely to produce septic infarcts at the site of embolization. *(2:108)*

34. **(B)** Shock is defined succinctly as inadequate tissue perfusion. All the other answers are common causes of inadequate tissue perfusion but do not define the single necessary criterion for shock. *(6:268–273)*

35. **(B)** The coagulation factors are proteins, not lipids. Each active factor activates other factors, with amplification at each step producing a cascade effect. The entire system is designed to produce a fibrin clot. Necessary cofactors are platelets and calcium. Genetic deficits, such as hemophilia (factor VIII), occur. *(2:97–99)*

36. **(B)** Adherence of platelets to the vessel wall is the earliest event in arterial thrombosis. This is followed by activation of Hageman factor of the intrinsic system and a cascade effect with subsequent activation of the rest of the intrinsic system components. The end result of intrinsic system activation is activation of the common pathway. Plasminogen activation is part of the fibrinolysin system and would dissolve clots, not form them. *(2:95–97)*

37. **(C)** A system of checks and balances in the body maintains the fine line between bleeding and thrombosis. *(2:93–104)*

38. **(D)** von Willebrand factor, a component of coagulation factor VIII, is made by endothelial cells and is a necessary cofactor for the adherence of platelets to subendothelial tissue. Although hepatocytes take many of the circulating protein coagulant factors, they do not produce von Willebrand factor. Platelets are crucial for coagulation but do not synthesize von Willebrand factor. Neutrophils and lymphocytes are not significantly involved in hemostasis. *(4:745)*

39. **(A)** A mural thrombus is a nonocclusive blood clot that forms on the wall of a large volume blood-filled organ, such as the heart or aorta. Small arteries, such as the cerebral and coronaries, form occlusive thrombi. Since the spleen is a solid organ, mural thrombi could not form. *(2:99–102)*

40. **(D)** A thrombus may be dissolved (lysis) by the fibrinolytic system. Other evolutions would include ingrowth of vascular channels (recanalization), ingrowth of granulation tissue (organization), or incorporation of additional thrombotic material (propagation). *(2:102)*

41. **(E)** An occlusive arterial thrombus, such as coronary thrombosis, is almost always at the site of a vessel abnormality. The most common abnormality is atherosclerosis. Rarer abnormalities include arteritis and trauma. An expected finding in coronary thrombosis is infarction of the myocardium, with ischemic (coagulative) necrosis. Thrombocytopenia is not expected in coronary thrombosis, since platelets must be present in adequate numbers and function to initiate a thrombus. A low platelet count would make thrombus formation unlikely. *(6:360–365)*

42. **(E)** TxA_2 is synthesized by platelets and is a crucial substance in platelet aggregation. Besides aggregating platelets, actions of TxA_2 are mediated through cAMP. Prostacyclin is a platelet antagonist, and by opposing the actions of TxA_2 it slows its effectiveness. *(2:95–97)*

43. **(A)** Factor VII is part of the extrinsic pathway. All the other choices are part of the intrinsic clotting mechanism. *(6:424)*

44. **(E)** The three major influences in thrombogenesis are injury to endothelium, alterations in normal blood flow (turbulent flow or stasis), and hypercoagulability (as in rare AT III-deficient people). A decrease in the clotting factors would make the blood potentially hypocoagulable, with subsequent thrombus formation unlikely. *(2:99–105)*

45. **(E)** Hemorrhagic infarcts, also called "red infarcts," are encountered usually with venous occlusions, in loose tissues, in tissues with a double circulation, and in tissues previously congested. The other type of infarct, white or anemic infarcts, is usually seen with arterial occlusion, single end-artery blood supply, and in solid tissues. The lungs

characteristically have hemorrhagic infarcts. *(2:99–105)*

46. **(E)** Occlusive arterial thrombi occur frequently in the coronary arteries, usually at the site of an atherosclerotic lesion. Other affected vessels include cerebral, iliac, and femoral arteries. Rarely, occlusive thrombi occur at sites of trauma or arteritis. Emboli almost never occur with occlusive arterial thrombi, since the artery's diameter decreases distally. Pulmonary emboli arise almost exclusively from the venous, not arterial, thrombi. *(2:99–108)*

47. **(D)** Paradoxical emboli are those from the venous system that gain access to the arterial circulation through a heart wall defect. Sudden death from a pulmonary embolus in healthy people is not common. These pulmonary emboli usually originate in the deep veins of the leg (deep venous thrombosis). Not all emboli cause infarcts. An organized embolism is one that has an ingrowth of young blood vessels and fibrous tissue. *(6:267)*

48. **(E)** Gas embolism is the abnormal occurrence of gas bubbles in the circulation. They gain entrance to the circulation by trauma (lung, chest wall, ruptured uterine veins) or by coming out of solution from fatty tissues (decompression sickness, or caisson disease). Hypertension, an elevation of blood pressure, predisposes to heart and kidney failure but not to gas embolism. *(2:108–111)*

49. **(B)** Shock, or inadequate tissue perfusion, commonly is associated with cardiogenic failure, hypovolemia, pooling of blood in periphery, anaphylaxis, and disseminated intravascular coagulation. Congestive heart failure is a compensatory mechanism of expanded intravascular volume, and shock rarely accompanies simple congestive heart failure. *(6:268–273)*

50. **(B)**

51. **(E)**

52. **(A)**

53. **(D)**

50 through 53. All of the listed choices are effectors of coagulation or fibrinolysis. The fibrinolytic system dissolves clots mainly through activation of plasmin. A potent inhibitor of plasmin activation is alpha$_1$-antitrypsin. A nonhuman source (exogenous) of plasmin activity is streptokinase, which is used therapeutically to dissolve thrombi, particularly those in the coronary circulation. Thrombin is the common name for factor II, an element of the common pathway. ADP is a platelet-aggregating factor. *(2:94–99)*

54. **(E)**

55. **(B)**

56. **(A)**

57. **(D)**

54 through 57. The major extracellular buffer is bicarbonate. It is the buffering salt of carbonic acid (H_2CO_3). Lactic acid is produced by anaerobic glycolysis in states of tissue anoxia. Aldosterone, a hormone, and antidiuretic hormone regulate sodium concentration in the body. Acetazolamide is an inhibitor of carbonic anhydrase, which is an enzyme present in lung and kidney and is involved in acid-base regulation. *(3:331–334)*

58. **(B)**

59. **(A)**

60. **(D)**

61. **(C)**

58 through 61. Total body water is about 60% of lean body weight (LBW). The total body water is two-thirds (40% LBW) intracellular and one-third (20% LBW) extracellular. Plasma, part of the extracellular component, makes up about 5% LBW. *(3:273–279)*

62. **(D)**

63. **(E)**

64. **(B)**

65. **(C)**

62 through 65. Abnormal collections of fluid in the body are named by both the site of occurrence and the character of fluid that accumulates. The most common sites include peritoneum, pericardium, thorax, joints, and fallopian tube. If the fluid that accumulates is watery or serous the prefix "hydro" is used. If the fluid is bloody the prefix "hemo" is used. Purulent collections are characterized by the prefix "py." For example, a collection of bloody fluid in the pericardium is termed "hemopericardium." Watery fluid accumulations in the pleural cavity of the chest are called "hydrothorax." Purulent expansions of the joint space are called "pyarthroses." *(6:263–265)*

66. **(B)**

67. **(C)**

68. (A)

69. (D)

66 through 69. Laboratory tests are commonly used to evaluate the hemostatic status of patients. The prothrombin time (PT) and partial thromboplastin time (PTT) are in vitro tests of the extrinsic and intrinsic clotting systems, respectively. Both employ activators (PT = thromboplastin, PTT = kaolin-cephalin) in the presence of added calcium to stimulate the patient's calcium-depleted plasma to produce a fibrin clot. The clot normally forms in about 12 seconds for the PT and about 25 seconds for the PTT. Decreased protein clotting factors or circulating anticoagulants will prolong these tests. The bleeding time is an in vivo test used to evaluate platelet and capillary function. After placing a blood pressure cuff at 40 mm Hg on the upper arm, a small incision is made on the forearm. Every 30 seconds thereafter the wound is gently touched with blotter paper to see if it is still bleeding. The time it takes the incision to stop bleeding is termed the "bleeding time." Normal values are usually less than 8 minutes. Abnormal platelet function, thrombocytopenia, or capillary abnormalities all can prolong the bleeding time. The clot retraction test is an in vitro test of platelet contraction. Normally, a clot will retract from 40% to 60% of its initial volume during 4 hours when incubated at 37°C. The clot lysis test is an in vitro test for fibrinolysis. If the fibrinolytic system is hyperactive (DIC, carcinomatosis), the clot will lyse in only a few hours, instead of the normal 18 to 24 hours. *(6:429)*

70. (E)

71. (B)

72. (A)

73. (D)

70 through 73. The draining suction of the terminal lymphatics and vascular oncotic pressure work together to maintain the interstitium in a dry, nonedematous state. Decreased oncotic pressure due to hypoalbuminemia can result in edema. Obstruction of the lymphatic channels occurs in filariasis and can produce edema. Urticaria is localized edema caused by histamine release, with increased endothelial permeability, and subsequent leakage of fluid into the interstitium. Congestive heart failure may produce edema via increased capillary hydrostatic pressure. *(2:87–90)*

74. (C)

75. (B)

76. (D)

77. (A)

74 through 77. The partial or complete obstruction of vascular channels from a traveling fragment of blood clot or other substance is termed "embolism." Amniotic embolism usually occurs during prolonged, strenuous labor due to the forceful introduction of amniotic fluid contents into the uterine venous sinuses. The pernicious nature of amniotic embolism results from DIC which amniotic fluid's potent thromboplastin activity initiates. Major boney fractures almost always release particles of fat into the venous circulation to embolize in brain, lung, and kidney. In certain instances adult respiratory distress syndrome and cerebral confusion may result. Decompression sickness is seen in divers that surface too rapidly after being submerged for long periods. As they ascend nitrogen gas comes out of solution as bubbles that act as emboli. Air embolism occurs when air enters the vascular system, usually due to thoracic trauma. Only about 150 ml of embolic air is fatal. *(1:144–150)*

78. (E)

79. (D)

80. (B)

81. (A)

78 through 81. As emboli travel through the vascular system, they may totally or partially occlude the vessel lumen. Ischemia, functional impairment, or infarction of the tissue may result from this luminal stenosis. For example, an embolic stenosis of the ophthalmic artery may produce transient monocular blindness (amaurosis fugax). Emboli to the middle cerebral artery often cause cerebral infarcts (strokes). Emboli to branches of the renal artery may result in a typical fan-shaped pale renal infarct of the end-artery type. "Angina pectoris" is the term used for chest pain due to myocardial ischemia. The usual etiology of angina pectoris is atherosclerosis with subsequent coronary artery stenosis. Ischemic leg pains that develop with exercise are called "intermittent claudication." Atherosclerotic stenosis of the femoral or popliteal artery is the usual cause of intermittent claudication. *(1:365–366, 729, 931–937)*

82. (C)

83. (E)

84. (D)

85. (A)

82 through 85. Cations are positively charged ions. Anions are negatively charged ions. The major intracellular and extracellular cations are potassium and sodium, respectively. The bicarbonate anion is the ionic component of the body's most important buffering mechanism. Calcium is a cation which is active in coagulation and muscle contraction. Chloride is an important extracellular anion. *(4:128–132, 3:333)*

86. (C)

87. (D)

88. (A)

86 through 88. In solving acid-base problems, first look at the pH. If the pH is less than 7.4, there is acidosis. If the pH is more than 7.4, there is alkalosis. Next look at the Pco_2 to see if there is a respiratory component. Pure acute metabolic processes will lack any contributing respiratory component and should demonstrate a normal Pco_2 of about 40 mm Hg. If there is a respiratory component present, the uncompensated acid-base disturbance should have an abnormal Pco_2.

Question 86 has a pH of 7.28 so the student is acidotic. The Pco_2 is abnormal so there is a respiratory component. Thus, the student has respiratory acidosis. It is acute because the experiment has had only a 10-minute duration and because there has not been sufficient time for compensatory renal actions to occur. Breathing air with an increased carbon dioxide concentration (respiratory failure, chronic lung disease, breath holding) will produce respiratory acidosis.

Question 87 has a pH of 7.51 so the child is alkalotic. The Pco_2 is abnormal so there is a respiratory component. Thus, the child has respiratory alkalosis. It is acute because of the immediate time frame of the hyperventilation and because there has not been sufficient time for compensatory renal actions to occur. Hyperventilation characteristically produces respiratory alkalosis.

Question 88 has a pH of 7.19 so there is acidosis. The Pco_2 is normal so there is no respiratory component. Thus, the man is in metabolic acidosis. The acidosis is acute because there is no evidence of compensatory respiratory actions. The ingestion of ethylene glycol will produce a marked metabolic acidosis with a large anion gap. Ingestion of sufficient ethylene glycol can be fatal. *(3:340–342)*

89. (E)

90. (B)

91. (H)

89 through 91. The first scenario depicts a young woman with a hypercoagulable state (antithrombin III deficiency). At autopsy the bowel is gangrenous in a segment drained anatomically by the superior mesenteric vein. A thrombosis of the vein is likely. Factors that predispose to thrombus formation include nonlaminal flow, hypercoagulable states, or damage to the endothelium. Mesenteric vein thrombosis is a common occurrence in antithrombin III deficient individuals. The second scenario describes diffuse intravascular coagulation resulting from amniotic fluid emboli. During prolonged labor, amniotic fluid material may enter the uterine venous sinuses and subsequently embolize to the lungs. Amniotic material is a potent thromboplastin which can initiate intravascular coagulation. The third scenario describes a man with Marfan's syndrome. Cystic medial necrosis and dissecting thoracic aneurysms are common complications seen in aged individuals with Marfan's syndrome. Proximal dissection into the pericardium invariably produces hemopericardium and cardiac tamponade. *(2:99–102, 108–109, 138–139)*

92. (C) Nitrogen embolism (acute decompression sickness) is seen in scuba divers who ascend too rapidly after a deep dive. While deeply submerged, inhaled compressed air becomes partially dissolved in the blood, tissue fluids, and fat. As the diver rapidly ascends, the dissolved air comes back out of solution as bubbles. The oxygen component of the bubbles is rapidly redissolved or metabolized. The nitrogen component, however, persists as minute bubbles that mechanically obstruct the minor vasculature with subsequent multifocal ischemia. Ischemia in the skeletal muscles produces severe pain (the bends). Mechanical blockage of pulmonary vessels impedes efficient respiratory exchange with resultant respiratory distress (the chokes). In the most serious cases, mechanical obstruction of cerebral vessels by nitrogen emboli may lead to obtundation, coma, or death. *(2:109–110)*

93. (A) Fractures of the major long bones or pelvis may produce fat embolization. Fatal fat embolism is rare, however, and is seen in only a small percentage of trauma cases. In fatal cases, microscopic fat and bone marrow globules are found in the small vessels of the brain, kidney, and lung. Brain microinfarcts and ischemia may result in confusion, decreased mental acuity, coma, or death. The lung emboli can produce adult respiratory distress syndrome and hypoxia. Kidney involvement may be documented by the premortem demonstration of fat globules in the urine. *(2:110–111)*

94. (B) Most pulmonary emboli arise from the large veins of the lower legs. Obesity, immobilization, estrogen usage, varicosities, and hypercoagulable states all predispose to venous thromboembolism. Most pulmonary emboli are too small to obstruct the main pulmonary artery and lodge further down the pulmonary arterial tree. Pulmonary infarction may complicate these smaller impacted emboli. The autopsy findings in this case revealed an obstructing saddle-type embolus in the main pulmonary artery. *(2:105–108)*

95. **(H)** The pleural effusion is a transudate. Transudates are typified as protein-poor collections of fluid devoid of inflammatory cells such as macrophages or neutrophils. The albumin levels are usually below 1 gm/dL and the specific gravity is usually less than 1.010. Transudates are seen in states of increased hydrostatic pressure or decreased plasma oncotic pressure. Congestive heart failure commonly produces pleural effusions that are transudative in nature. *(2:41–42)*

96. **(G)** The pleural effusion is an exudate. Exudates occur in inflammatory states. There is leakage of protein-rich fluid into body spaces with accompanying cellular elements. Usually the exudate has an albumin level greater than 2 gm/dL and a specific gravity of more than 1.010. Neutrophils, red blood cells, macrophages, tumor cells, mast cells, and eosinophils may populate the exudate. Cellular disruption may produce elevations in clinically significant enzymes such as lactate dehydrogenase. Malignant tumors metastatic to the pleural cavity characteristically produce exudative effusions. *(2:41–42)*

REFERENCES

1. Chandrasoma P, Taylor CR: Concise Pathology, Norwalk, Appleton and Lange, 1991
2. Cotran RS, Kumar V, Robbins SL: Robbins Pathologic Basis of Disease, 4th edition, Philadelphia, Saunders, 1989
3. Guyton AC: Textbook of Medical Physiology, 8th edition, Philadelphia, Saunders, 1991
4. Henry JB (ed): Clinical Diagnosis and Management by Laboratory Methods, 18th edition, Philadelphia, Saunders, 1991
5. Kissane JM (ed): Anderson's Pathology, 9th edition, St. Louis, Mosby, 1990
6. Rubin E, Farber JL: Pathology, Philadelphia, Lippincott, 1988

CHAPTER 4

Immunopathology

Recent advances in the field of immunology have produced an explosion of knowledge about the immune system. This chapter deals with the basic concepts of immunology and the immunologic mechanisms involved in disease states of excess or deficient immunity.

BASIC FACTS AND CONCEPTS

The immune system is designed to produce humoral or cellular immunity. The salient features of both are shown in Table 4–1. The immunoglobulins (Ig) produced by plasma cells share a common double heavy-double light chain disulfide bonded structure with a Fab antibody end and an opposite Fc cell-binding end. The type of heavy chain involved defines the Ig into one of five major classes: IgG, IgM, IgA, IgE, or IgD. Each class has peculiarities (Table 4–2).

The hypersensitivity reactions are ordinary cellular or humoral immunity to foreign antigens carried to the point of damage to the person. The cogent features are listed in Table 4–3. Other instances of hyperimmunity are demonstrated by the autoimmune disorders (Table 4–4). In these diseases, the inciting antigen is a natural bodily substance, not an outside (nonself) antigen, as was the case in the hypersensitivity reactions. Some people suffer from deficient immune systems, either congenital or acquired. The major hereditary immunodeficiency states are shown in Table 4–5. Common acquired immunodeficiency states include acquired immunodeficiency syndrome (AIDS) and those resulting from immunosuppressive therapy for transplantation or neoplasia.

TABLE 4–1. FEATURES OF HUMORAL AND CELLULAR IMMUNITY

	Humoral Immunity	Cellular Immunity
Principal cell	B cell lymphocyte	T cell lymphocyte
Assisting cells	Macrophages T helper cells	? Macrophages
End result	Immunoglobulin	Lymphokines Cytotoxic T cells
Effective against	Bacteria toxins	Viruses, fungi, transplants, tumor cells

TABLE 4–2. CHARACTERISTICS OF IMMUNOGLOBULINS

Class	Heavy Chain	Principal Location	Construction	Peculiar Function
IgG	Gamma	Serum	Monomer	Secondary (anamnestic) immune response
IgM	Mu	Serum	Pentamer	Primary immune response
IgA	Alpha	Secretions	Dimer	Immunity against luminal antigens(?)
IgE	Epsilon	Mast cells	Monomer	Type I hypersensitivity Anaphylaxis
IgD	Delta	B lymphocytes	Monomer	Immune modulation

TABLE 4-3. HYPERSENSITIVITY REACTIONS

Type of Reaction		Humoral or Cellular Immunity	Function
Type I	Anaphylactic	Humoral IgE	Antigen causes mast cell degranulation with resultant local or systemic anaphylaxis
Type II	Cytolytic (erythroblastosis)	Humoral IgG IgM complement	Antigen causes Ig and complement binding with cell lysis
Type III	Immune complex (systemic: serum sickness; localized: Arthus reaction)	Humoral IgG IgM ± complement	Antigen-antibody complexes deposited at sites and via active intermediates produce tissue injury
Type IV	Cell-mediated (tuberculin reaction)	Cellular	Cell-mediated immunity produces lymphokines and cell-mediated cytotoxicity

TABLE 4-4. MAJOR AUTOIMMUNE DISEASES AND PRINCIPAL FEATURES

Disease	Probable Antigen	Symptoms
Systemic lupus erythematosus	Nuclear components	Facial rash, renal failure, serositis, arthritis
Rheumatoid arthritis	IgG	Arthritis
Scleroderma	Nuclear components	Cutaneous atrophy, dysphagia
Sjögren's syndrome	Salivary gland	Dry eyes, dry mouth, salivary destruction
Hashimoto's thyroiditis	Microsomes, thyroglobulin	Hypothyroidism
Myasthenia gravis	Acetylcholine receptors	Muscular weakness
Pemphigus vulgaris	Keratinocytes	Cutaneous bullae
Primary biliary cirrhosis	Mitochondria	Jaundice, cirrhosis

TABLE 4-5. MAJOR HEREDITARY IMMUNODEFICIENCY STATES

Type	Deficit	Characteristics
DiGeorge's immunodeficiency	Cellular	Thymic hypoplasia, tetany (parathyroid hypoplasia)
Bruton's immunodeficiency	Humoral	X-linked inheritance, agammaglobulinemia
Severe combined immunodeficiency	Cellular and humoral	Stem cell absence
Isolated IgA deficiency	IgA protein	Sinopulmonary infections
Wiskott-Aldrich syndrome	Cellular and humoral	X-linked inheritance, thrombocytopenia, eczema

Questions

DIRECTIONS (Questions 1 through 47): Each of the numbered items or incomplete statements in this section is followed by answers or by completions of the statement. Select the ONE lettered answer or completion that is BEST in each case.

1. The principal cell involved in immunity is

    (A) red blood cell
    (B) lymphocyte
    (C) endothelial cell
    (D) pancreatic acinar cell
    (E) adipose cell

2. Identify the INCORRECT statement about B cell lymphocytes

    (A) found in white pulp of spleen
    (B) constitute 70 to 80% of circulating lymphocytes
    (C) express surface immunoglobulin
    (D) express a receptor for complement 3b (C3b)
    (E) found in germinal follicles in lymph nodes

3. Which statement about T cell lymphocytes is true?

    (A) not found in the peripheral circulation
    (B) unable to bind to sheep erythrocytes
    (C) play a key role in cellular immunity
    (D) mature into plasma cells
    (E) have a receptor for Fc

4. Thymosin is

    (A) a pituitary hormone that regulates thymic development
    (B) a glycoprotein that confers passive immunity to nonsensitized hosts
    (C) an antiserum against thymocytes
    (D) a thymic hormone that induces maturation of pre-T cells
    (E) a lymphokine elaborated by activated thymocytes

5. Which statement about macrophages is FALSE?

    (A) they help process and present antigen to immunocompetent cells
    (B) they act as mediators in certain cell-mediated immune reactions
    (C) they can have Fc receptors
    (D) they can have complement 3 (C3) receptors
    (E) they can produce immunoglobulin

6. Cell-mediated immunity is an important host defense mechanism against all EXCEPT

    (A) deep-seated mycotic infections
    (B) pyogenic bacterial infections
    (C) *Mycobacterium tuberculosis*
    (D) schistosomiasis
    (E) measles

7. The fusion of a myeloma cell with an antigensensitized B cell lymphocyte is termed

    (A) dendritic cell
    (B) opsonization
    (C) natural killer cell
    (D) null cell
    (E) hybridoma

8. Which cell is LEAST LIKELY to contain human leukocyte antigens (HLA)?

    (A) T lymphocytes
    (B) macrophages
    (C) B lymphocytes
    (D) endothelial cells
    (E) red blood cells

9. Which human chromosome contains the HLA complex?

    (A) chromosome 11
    (B) chromosome 23
    (C) chromosome 48
    (D) chromosome 6
    (E) sex chromosome

10. The chance that any two siblings will inherit an identical set of HLA antigens is

    (A) 100%
    (B) 25%
    (C) 50%
    (D) less than 1%
    (E) 33%

11. Mixed lymphocyte culture is useful in testing for

    (A) HLA-A
    (B) HLA-B
    (C) HLA-C
    (D) HLA-D
    (E) HLA-E

12. Specific HLA have been associated with all the diseases listed EXCEPT

    (A) Reiter's disease
    (B) ankylosing spondylitis
    (C) Addison's disease
    (D) multiple myeloma
    (E) acute anterior uveitis

13. The immunoglobulin most likely to be found in secretions is

    (A) IgA
    (B) IgD
    (C) IgE
    (D) IgG
    (E) IgM

14. Identify the INCORRECT statement about immunoglobulins

    (A) the Fc contains the site of antigen-antibody interaction
    (B) can exist as monomers, dimers, and pentamers
    (C) consist of heavy and light chains
    (D) reagin antibodies are IgE
    (E) macrophages possess receptors for Fc

15. A delta heavy chain would be expected in

    (A) IgA
    (B) IgD
    (C) IgE
    (D) IgG
    (E) IgM

16. The major immunoglobulin produced in a primary immune response is

    (A) IgG
    (B) IgM
    (C) IgE
    (D) IgD
    (E) IgA

17. When pepsin acts on an immunoglobulin, the result is

    (A) Fc and heavy chains
    (B) heavy chains and light chains
    (C) Fc and Fab
    (D) Fab and light chains
    (E) Fc and light chains

18. An anamnestic immunologic response would be expected to occur with

    (A) immunodeficient populations
    (B) Bruton's hypogammaglobulinemia
    (C) rechallenge of a sensitized host with the sensitizing antigen
    (D) neurologically damaged patients with immune defects
    (E) common variable immunodeficiency

19. Anaphylactic reactions involve all of the following EXCEPT

    (A) IgE
    (B) Langhans' giant cells
    (C) histamine release
    (D) basophils
    (E) mast cells

20. Identify the INCORRECT statement about the complement (C) system

    (A) may result in cell lysis
    (B) properdin is crucial to classic pathway
    (C) components are mostly glycoproteins
    (D) C3b fragment is active in opsonization
    (E) classic pathway starts at sites of immunoglobulin attachment

21. Which cation is important to the function of complement 3 (C3) convertase?

    (A) sodium
    (B) chloride
    (C) bicarbonate
    (D) calcium
    (E) magnesium

22. Identify the complement (C) factor with chemotactic activity

    (A) C5b67
    (B) C9
    (C) C8
    (D) C3a
    (E) C1

23. The ultimate function of the completed complement pathway onto a cell is to promote

    (A) mitosis
    (B) immunocompetency

(C) lysis
(D) immunoglobulin synthesis
(E) immune tolerance

24. Eight to twelve days after injection of a foreign antigen, an individual experiences fever, lymphadenopathy, glomerulonephritis, arthritis, and malaise. The most likely diagnosis would be

   (A) type I hypersensitivity reaction
   (B) type II hypersensitivity reaction
   (C) type III localized hypersensitivity reaction
   (D) type III generalized hypersensitivity reaction
   (E) type IV hypersensitivity reaction

25. An example of type IV hypersensitivity is

   (A) tuberculin reaction
   (B) Arthus reaction
   (C) serum sickness
   (D) immune agranulocytosis
   (E) hemolytic transfusion reaction

26. Which substance is not a lymphokine?

   (A) macrophage migration-inhibiting factor (MMIF)
   (B) interferon
   (C) transfer factor
   (D) interleukin II
   (E) histamine

27. Which item is not a structural component of IgG?

   (A) kappa light chain
   (B) Fc region
   (C) variable region
   (D) Fab region
   (E) alpha heavy chain

28. Immune surveillance as a mechanism of host protection against tumorigenesis is best supported by

   (A) increased levels of cancer in immunodeficient populations
   (B) low levels of immune complexes
   (C) increased levels of antibody
   (D) abnormal lymphocytes
   (E) decreased levels of cancer in transplantation populations

29. An enlarged spleen is found to contain abundant acellular eosinophilic hyaline material by light microscopy. A Congo red stain demonstrates green birefringence. The most likely identity is

   (A) amyloid
   (B) edema fluid
   (C) bacteria
   (D) talc
   (E) none of the above

30. On Southern blot examination the DNA of a malignant tumor is found to have a clonal immunoglobulin gene rearrangement. From what type of cell is the tumor derived?

   (A) fibroblast
   (B) T lymphocyte
   (C) squamous epithelium cell
   (D) cuboidal epithelium cell
   (E) B lymphocyte

31. Goodpasture's syndrome is characterized by autoantibodies to

   (A) basement membrane
   (B) platelet surface antigens
   (C) parietal cell antigens
   (D) acetylcholine receptors
   (E) colonic mucosal cells

32. Antimicrosomal antibodies are commonly seen in

   (A) rheumatoid arthritis
   (B) systemic lupus erythematosus (SLE)
   (C) Hashimoto's thyroiditis
   (D) scleroderma
   (E) mixed connective tissue disease

33. Autoantibodies against acetylcholine receptors characterize

   (A) pernicious anemia
   (B) myasthenia gravis
   (C) dermatomyositis
   (D) rheumatoid arthritis
   (E) scleroderma

34. A fluorescent antinuclear antibody (FANA) test may be helpful in diagnosing

   (A) Hashimoto's thyroiditis
   (B) primary biliary cirrhosis
   (C) isolated IgA deficiency
   (D) Wiskott-Aldrich syndrome
   (E) systemic lupus erythematosus (SLE)

35. Nonbacterial verrucous endocarditis most commonly is associated with

   (A) systemic lupus erythematosus (SLE)
   (B) pneumocystis pneumonia
   (C) complement 1 (C1) inhibitor deficiency
   (D) Epstein-Barr virus (EBV) infection
   (E) cytomegalovirus (CMV) infection

36. Identify the incorrect statement concerning Sjögren's syndrome

    (A) may have keratoconjunctivitis sicca
    (B) may have xerostomia
    (C) has lymphocytic infiltration of salivary glands
    (D) has an increased risk for malignant lymphoma
    (E) rheumatoid factor, ANA, and LE cell preparations are always negative

37. A 35-year-old woman complains of dysphagia, symmetrical edema and thickening of the fingers, and Raynaud's phenomenon. Which immunologic disease is most likely?

    (A) *Vibrio cholera* infection
    (B) shigellosis
    (C) polyarteritis nodosa
    (D) scleroderma
    (E) Hashimoto's thyroiditis

38. Severe combined immunodeficiency (SCID) can include all of the following EXCEPT

    (A) poor cell-mediated immunity
    (B) autosomal or sex-linked inheritance
    (C) 80% 10-year survival
    (D) low levels of adenosine deaminase
    (E) poor humoral immunity

39. Chronic granulomatous disease includes all of the following EXCEPT

    (A) poor bacterial killing by neutrophils
    (B) usually afflicts males
    (C) symptoms of pneumonia, lymphadenitis, or splenomegaly
    (D) usually manifest in the first 2 years of life
    (E) increased nitroblue tetrazolium (NBT) reduction

40. Hereditary deficiency of complement 1 (C1) inhibitor is characterized by

    (A) recurrent angioedema
    (B) mild adolescent disease, crippling adult disease
    (C) high levels of C1 inhibitor
    (D) systemic lupus erythematosus (SLE)
    (E) sex-linked inheritance

41. A 6-year-old boy with a history of recurrent bacterial infections, partial albinism, and central nervous system disorders is found to have an unusual peripheral blood smear characterized by giant cytoplasmic granular inclusions in white cells and platelets. The most likely diagnosis is

    (A) selective IgM deficiency
    (B) selective IgA deficiency
    (C) Wiskott-Aldrich syndrome
    (D) Chediak-Higashi syndrome
    (E) selective deficiency of IgG subclass

42. A marked decrease in T helper cells is a characteristic feature of

    (A) systemic lupus erythematosus (SLE)
    (B) acquired immunodeficiency syndrome (AIDS)
    (C) erythroblastosis fetalis
    (D) autoimmune hemolytic anemia
    (E) pernicious anemia

43. The causative agent of acquired immunodeficiency syndrome (AIDS) is

    (A) a virus
    (B) *Pneumocystis carinii*
    (C) a protozoan parasite
    (D) Kaposi's sarcoma
    (E) lymphadenopathy

44. Usual findings in acquired immunodeficiency syndrome (AIDS) may include all the following EXCEPT

    (A) fever, weight loss, and lymphadenopathy
    (B) *Pneumocystis carinii* infections
    (C) increased cell-mediated immunity
    (D) cytomegalovirus (CMV) infection
    (E) Kaposi's sarcoma

45. A transfer of immunocompetent cells into an antigenically different recipient who is immunocompromised is likely to produce

    (A) Bruton's agammaglobulinemia
    (B) graft-vs-host disease
    (C) type I hypersensitivity reactions
    (D) clonal deletion
    (E) DiGeorge's syndrome

46. Identify the FALSE statement about hyperacute renal transplantation rejection

    (A) classic example of type IV hypersensitivity reaction
    (B) involves recipient's preformed circulating antibodies
    (C) usually occurs within minutes after transplantation
    (D) early lesions are at vascular endothelium
    (E) grossly appears as a flaccid, mottled, cyanotic kidney

47. Which statement is FALSE?

    (A) amyloid can occur in both systemic and localized forms
    (B) amyloid is more common in infants than in geriatric populations

(C) amyloid's peculiar chemical properties result in part from a beta-pleated sheet construction
(D) genetic forms of amyloidosis exist
(E) amyloid may be seen in lymphoproliferative disorders

DIRECTIONS (Questions 48 through 99): Each group of items in this section consists of lettered headings followed by a set of numbered words or phrases. For each numbered word or phrase, select the ONE lettered heading that is most closely associated with it. Each lettered heading may be selected once, more than once, or not at all.

Questions 48 through 51

(A) HLA-B8
(B) HLA-Bw47
(C) HLA-B27
(D) HLA-C4
(E) HLA-C6

48. Ankylosing spondylitis

49. Celiac disease

50. Acute anterior uveitis

51. Reiter's disease

Questions 52 through 55

(A) type I hypersensitivity
(B) type II hypersensitivity
(C) type III hypersensitivity
(D) type IV hypersensitivity
(E) type V hypersensitivity

52. Cell-mediated type   D

53. Immune complex disease   C

54. Anaphylactic type   A

55. Cytotoxic type   B

Questions 56 through 59

(A) Hashimoto's thyroiditis
(B) autoimmune hemolytic anemia
(C) Goodpasture's syndrome
(D) systemic lupus erythematosus (SLE)
(E) pemphigus vulgaris

56. Antibodies against red blood cells   B

57. Antibodies against microsomal components   A

58. Antibodies against basement membranes   C

59. Antibodies against nuclear antigens   D

Questions 60 through 63

(A) xenograft
(B) isograft
(C) autograft
(D) allograft
(E) avascular graft

60. Retransplantation of a host's own tissue   C

61. Transplantation from a genetically identical twin   B

62. Transplantation from a genetically dissimilar member of the same species   D

63. Transplantation from a different species   A

Questions 64 through 67

(A) platelets
(B) Langerhans' cells
(C) T cell lymphocytes
(D) B cell lymphocytes
(E) NK cells

64. Progenitor of plasma cells   D

65. Have helper (CD4) and suppressor (CD8) subsets   C

66. Antigen-processing cells usually found in skin   B

67. Cytotoxic cells lacking well-defined T or B cell markers   E

Questions 68 through 71

(A) IgM
(B) IgA
(C) IgG
(D) IgE
(E) IgD

68. Fc portion can bind to mast cells   D

69. Usually a dimer found in secretions   B

70. Gamma heavy chain   C

71. Usually found as pentamers   A

Questions 72 through 75

(A) DiGeorge's syndrome
(B) Bruton's agammaglobulinemia
(C) Wiskott-Aldrich syndrome
(D) myasthenia gravis
(E) isolated IgA deficiency

72. Thymic hypoplasia, tetany, and deficient cellular immunity   A

73. X-linked hereditary disorder of humoral and cellular immunity with thrombocytopenia and eczema *C*

74. X-linked hereditary disorder of humoral immunity with absent gamma globulin *B*

75. Reduced IgA levels with recurrent sinopulmonary infections *E*

Questions 76 through 79

(A) class I major histocompatibility complex
(B) class II major histocompatibility complex
(C) class III major histocompatibility complex
(D) class IV major histocompatibility complex
(E) class V major histocompatibility complex

76. HLA-DR *B*

77. HLA-A *A*

78. Complement proteins *C*

79. HLA-B *A*

Questions 80 through 83

(A) type I hypersensitivity reaction
(B) type II hypersensitivity reaction
(C) type III hypersensitivity reaction
(D) type IV hypersensitivity reaction

80. Erythroblastosis fetalis *B*

81. Tuberculin skin test *D*

82. Anaphylaxis following an insect sting *A*

83. Serum sickness *C*

Questions 84 through 87

(A) systemic lupus erythematosus (SLE)
(B) primary biliary cirrhosis
(C) pemphigus vulgaris
(D) myasthenia gravis
(E) Hashimoto's thyroiditis

84. Autoantibodies to thyroglobulin *E*

85. Autoantibodies to mitochondria *B*

86. Autoantibodies to keratinocytes *C*

87. Autoantibodies to acetylcholine receptors *D*

Questions 88 through 91

(A) properdin
(B) C3a
(C) C6
(D) C5b6789 complex
(E) C1

88. Causes focal cell membrane lysis *D*

89. Binds to Fc initiating the classic pathway *E*

90. Initiator of the alternative pathway *A*

91. Anaphylatoxic *B*

Questions 92 through 95

(A) systemic lupus erythematosus (SLE)
(B) scleroderma
(C) Sezary's syndrome
(D) DiGeorge's syndrome
(E) rheumatoid arthritis
(F) myasthenia gravis
(G) secondary amyloidosis
(H) Hashimoto's thyroiditis

92. A 47-year-old female has noticed that in the mornings the small joints of her hands are swollen, painful, and stiff. Her rheumatoid factor is reported as strongly positive. What disease is she most likely to have? *E*

93. A 51-year-old man has had a generalized erythroderma with intense itching for about 2 months. Numerous atypical lymphoid cells with cerebriform convoluted nuclei are evident in his peripheral blood. These atypical cells have T cell markers. What disease is he most likely to have? *C*

94. A 76-year-old male with a long history of chronic osteomyelitis gradually develops cardiac arrhythmias and splenomegaly. A rectal biopsy shows abundant eosinophilic acellular material which by polarized light examination displays apple green birefringence after staining with Congo red. What disorder is he most likely to have? *G*

95. A 32-year-old woman complains of diplopia and drooping eyelids. A trial dose of edrophonium produces an immediate transient improvement of her ocular muscle weakness. A serum assay for acetylcholine receptor antibodies is reported as positive. What disease is she most likely to have? *F*

Questions 96 through 99

(A) neoplasm of B lymphocytes
(B) neoplasm of T lymphocytes
(C) tumor of Langerhans' cells
(D) neoplasm of myeloid cells
(E) neoplasm of erythroid cells
(F) neoplasm of thrombocytes
(G) neoplasm of epithelial cells
(H) neoplasm of muscle cells

96. A 77-year-old female is noted to be anemic. Her serum protein electrophoresis demonstrates a large monoclonal IgG kappa protein. In her bone marrow are increased numbers of atypical plasma cells. Her skull x-rays show multiple lytic areas.

97. A 12-year-old African boy develops a large disfiguring tumor of the jaw. Histologically, the tumor is composed of small actively mitotic undifferentiated cells in a "starry sky" background. The scant cytoplasm of the cells is positive for Oil red O vacuoles. The majority of the cells have surface immunoglobulin.

98. A 45-year-old male has noticed an erythematous skin rash for about 2 months. On biopsy the skin demonstrates Pautrier's microabscesses and tumor cells. The tumor cells are positive for CD4 and CD3. No surface immunoglobin is present on the tumor cells.

99. A 15-year-old female complains of rib pain. An x-ray demonstrates a solitary lytic rib lesion. The biopsy contains eosinophils and tumor cells. The tumor cells are large, have nuclear groves, contain S100 antigen, and on electron microscopy are shown to possess Birbeck bodies.

Answers and Explanations

1. **(B)** Lymphocytes (both T and B cell types) are the principal cells involved in immunity. Macrophages and neutrophils also are helpful in modulating the immune response. Red cells, endothelial cells, pancreatic acinar cells, and adipose cells are not significantly involved in immunity. *(2:163–167)*

2. **(B)** B lymphocytes make up only about 10 to 20% of lymphocytes in the peripheral blood. T lymphocytes are the subset that constitute 79 to 80% of circulating lymphocytes. *(2:163–167)*

3. **(C)** T cells play a pivotal role in cellular immunity. They are present in the peripheral blood and readily bind sheep erythrocytes (rosetting). B cells, not T cells, have Fc receptors and mature into plasma cells. *(2:165–167)*

4. **(D)** Thymosin is a thymic hormone that regulates pre-T cell development. It is not released from the pituitary. Antithymocyte antibodies are not thymosin but are useful in transplantation rejection therapy. Lymphokines are released from T cells, but thymosin is a thymic hormone, not a lymphokine. *(4:98–99)*

5. **(E)** Macrophages are crucial effectors and affectors of immunity. They can produce soluble factors to influence the growth and function of lymphoid and nonlymphoid tissue, as well as responding to certain lymphokines. Plasma cells, derived from B lymphocytes, not macrophages, secrete immunoglobulin. *(4:98–102)*

6. **(B)** Cell-mediated immunity is an important host mechanism against infection by obligatory intracellular pathogens, fungi, and parasites. Humoral immunity, not cellular immunity, is more important in containment of infections caused by pyogenic bacteria. *(1:52–61)*

7. **(E)** The usefulness of hybridomas arises from their ability to produce abundant monoclonal antibody to specific antigens. Natural killer and null cells are types of lymphoid cells. Dendritic cells may possess weak phagocytic activity and may be helpful in antigen presentation. Opsonization is the coating of antigens, usually bacterial, with complement fragments to enhance phagocytosis. *(2:163–168)*

8. **(E)** The human leukocyte antigens (HLA) are glycoproteins present on the surface of virtually all nucleated cells. Of the given choices, only red blood cells are nonnucleated and could be expected to have little or no leukocyte antigens. *(4:102–104)*

9. **(D)** The HLA system is present on chromosome 6. Beta-hemoglobin production is present on chromosome 11, making it the site of thalassemias and beta-hemoglobinopathies. Chromosome 23 and the sex chromosome are identical. Since humans have only 23 chromosome pairs, there is no chromosome 48. *(4:102–104)*

10. **(B)** Half of each parental HLA genotype is transmitted to each offspring. Since each child possesses half of the mother's and half of the father's HLA antigens, the chance of any two siblings possessing the same HLA genotype (identical HLA antigens), is 0.5×0.5, or 25%. *(1:120)*

11. **(D)** Mixed lymphocyte cultures demonstrate the approximately 12 subsets of HLA-D. Mixing non-D identical lymphocytes will result in a proliferation of the lymphocytes indicating nonidentity. HLA-A, HLA-B, and HLA-C usually are determined by serologic procedures. There is no HLA-E. *(3:774–776)*

12. **(D)** Ankylosing spondylitis, Reiter's disease, and acute anterior uveitis are all associated with HLA-B27. Addison's disease is associated with HLA-B8. Multiple myeloma is not associated with any specific HLA type. *(2:171–172)*

13. **(A)** IgA has its major role in secretions. It is secreted as a dimer with some linking pieces and a secretory piece made by epithelial cells in the vicinity of the plasma cells in which IgA is made. IgM is predominantly intravascular. IgG is both intravascular and extravascular. IgE is bound to mast

cells or basophils. IgD is present throughout the body in very scant quantity. *(3:809–824)*

14. **(A)** The Fab portion contains the site of antibody–antigen interaction. The Fc portion is the site of macrophage receptor binding. Immunoglobulins are Y-shaped and occur as monomers, dimers, and pentamers. They consist of both light and heavy chains. Reagin antibodies are another term for immunoglobulins of the IgE class. *(3:809–824)*

15. **(B)** The heavy chains are specific for each of the five major classes of immunoglobulins. The heavy chains are alpha, delta, epsilon, gamma, and mu for IgA, IgD, IgE, IgG, and IgM, respectively. *(3:819)*

16. **(B)** IgM is the effector of the primary immune response. The primary response follows the antigen encounter by 4 to 7 days and results in sensitization in the immunocompetent host. Rechallenge by the same antigen in a sensitized host will produce a secondary immune response with IgG. *(1:67–69)*

17. **(C)** An immunoglobulin is composed of four peptide chains linked by disulfide bonds. Pepsin splits the immunoglobulin into Fc (crystallizable) and Fab (antigen-binding) fragments. Free heavy or free light chains are not produced by pepsinolytic activity. *(1:61–63)*

18. **(C)** An anamnestic immune response, also called the "secondary immune response," occurs in immunocompetent and sensitized individuals rechallenged by the sensitizing antigen. The word *anamnestic* has origin from the Greek, meaning to recall or recollect. The other four listed choices are states of immunodeficiency and would be unlikely to mount an anamnestic response. *(1:67–69)*

19. **(B)** Anaphylactic (type I hypersensitivity) reactions involve formation of IgE cytotropic antigen binding to mast cells or basophils. Appropriate antigens react with the IgE antibodies to cause cell degranulation, histamine release, and anaphylaxis. Langhans' foreign body giant cells are seen in type IV hypersensitivity reactions, not type I. *(2:173–177)*

20. **(B)** The complement system is composed predominantly of glycoproteins. It can be activated by either antigen–antibody reactions (classic pathway) or by properdin stabilization (alternate pathway). Properdin does not play a role in the classic pathway. Fragments generated in the pathway may become chemical mediators, such as C3b for opsonization. The ultimate goal of the complement system, when fully activated, is to produce cellular lysis. *(1:65–67)*

21. **(E)** Magnesium is a cofactor in C3 convertase, allowing cleavage of C3 and yielding C3a and C3b fragments. Cations must have positive electrical charges. HCO_3 and chloride are anions. *(3:831–833)*

22. **(A)** The complement factor $\overline{C5b67}$ is chemotactic and induces migration of neutrophils and monocytes. The C3a and C5a factors are anaphylatoxins, increasing vascular permeability and causing smooth muscle contraction. C9 and C8 are final proteins in the complement pathway and are needed for complement-mediated cell lysis. *(3:834–835)*

23. **(C)** The complement pathway has cell lysis as its ultimate goal. In the process, numerous chemotactic, opsonin, and spasmogenic products are produced. *(3:830–837)*

24. **(D)** The clinical history is a classic description of one-shot serum sickness, a generalized type III hypersensitivity reaction. The localized type III hypersensitivity reaction is the Arthus complex and usually is characterized by swelling and fibrinoid vasculitis at a subcutaneal injection site. *(4:109–113)*

25. **(A)** Type IV hypersensitivity reactions involve cell-mediated immunity, with the tuberculin reaction being the classic example. Serum sickness and the Arthus reaction are examples of generalized and localized type III hypersensitivity, respectively. Immune agranulocytosis and hemolytic transfusion reactions are examples of type II hypersensitivity. *(4:104–116)*

26. **(E)** Lymphokines are substances produced by lymphocytes to assist in cell-mediated immunity and type IV hypersensitivity reactions. They include MMIF, interferon, chemotactic factors, interleukin II, and transfer factor. Histamine is not a lymphokine. It is present in basophils and mast cells and plays a major role in anaphylaxis (type I hypersensitivity). *(4:98–102)*

27. **(E)** The IgG molecule is composed of either two gamma heavy chains and two kappa light chains, or two gamma heavy chains and two lambda light chains. The heavy chains are located centrally within the molecule and bound together by disulfide linkages. The two identical light chains are located peripherally and opposite each other: one bound to each heavy chain by disulfide linkages. Conceptually, the immunoglobulin molecule can be viewed as a "Y." The open branched end contains variable regions of the heavy and light chains that are termed "Fab." The Fab portion of the molecule is the site of antigen recognition and antibody–antigen binding. The other end of the immunoglobulin molecule contains the Fc region, constructed only by the two heavy chains. The Fc component can fix complement and has chemotactic properties. The intact whole immunoglobulin molecule can be

split into Fab (fragment antibody) and Fc (fragment complement) by enzymatic digestion. *(3:809–820)*

28. **(A)** Immune surveillance is the mechanism whereby a host mounts an immune response against antigens expressed by the tumor. The increased level of tumorigenesis seen in immunodeficient populations supports the concept of immune surveillance. Low levels of immune complexes, increased levels of antibody, and abnormal lymphocytes are not central concepts to immune surveillance. There are increased, not decreased, levels of tumorigenesis in transplant populations. *(2:297–299)*

29. **(A)** Amyloid is acellular material that by routine light microscopy appears eosinophilic and hyaline. Special stains, such as Congo red, produce a diagnostic green birefringence. An additional aid is that the spleen is a likely systemic site for amyloid deposition. *(2:210–220)*

30. **(E)** The Southern blot technique is a very potent laboratory test for identifying the lineage of lymphomatous tumor cells. Very early in their ancestry B lymphocytes and T lymphocytes undergo physical rearrangement of their immunoglobulin genes and T cell receptor genes, respectively. Identification of rearranged monoclonal immunoglobulin genes in a tumor points to a B cell lineage. Likewise, tumors that demonstrate monoclonal T cell receptor genes are T lymphocyte derived. The Southern blot technique involves the initial fragmentation of tumor DNA by endonucleases. The fragmented DNA is then sorted by size through electrophoresis. Labelled complementary DNA probes to immunoglobulin genes or T cell receptor genes are then hybridized with the tumor sample. Monoclonal binding indicates the appropriate lineage. If there is binding only to the germline (nonrearranged) DNA component, then the tumor cells are of nonlymphoid origin, such as fibroblasts or epithelial cells, or the tumor is not a clonal proliferation (benign). *(3:298–300)*

31. **(A)** Goodpasture's disease is characterized by antibasement antibodies, with the lung and kidneys bearing the brunt of the damage. Antibodies against platelet surface antigens, parietal cells, acetylcholine receptors, and colonic mucosal cells are seen in autoimmune thrombocytopenia, pernicious anemia, myasthenia gravis, and ulcerative colitis, respectively. *(1:122–126)*

32. **(C)** Antimicrosomal antibodies are commonly seen in Hashimoto's thyroiditis. Parenchymal immune destruction of the thyroid gland can produce clinical hypothyroidism. Antinuclear antibodies are associated with SLE, scleroderma, and Sjögren's syndrome. Mixed connective tissue disease is characterized by antiribonuclear protein antibodies. *(1:122–126)*

33. **(B)** Autoantibodies against acetylcholine receptors characterize myasthenia gravis. Antinuclear antibodies are found in scleroderma and dermatomyositis. Pernicious anemia is the result of antiparietal and anti-intrinsic factor antibodies. Rheumatoid arthritis is characterized by anti-Ig antibodies, usually of the IgM type. *(1:122–126)*

34. **(E)** A FANA test is used to detect antibodies against nuclear cellular components. Only SLE of the choices listed characteristically has a positive FANA. Antibodies against thyroglobulin and microsomal antigens characterize Hashimoto's thyroiditis. Antibodies against mitochondria are seen in primary biliary cirrhosis. Wiscott-Aldrich syndrome and isolated IgA deficiency are immunodeficiency states. *(2:193–202)*

35. **(A)** Nonbacterial verrucous endocarditis, also called Libman-Sacks endocarditis, is associated with SLE and is characterized by sterile excrescences on the mitral and tricuspid valves with fibrinoid necrosis. C1 inhibitor deficiency is characterized by bouts of episodic angioedema. Pneumocystis, EBV, and CMV infections are features of acquired immunodeficiency syndrome (AIDS). Neither AIDS nor C1 inhibitor deficiency has a strong association with nonbacterial verrucous endocarditis. *(2:193–202)*

36. **(E)** Sjögren's syndrome is characterized by lymphocytic infiltration and fibrosis of lacrimal and salivary gland tissue, producing a clinical picture of dry eyes (keratoconjunctivitis) and dry mouth (xerostomia). Other autoimmune diseases, such as rheumatoid arthritis, systemic lupus erythematosus, polymyositis, scleroderma, vasculitis, and thyroiditis, are seen in a fair number of Sjögren's patients. Because of this, many patients have positive rheumatoid factor, ANA, and LE cell preparations. The risk factor for subsequent lymphoma is estimated as 40 times higher in Sjögren's patients. *(2:202–204)*

37. **(D)** The clinical history provides the classic presentation of scleroderma, also called progressive systemic sclerosis. Hashimoto's thyroiditis, an autoimmune disorder, usually occurs with hypothyroidism and goiter. Cholera and shigellosis are bacterial infections with severe diarrhea. Polyarteritis nodosa is a noninfectious necrotizing vasculitis of possible autoimmune origin, with a protean clinical appearance. *(2:204–207)*

38. **(C)** Most children with SCID die in the first 2 years of life; long-term survival is exceptional. SCID re-

sults in impaired cellular and humoral immunity. Autosomal recessive and sex-linked inheritance have been described. In the autosomal recessive form, adenosine deaminase levels are markedly reduced in some patients. *(4:123–124)*

39. **(E)** Chronic granulomatous disease is most often X-linked and associated with a decreased ability of neutrophils and other phagocytic cells to kill bacteria. As a result, by 2 years of age, signs of chronic low-grade infections appear, such as lymphadenopathy, splenomegaly, pneumonia, and sinusitis. The NBT test shows markedly decreased, not increased, chemical reduction and helps confirm the diagnosis, since lack of NBT reductive capacity correlates with poor bactericidal activity. *(1:93, 413)*

40. **(A)** Hereditary deficiency of C1 inhibitor is characterized by angioedema. The mode of inheritance is autosomal dominant, not sex-linked. There is a marked decrease in the levels of C1 inhibitor, which is worse in adolescents and gradually subsides in about the fifth decade. SLE is associated with genetic deficiency of C2 inhibitor. *(4:46)*

41. **(D)** The clinical description as well as the peripheral blood findings are classic for Chediak–Higashi syndrome. Selective immunoglobulin deficiencies are not associated with albinism, and the leukocytes and platelets both are morphologically normal. Wiskott–Aldrich syndrome is immunodeficiency with eczema and thrombocytopenia. *(3:726)*

42. **(B)** AIDS is characterized by a relative decrease in T helper cells. The usual ratio of helper/suppressor cells is about 2. In AIDS patients, ratios of 0.7 to 0.4 are not uncommon. *(4:98–103)*

43. **(A)** AIDS is caused by the human immunodeficiency virus (HIV, formerly called HTLV III). The other listed choices are opportunistic infections, neoplasms, or symptoms associated with AIDS. *(4:98–103)*

44. **(C)** The basic problem in AIDS is decreased cellular immunity, due in part to destruction of T helper (T4) cells. As a result of poor cellular immunity, opportunistic infections and exotic tumors, such as *Pneumocystis carinii*, CMV, and Kaposi's sarcoma are common. Usual findings in the AIDS patient include weight loss, fever, diarrhea, and generalized lymphadenopathy. *(4:98–103)*

45. **(B)** A transfer of immunocompetent cells into an antigenically different immunodeficient host is likely to produce graft-vs-host disease. The term "clonal deletion" refers to Burnet's theory of how self-antigens are eliminated from the lymphoid system during development. Bruton's agammaglobulinemia and DiGeorge's syndrome are genetic immunodeficiency states. *(2:188–189)*

46. **(A)** Hyperacute renal transplantation rejection usually occurs minutes after re-establishing blood flow to the donor organ. Preformed circulating antibodies attach to endothelial sites, causing vascular injury. This is reflected grossly by a cyanotic, mottled, flaccid kidney. There is no involvement of cell-mediated immunity, as in type IV hypersensitivity reactions, in hyperacute rejection. Type IV reactions are important in chronic transplant rejection. *(2:183–187)*

47. **(B)** Amyloid is more common in a geriatric population than in infants. The finding of amyloid in older populations is called "senile amyloidosis" or "amyloidosis of aging" and is a fairly frequent occurrence. *(2:210–220)*

48. **(C)**

49. **(A)**

50. **(C)**

51. **(C)**

48 through 51. Some autoimmune and immunologic disorders have been associated with certain HLA types. The close spatial relationship of the Ir genes and the HLA locus may be the operative factor. HLA-B27 is strongly associated with ankylosing spondylitis, Reiter's disease, and acute anterior uveitis. HLA-B8 and HLA-DR3 are associated with celiac disease (gluten-induced enteropathy). The HLA-DR3 locus is also linked to myasthenia gravis, systemic lupus erythematosus, and insulin-dependent diabetes mellitus. HLA-DR2 is associated with multiple sclerosis and Goodpasture's syndrome. HLA-DR4 is seen with rheumatoid arthritis and pemphigus vulgaris. HLA-DR5 occurs in many individuals with Hashimoto's thyroiditis, pernicious anemia, and juvenile rheumatoid arthritis. *(1:124–126, 589)*

52. **(D)**

53. **(C)**

54. **(A)**

55. **(B)**

52 through 55. Type I, or anaphylactic, hypersensitivity involves a rapid release of vasoactive amines from cytotropic mast cells and basophils. Type II, or cytotoxic, hypersensitivity involves immune-facilitated phagocytosis or cell lysis. Type III, or immune complex, hypersensitivity involves the activation of neutrophils through antigen–antibody complexes and complement. Type IV, or cell-mediated, hypersensitivity involves sensitized T lymphocytes. *(4:104–116)*

56. **(B)**
57. **(A)**
58. **(C)**
59. **(D)**

56 through 59. A number of disease states are characterized by autoantibodies against specific cellular components. Antibodies against red blood cells are the characteristic alteration in autoimmune hemolytic anemia. Hashimoto's thyroiditis has autoantibodies against thyroglobulin and microsomal antigens. Autoantibodies against lung and kidney basement membranes are features of Goodpasture's syndrome. SLE produces antibodies against numerous nuclear components. *(1:122–126)*

60. **(C)**
61. **(B)**
62. **(D)**
63. **(A)**

60 through 63. The body's acceptance or rejection of transplanted tissue is determined by the antigenic similarity of the transplanted tissue to the host's native tissue as well as the host's immune competency. Autotransplantation involves retransplantation of a host's own tissue, such as using an individual's own saphenous leg vein in a coronary bypass operation. Isografts are transplants between genetically identical twins. Autografts and isografts do not evoke an immune rejection response. Allografts are transplants derived from genetically dissimilar individuals of the same species, such as a human cadaveric kidney transplantation. The degree of rejection is dependent on the antigenic dissimilarity between donor and host, and the immune status of the host. Xenografts are transplants between species. They evoke a strong immune rejection response. Avascular grafts refer to sites, such as the cornea, that are unable to mount an immune rejection response to antigenically foreign material because immunocompetent cells have no vascular access to the site. *(1:17–18)*

64. **(D)**
65. **(C)**
66. **(B)**
67. **(E)**

64 through 67. A wide variety of cells are involved in the immune system. T cell lymphocytes constitute about 75% of the circulating peripheral blood lymphocytes. T cells are a critical element in cellular immunity. Further, the helper and suppressor subsets of T lymphocytes help to modulate varied immune processes. B cell lymphocytes are the progenitors of plasma cells. Plasma cells secrete immunoglobulin, the effector protein of humoral immunity. The Langerhans' cells are usually found scattered in the middle strata of the epidermis. These bone marrow derived dendritic cells have monocytic–macrophagic properties, are S100 antigen positive, and by electron microscopy possess a unique racquet-shaped pentalaminar Birbeck body. The Langerhans' cells are believed to play a role in antigen processing. The NK cells are large granular lymphocytes which lack well-defined mature T cell or B cell markers. Many NK (natural killer) cells have cytotoxic ability. Platelets are bone marrow derived elements and are a vital component of blood clotting. They are not believed to have any immune function. *(4:98–102)*

68. **(D)**
69. **(B)**
70. **(C)**
71. **(A)**

68 through 71. There are five major classes of immunoglobulins synthesized by plasma cells. Their characteristics are outlined in Table 4–2 at the beginning of this chapter. The IgA molecule is unusual in that it is first synthesized as a monomer by plasma cells located in luminal mucosa and submucosa. As the monomer travels through the surface epithelium, a dimer is formed by joining two IgA molecules with an epithelial synthesized J (joining) protein. The dimer is then bound additionally to a secretory component, also produced by epithelial cells, to facilitate passage of the dimer complex out into the lumen. The IgE class of immunoglobulins is avidly bound to mast cells and basophils so that the free (nonbound) serum IgE concentration is usually very low. In states of prolonged allergenic challenge, such as asthma, free serum IgE levels may be markedly elevated. In these cases the specific offending allergen may be identified by radioallergosorbent testing (RAST). *(1:61–63,125)*

72. **(A)**

73. (C)

74. (B)

75. (E)

72 through 75. DiGeorge's syndrome is characterized by disembryogenesis of the third and fourth brachial pouch. This developmental failure usually results in an absence of the parathyroids and thymus gland. Hypocalcemic tetany can result from hypoparathyroidism. There is deficient T cell immune function because of thymic aplasia. The mode of inheritance is autosomal recessive. Bruton's agammaglobulinemia is an x-linked hereditary disorder in which there are no B cells or their B cell precursors. Repeated bacterial infections develop due to the lack of immunoglobulin production. Most of the offending bacterial organisms are pyogenic (streptococci, staphylococci) and the common sites of infection include pharynx, conjuctiva, inner ear, lung, and skin. Wiskott–Aldrich syndrome is an x-linked recessive hereditary disorder characterized by decreased platelet aggregation, thrombocytopenia, eczema, and a combined deficiency of antibody production and cellular immunity. Clinically, there are repeated infections with bacterial and viral organisms. Most Wiskott–Aldrich individuals die before age 5. Selective IgA deficiency is the most common of the isolated immunoglobulin deficiencies. Patients lacking IgA suffer from recurrent sinopulmonary bacterial infections. Isolated IgA deficiency is also associated with gluten-sensitive enteropathy, allergies, and arthritis. *(2:220–223)*

76. (B)

77. (A)

78. (C)

79. (A)

76 through 79. The major histocompatibility complex (MHC) in humans is located on the short arm of chromosome 6. The MHC is presently divided into three classes. Class I antigens include HLA-A, HLA-B, and HLA-C. These genes code for transmembrane glycoproteins which are noncovalently linked to beta$_2$-microglobulin. These class I antigens are present on almost all nucleated cells in the body. Because of their highly polymorphic nature they provide a unique immunologic marker for "selfness." The class II MHC genes code for HLA-DR, HLA-DQ, and HLA-DP molecules. These molecules are found mainly on macrophages and B cell lymphocytes. Class II antigens consist of two noncovalently linked transmembrane glycoprotein chains. The larger is termed "alpha" and is about 34,000 daltons. The smaller is termed "beta" and is about 29,000 daltons. Class II molecules help with antigen presentation to the T cells. The class III MHC region codes for complement proteins C2, factor B, and C4. At present there are no class IV or class V MHC antigens. *(3:761–771)*

80. (B)

81. (D)

82. (A)

83. (C)

80 through 83. Erythroblastosis fetalis (hemolytic disease of the newborn) is a type II hypersensitivity reaction in which maternal IgG antibodies cross the placenta to lyse fetal erythrocytes. The provoking fetal antigen is usually Rh D (Rh positive) reoccurring in a previously sensitized mother. In the most severe instances, there is fetal hydrops with intrauterine demise, anasarca, and maceration. The tuberculin skin test is an example of a type IV hypersensitivity reaction. Immunologically competent and sensitized lymphocytes produce a granulomatous response to the tuberculin antigen. Anaphylaxis following an insect bite is an example of a type I hypersensitivity reaction. The insect venom antigens reacting with IgE antibodies bound to basophils and mast cells stimulate these cells to release vasoactive amines into the peripheral circulation. These vasoactive amines can bring about circulatory collapse and anaphylactic shock through generalized vasodilation, increased vascular permeability, and reduced intravascular volume. Serum sickness is an example of an immune complex injury. Following exposure to a large dose of foreign antigen circulating immune complexes form in the blood. These immune complexes may be trapped in the endothelial pores in blood vessels causing vasculitis, or in the kidney causing glomerulonephritis. Complement may exacerbate the tissue damage by recruiting inflammatory cells. Serum sickness is a Type II hypersensitivity reaction. *(4:104–116)*

84. (E)

85. (B)

86. (C)

87. (D)

84 through 87. Autoantibodies directed against native components of the body can produce a wide range of clinical disease states. Hashimoto's thyroiditis is an autoimmune disorder in which there is immunologic destruction of the thyroid gland with resultant hypothyroidism. The antibodies produced act

against thyroglobulin and microsomal follicular cell fractions. Histologically, the thyroid gland demonstrates a mixed lymphocytic and plasmacytic inflammatory infiltrate, germinal follicle formation, and reactive epithelial changes. Another autoimmune disorder, primary biliary cirrhosis, typically has high titers of antibodies that react with mitochondria. In this disorder there is immune-mediated destruction of hepatic bile ductules, with subsequent cirrhosis. Pemphigus vulgaris is a disease of autoimmunity in which there are antibodies produced against keratinocytes and their desmosomal attachment sites. Clinically, skin bullae occur because of autoimmune-mediated disattachment of affected keratinocytes. Myasthenia gravis is an autoimmune disorder in which acetylcholine receptor autoantibodies are produced. The immunologic impairment of the acetylcholine receptors is observed clinically as diminished muscular endurance, particularly noticeable in the periorbital and eyelid muscles. *(4:760–764,1138–1139,1211–1214)*

88. (D)

89. (E)

90. (A)

91. (B)

88 through 91. Complement may be activated either through the classical pathway or through the properdin alternative pathway. In the classic pathway IgG or IgM first binds to an antigen. The C1 fraction of complement then attaches to the Fc portion of the immunoglobulin molecule. Cleavage of bound C1 initiates the complement cascade. In the alternative pathway properdin and other cofactors (D, B, and magnesium) can cleave C3 independent of antibody binding and independent of the early classic pathway complement proteins (C1, C2, and C4). As the complement cascade builds, a number of biologically active fractions are released. For example, the C3a and C5a fragments are anaphylatoxins. C3b encourages immune phagocytosis by macrophages and neutrophils due to its opsonic properties. C5b67 is chemotactic. The final product of the complement cascade is a C5b6789 complex which is capable of inducing focal cell membrane lysis. *(1:65–68)*

92. (E) In this scenario the patient most likely has rheumatoid arthritis, an immunologic disorder of the joints. The disease is usually seen in Western European and North American white females between the ages of 30 and 50 years old. The clinical hallmark of the disease is symmetric swelling of the small joints of the hands and feet, particularly at the proximal interphalangeal joint. Swelling, pain, and stiffness is most severe in the morning. Pathologically, a pannus of hypertrophic inflamed synovium is produced that may eventually erode the articular cartilage with subsequent fibrosis, restriction of movement, and deformity. Most individuals with rheumatoid arthritis demonstrate a serum rheumatoid factor, an IgM molecule with anti-IgG specificity. *(1:988–989)*

93. (C) Sezary's syndrome is a lymphoproliferative disorder of T cell lymphocytes. Sezary cells are found circulating in the peripheral blood and are characterized as convoluted lymphocytic cells with cerebriform nuclei. T cell markers are invariable present on these cells, usually of the helper (T4, CD4) subset. Most individuals have erythroderma or eczema concomitant with the circulating cerebriform lymphocytes. The median survival rate is about 9 years. In the late stages of the disorder, there is extensive involvement of the visceral organs and lymph nodes by lymphomatous cells. *(2:716–717)*

94. (G) The elderly gentleman in this scenario is most likely to have secondary amyloidosis. Amyloid is a pathologic proteinaceous material deposited in the interstitial spaces. It is an acellular eosinophilic material with the biochemical ability to produce apple green birefringence when examined under polarized light in Congo red stained histologic material. This peculiar optical feature is due to the beta-pleated sheet arrangement of the amyloid molecules. Clinically, amyloidosis occurs in both localized and systemic forms. It is not uncommon to see amyloidosis follow longstanding inflammatory or infectious disorders, such as chronic osteomyelitis or tuberculosis. In these cases, the amyloidosis is almost always systemic in nature and deposited throughout the body. The heart interstitium, spleen interstitium, and perirectal blood vessels are preferential sites of systemic amyloid deposition. *(2:210–220)*

95. (F) The woman most likely has myasthenia gravis. This is an immunologic disorder most commonly occurring in women between the ages of 20 to 40 years old. Individuals with myasthenia gravis have muscle weakness that worsens as the muscle is exercised. The periorbital and lid muscles are likely to be involved, with affected individuals complaining of drooping eyelids and double vision (diplopia). Antibodies to acetylcholine receptors are present in myasthenia gravis and thought to be the most sensitive and specific method of diagnosing the disorder in patients with the appropriate clinical symptoms. Another diagnostic technique is to administer edrophonium, a short-acting anticholinesterase drug, to suspected myasthenic individuals. Those with myasthenia gravis will demonstrate a transient immediate improvement of muscular endurance and strength. Untreated, about 40% of myasthenic patients will die of their disease within 10

years, usually due to respiratory complications. Thymic abnormalities (hyperplasia and thymomas) may be seen in association with myasthenia gravis. *(1:965–966)*

96. **(A)** The elderly woman has multiple myeloma, a malignant tumor of plasma cells. Plasma cells are derived from B cell lymphocytes. Multiple myeloma is a disease rarely seen before age 50. The clinical features include anemia, bone pain, renal disease, hypercalcemia, infections, bleeding diatheses, and neuropathy. The bones may demonstrate multiple lytic defects when examined radiographically. The bone marrow contains increased numbers of atypical plasma cells. A monoclonal intact immunoglobulin, heavy chain, or light chain can be found in serum, urine, or both serum and urine. The mean survival is about 3 years. Death is usually due to hemorrhagic or infectious complications. *(1:460–463)*

97. **(A)** The child has Burkitt's lymphoma (small noncleaved cell lymphoma), a malignancy of B cell lymphocytes. Burkitt's lymphoma is a common tumor of African children. It usually occurs as a large disfiguring mass of the jaw. In North America the disease is infrequent. The North American variety is characterized by abdominal masses in childhood. Both the tropical and temperate varieties share similar histology: sheets of small undifferentiated cells with an elevated mitotic rate and a "starry sky" background of phagocytic macrophages filled with debris. Histochemically, the cytoplasm of the tumor cells contains Oil red O vacuoles. There is surface immunoglobulin on the Burkitt's cells confirming their B cell lineage. Burkitt's lymphoma is an aggressive high grade lymphoma. *(4:1104)*

98. **(B)** The man has mycosis fungoides (cutaneous T cell lymphoma), a malignancy of T cell lymphocytes. This neoplasm is a primary lymphoreticular malignancy that originates in the skin. The early stages of the disease may have only nonspecific erythroderma. Later stages of the disorder are plaque-like and demonstrate the diagnostic histology of Pautrier's microabscesses and Sezary–Lutzner tumor cells. The tumor cells are CD4 positive (T-helper subset) and have a folded cerebriform nucleus. A leukemic variety of this disorder is termed "Sezary's syndrome." Most individuals with mycosis fungoides eventually die from widespread visceral lymphoma, hemorrhagic complications, or infections. *(2:1293–1294)*

99. **(C)** The adolescent has an eosinophic granuloma, a tumor of Langerhans' cells. The disorder usually occurs in individuals under the age of 20. There is bone pain with one or two lytic areas noted radiographically. The ribs and vertebral bones are most commonly affected. If these lytic areas are biopsied, they are found to contain a polymorphous mixture of inflammatory cells, eosinophils, fibrous tissue, and Langerhans' cells. The Langerhans' cells can be identified with certainty by demonstrating their S100 protein positivity and the presence of pentalaminar Birbeck bodies. Eosinophilic granuloma is a benign self-limited disorder in the bones. Biopsy or curretage is usually curative. More aggressive diseases of Langerhans' cells include Hand–Schuller–Christian disease and Letterer-Siwe disease. *(4:1336–1338)*

REFERENCES

1. Chandrasoma P, Taylor CR: Concise Pathology, Norwalk, Appleton and Lange, 1991
2. Cotran RS, Kumar V, Robbins SL: Robbins Pathologic Basis of Disease, 4th edition, Philadelphia, Saunders, 1989
3. Henry JB (ed): Clinical Diagnosis and Management by Laboratory Methods, 18th edition, Philadelphia, Saunders, 1991
4. Rubin E, Farber JL: Pathology, Philadelphia, Lippincott, 1988

CHAPTER 5

Infectious Diseases

Although man can build a better mousetrap, nature always seems to build a better mouse.

—Alto E. Feller (1953)

BASIC FACTS AND DEFINITIONS

This chapter emphasizes the interactions and the host responses to invasion by microbiologic organisms. There are complicated interactions between host and parasite mediated through the immune system. There is an important distinction among symbiosis, commensalism, and parasitism.

The outcome and resultant disease processes that occur in response to invasion by pathogenic organisms depend on the balance between host factors and properties of the organism (Fig 5–1). Some examples of defense mechanisms and their failure to prevent microorganism-related diseases are seen in Table 5–1. Table 5–2 summarizes some of the more important characteristics of the various types of pathogenic organisms in human disease.

An important aspect of disease associated with protozoa and metazoa is the life cycle of the parasites. Examples are shown in Figure 5–2 and Table 5–3 to demonstrate how humans may occupy different positions in such life cycles.

Examples of bacteria that produce some of their effects through the production of toxins are shown in Table 5–4. Fungal or mycotic infections can produce superficial (most frequent) or deep and widespread lesions. Table 5–5 summarizes some of the more important causes of deep fungal infections for quick reference. There are many more fungal infections, with specialized geographic distribution.

Many and varied types of protozoa are pathogenic to humans. Table 5–6 summarizes some of these.

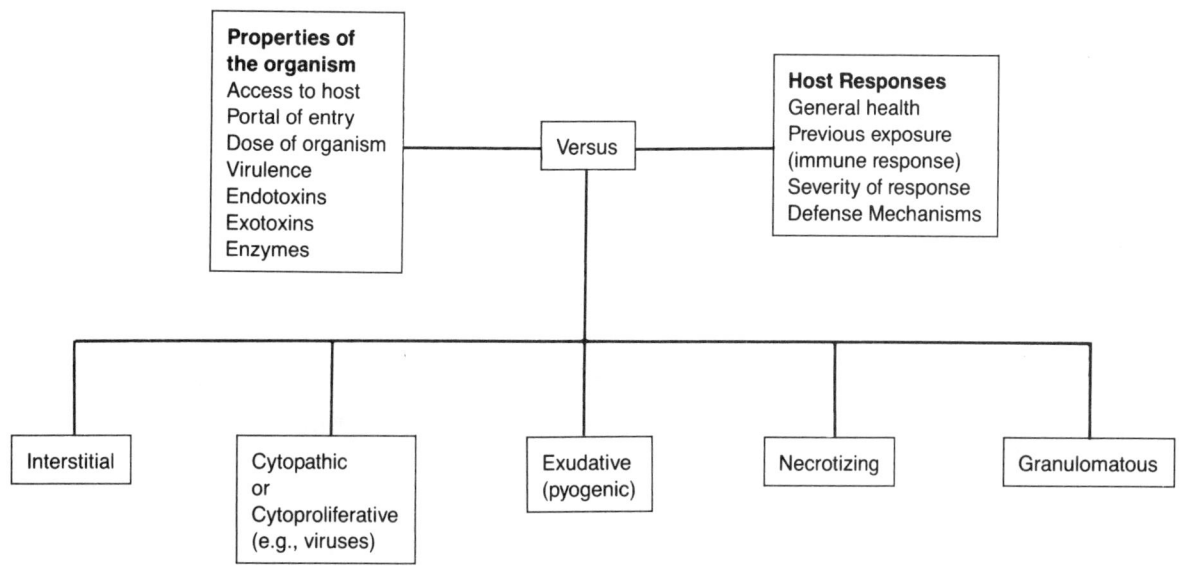

Figure 5–1. Pathogenesis of infectious diseases.

TABLE 5–1. SOME EXAMPLES OF DEFENSE MECHANISMS IN INFECTIOUS DISEASES

Portal of Entry	Defense Mechanisms	Examples of Failure or Breakdown of Defenses
Skin	Layers of stratified squamous epithelium Antimicrobial effects of secretions	Wounds, abrasions, burns, ulceration, pre-existing dermatoses
Respiratory tract	Nasal–oral secretions, pharyngeal lymphoid ring Mucociliary mechanism, cough reflex	Trauma, aspiration of material, obstruction, loss of cough reflex, failure of mucociliary action, low temperature, noxious gases, viral infection, destruction of epithelium
Gastrointestinal tract	Oral secretions, pharyngeal lymphoid ring, epithelium of esophagus and stomach acid, lymphoid tissue with secretion IgA of intestine, resident normal bacterial flora	Ingestion of infected material, food in nasopharynx or sputum, loss of gastric acid, ulceration of mucosa, obstruction, trauma, perforation, loss of flora due to stagnation or broad-spectrum antibiotics
Urinary tract	Flow of urine, pH of urine, transitional epithelium	Obstruction, stagnation of urine, stones, catheters, alteration of pH, penetrating injuries, ulceration
Female genital tract	Stratified squamous epithelium of vagina, acid and normal flora of vagina, mucous plugs of cervix	Hormonal loss with epithelial regressive changes, lowering of acidity and flora, trauma, parturition, foreign bodies (tampons), tumors, ulceration
Eyes (conjunctiva)	Secretions, tears, intact epithelium	Direct inoculation with infected material, lack of tears and secretions, trauma
Bloodstream and lymphatics	Usual inaccessability and immune factors	Extension from any of the above mechanisms, direct inoculation—intravenous or intra-arterial fluids, failure of immune mechanism, loss of leukocytes of various types

TABLE 5–2. SUMMARY OF IMPORTANT CHARACTERISTICS OF SOME PATHOGENIC ORGANISMS

Bacteria (0.8–15 μm)	Viruses (20–30 nm)	Rickettsia (300–1200 nm)	Mycoplasma (25–35 μm)	Fungi (2–200 μm)	Protozoa (1–50 mm)	Metazoa (including helminth) (3–10 mm)	Chlamydiae (20–1000 nm)
Facultative, Intracellular, or extra-cellular	Mostly obligate Intracellular	Mostly obligate Intracellular	Extracellular	Facultative, Intracellular, or extra-cellular	Variable, Extracellular, or intra-cellular	Variable, intracellular, or extra-cellular	Mostly obligate Intracellular

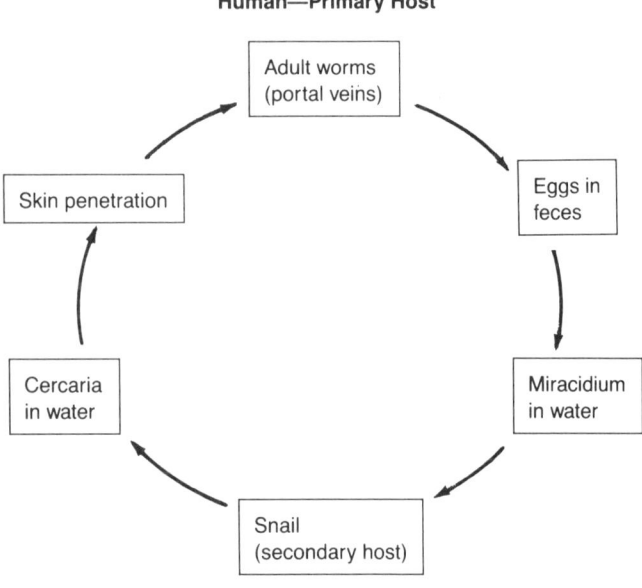

Figure 5-2. Schematic representation of the life cycle of *Schistosoma mansoni*.

TABLE 5–3. TYPES OF PARASITIC LIFE CYCLES

Parasite	Primary Host (Adult Form of Parasite)	Secondary Host	Intermediate Host (Often Accidental)
Schistosoma	Human	Snail	—
Plasmodium (malaria)	Mosquito	Human	—
Taenia solium (pig tapeworm)	Human	Pig	—
Echinococcus	Dog	Sheep	Human
Hookworm	Human	—	—

TABLE 5-4. EXAMPLES OF BACTERIAL TOXINS AND THEIR EFFECTS ON THE HOST

Type of Organism	Type of Toxin	Effect
Staphylococcus aureus	Enterotoxin	Gastrointestinal tract; food poisoning
	Alpha toxin	Necrosis of tissue; abscess formation
	Exfoliation	Exfoliation of skin
	Pyrogens	Fever
Streptococcus pyogenes	Streptolysins	Cellulitis
	Erythrogenic toxin	Vascular injuries: scarlet fever
Escherichia coli	Enterotoxin	Damage to intestinal epithelium, diarrhea, dehydration
Vibrio cholerae	Enterotoxin	Damage to intestinal epithelium, diarrhea, dehydration
Clostridium difficile	Enterotoxin	Epithelial damage: pseudomembranous colitis
Clostridium perfringens	Alpha toxin	Necrosis and hemolysis
Clostridium botulinum	Botulinim toxin	Neurotoxic, causes paralysis
Clostridium tetani	Tetanus toxin	Neurotoxic
Corynebacterium diphtheriae	Diphtheria toxin	Neurotoxic

TABLE 5-5. SUMMARY OF DEEP MYCOTIC INFECTIONS

Species of Fungus	Usual Port of Entry	Distribution of Lesions in Body
Sporothrix schenckii	Skin	Skin, occasionally lymph nodes
Torulopsis glabrata	Oral	Systemic
Candida subspecies	Skin, gastrointestinal tract, intravenous	Skin or mucus membranes, systemic: various organs
Cryptococcus neoformans	Respiratory tract	Lung, meninges, systemic
Aspergillus subspecies	Respiratory tract	Lung localized, lung diffuse, systemic
Mucor species	Respiratory tract	Upper respiratory, lung, systemic
Blastomyces dermatitidis	Respiratory tract	Lung, systemic with skin lesions
Coccidioides	Respiratory tract	Lung, systemic with meninges
Histoplasma capsulatum	Respiratory tract	Lung, systemic with widespread locations

TABLE 5-6. EXAMPLES OF PATHOGENIC PROTOZOA

Species	Usual Site of Disease	Usual Pathologic Disorder
Luminal		
Entamoeba histolytica	Colon	Amebic dysentery, liver or lung abscess
Balantidium coli	Colon	Dysentery
Giardia lamblia	Small intestine	Diarrhea with malabsorption
Cryptosporidium	Small and large intestine	Enterocolitis with malabsorption
Trichomonas vaginalis	Vagina and urethra	Vaginitis and urethritis
Pneumocystis carinii	Bronchial tree	Opportunistic lung infections
Bloodstream		
Plasmodium species	Red cells and blood stream, some in liver	Malaria
Trypanosoma species	Bloodstream	African sleeping sickness
Intracellular		
Trypanosoma cruzi	Various parenchymal cells, including myocardial cells	Chagas disease
Leishmania donovani	Macrophages	Kala-azar
Leishmania species	Macrophages	Cutaneous and mucocutaneous leishmaniasis
Toxoplasma gondii	Various parenchymal cells	Toxoplasmosis

Questions

DIRECTIONS (Questions 1 through 17): Each of the numbered items or incomplete statements in this section is followed by answers or by completions of the statement. Select the ONE lettered answer or completion that is BEST in each case.

1. The relationship between the human host organism and the normal bacterial flora (indigenous microbiota) is best called

    (A) saphrophytic
    (B) commensal
    (C) symbiotic
    (D) parasitic
    (E) facultative

2. Infection by all of the following characteristically produce diarrhea EXCEPT

    (A) rotavirus
    (B) enteropathogenic *Escherichia coli*
    (C) *Shigella dysenteriae*
    (D) *Vibrio cholerae*
    (E) *Klebsiella rhinoscleromatis*

3. Which organism is an obligate intracellular parasite?

    (A) *Mycobacterium tuberculosis*
    (B) *Mycobacterium kansasii*
    (C) *Mycobacterium leprae*
    (D) *Histoplasma capsulatum*
    (E) *Legionella pneumophila*

4. The pathogenicity of each of the following organisms involves endothelial or mural vascular invasion EXCEPT

    (A) rickettsiae
    (B) *Pseudomonas*
    (C) *Aspergillus*
    (D) *Treponema pallidum*
    (E) *Actinobacillus*

5. Which of the following ectoparasites has no intermediate host?

    (A) *Loa loa*
    (B) *Trichuris trichiura*
    (C) *Paragonimus westermani*
    (D) *Dracunculus medinensis*
    (E) *Clonorchis sinensis*

6. Stellate microabscesses with a granulomatous rim of epithelioid histiocytes may be seen in biopsies of lymphoid tissue from patients with

    (A) *Yersinia enterocolitica* infection
    (B) lymphogranuloma venereum (LGV)
    (C) *Brucella suis* infection
    (D) cat-scratch disease
    (E) all of the above

7. Genital skin ulcers are common in the acute presentation of each of the following venereal diseases EXCEPT

    (A) syphilis
    (B) granuloma inguinale
    (C) *Ureaplasma ureolyticum* infection
    (D) chancroid
    (E) herpes simplex virus type 2 infection

8. Acute inflammation, suppuration, and abscess formation are common features of infections caused by which organism?

    (A) *Staphylococcus aureus*
    (B) *Sporothrix schenckii*
    (C) *Blastomyces dermatiditis*
    (D) *Coccidiodes immitis*
    (E) *Cryptococcus neoformans*

9. The prognosis is best in rapidly progressive (crescentic) golmerulonephritis associated with

    (A) poststreptococcal glomerulonephritis
    (B) systemic lupus erythematosus (SLE)
    (C) Henoch-Schoenlein purpura
    (D) polyarteritis nodosa
    (E) Goodpasture's syndrome

10. The most common cause of parasitic endophthalmitis is

    (A) *Cysticercus cellulosae*
    (B) *Toxacara* species
    (C) *Toxoplasma gondii*
    (D) *Oncocerca volvulus*
    (E) *Loa loa*

11. The only ciliated pathogen of humans is

    (A) *Giardia lamblia*
    (B) *Trichomonas vaginalis*
    (C) *Chilomastix mesnili*
    (D) *Balantidium coli*
    (E) *Acanthamoeba culbertsoni*

12. Which of the following diseases is transmitted by *Culex* mosquitoes?

    (A) filariasis caused by *Onchocerca volvulus*
    (B) filariasis caused by *Wuchereria bancrofti*
    (C) leishmaniasis
    (D) malaria
    (E) all of the above

13. Which of the following is true of mumps?

    (A) humans are the only natural host
    (B) commonly occurs in infants
    (C) commonly causes orchitis and consequent sterility
    (D) produces intracellular inclusions in vivo in infected parotid acinar cells
    (E) optimum prevention is by administration of killed mumps virus

14. The fungus most frequently isolated by the clinical laboratory from patient blood cultures is

    (A) *Aspergillus* species
    (B) *Actinomyces* species
    (C) *Cryptococcus* species
    (D) *Candidia* species
    (E) *Mucor* species

15. Each of the following descriptions is true of *Plasmodium falciparum* EXCEPT

    (A) the sporozoites form more merozoites than the sporozoites of other malarial plasmodia
    (B) the merozoites parasitize both young and old red blood cells (RBC)
    (C) parasitized erythrocytes have increased adherence to vascular endothelium
    (D) infection is more frequently fatal than is infection with the other malarial plasmodia
    (E) persistent exoerythrocytic stage may result in relapse

16. The adult population groups that currently have a greatly increased risk of infection with human immunodeficiency virus (HIV) are homosexual or bisexual men, intravenous drug abusers, and their sexual contacts. What percentage of adult acquired immunodeficiency syndrome (AIDS) patients in the United States is classified as having none of these risk factors?

    (A) 3%
    (B) 10%
    (C) 15%
    (D) 20%
    (E) 25%

17. Enzyme immunoassay (EIA) screening tests are the standard method used to detect the presence of serum antibody to human immunodeficiency virus (anti-HIV). The sensitivity and specificity of EIA for anti-HIV are both

    (A) 1%
    (B) 10%
    (C) 50%
    (D) 90%
    (E) 99%

DIRECTIONS (Questions 18 through 76): Each group of items in this section consists of lettered headings followed by a set of numbered words or phrases. For each numbered word or phrase, select the ONE lettered heading that is most closely associated with it. Each lettered heading may be selected once, more than once, or not at all.

Questions 18 through 22

(A) pathogenicity does not involve mucosal invasion but is caused by an enterotoxin
(B) an enteroinvasive, flagellated gram-negative bacillus
(C) recovery from stool culture enhanced by cold enrichment
(D) pulmonary and cutaneous transmission by spores
(E) pathogenicity involves attachment of surface pili to host mucosal cell surface

18. *Neisseria gonorrhoeae*

19. *Vibrio cholerae*

20. *Campylobacter jejuni*

21. *Yersinia enterocolitica*

22. *Bacillus anthracis*

Questions 23 through 25

(A) the mature egg is an infective agent
(B) infective larvae are injected into humans by infected black fly or buffalo gnat
(C) larvae reaching soil via human feces may develop into a parasitic infective phase or a nonparasitic free-living phase
(D) the only tapeworm with humans as both intermediate and definitive hosts
(E) larvae become encysted in muscles of pigs or carnivores

23. *Onchocerca volvulus* B

24. *Hymenolepsis nana* D

25. *Ascaris lumbricoides* A

Questions 26 through 29

(A) entry into host cell involves fusion of viral coat with cell membrane
(B) entry into host cell involves release of nucleocapsid from endosome into cytosol
(C) entry into host cell involves release of nucleocaspid from endosome into cell nucleus
(D) entry into cell host involves fusion with T4 receptor on host cell surface
(E) an enveloped double-stranded DNA virus that replicates in the host cell cytoplasm

26. Influenza A virus B

27. Polyoma virus C

28. Human immunodeficiency virus (HIV) D

29. *Paramyxovirus* A

Questions 30 through 35

These questions refer to the microscopic examination of a stained smear of stool or diarrhea contents from a patient to ascertain the presence and type of inflammatory cells as a diagnostic test for pathogenesis of enteritis.

(A) many basophils
(B) many mononuclear leukocytes
(C) no (or rare) leukocytes
(D) many polymorphonuclear leukocytes
(E) many multinucleated giant cells

30. Typhoid fever B

31. Shigellosis D

32. Cholera C

33. Enterotoxigenic *Escherichia coli* C

34. Salmonellosis D

35. Ulcerative colitis D

Questions 36 through 39

Studies have shown that most patients in the United States with acquired immunodeficiency syndrome (AIDS) fall into four common categories. What is the approximate percentage of AIDS patients in each numbered category?

(A) 17%
(B) 1%
(C) 4%
(D) 73%
(E) 100%

36. Homosexual or bisexual men D

37. Hemophiliacs B

38. Intravenous drug abusers A

39. Haitians living in the United States C

Questions 40 through 44

(A) *Streptococcus pyogenes*
(B) *Clostridium perfringens*
(C) *Clostridium botulinum*
(D) *Clostridium tetani*
(E) *Clostridium difficile*

40. Tetanus D

41. Scarlet fever A

42. Pseudomembranous enterocolitis E

43. Gas gangrene B

44. Botulism C

Questions 45 through 49

(A) *Coxiella burnetti*
(B) *Rickettsia rickettsii*
(C) *Chlamydia psittaci*
(D) *Chlamydia trachomatis*
(E) *Rickettsia prowazekii*

45. Epidemic typhus E

46. Rocky Mountain spotted fever B

47. Blindness D

48. Q fever A

49. Ornithosis C

Questions 50 through 54

(A) *Trypanosoma cruzi*
(B) *Entamoeba histolytica*
(C) *Borrelia burgdoferi*
(D) *Leishmania donovani*
(E) *Plasmodium* species

50. Chagas' disease A

51. Malaria E

52. Lyme disease C

53. Amebiasis B

54. Kala-azar D

Questions 55 through 59

(A) *Wuchereria bancrofti*
(B) *Enterobius vermicularis*
(C) *Taenia solium*
(D) *Necator americanus*
(E) *Toxocara canis*

55. Filariasis A

56. Visceral larva migrans E

57. Hookworm D

58. Pork tapeworm C

59. Pinworm B

Questions 60 through 64

(A) Epstein-Barr virus
(B) human papillomavirus
(C) rubella virus
(D) coxsackievirus type A
(E) rhinovirus

60. Common cold E

61. Infectious mononucleosis A

62. Herpangina D

63. Infection in the female genital tract may be associated with cervical dysplasia B

64. German measles C

Questions 65 through 69

(A) Anopheles mosquitoes
(B) fleas
(C) Ixodid ticks
(D) tsetse flies
(E) no insect vector known

65. Vector of sleeping sickness D

66. Vector of Lyme disease C

67. Vector of plague B

68. Vector of smallpox E

69. Vector of malaria A

Questions 70 through 72

(A) aerobic bacteria
(B) anaerobic bacteria
(C) toxigenic bacteria
(D) fungal organism
(E) obligate intracellular virus
(F) obligate extracellular virus
(G) protozoan organism
(H) blastogenic infection

70. A 45-year-old insulin-dependent diabetic male develops a sore throat. On examination the pharynx is coated by a superficial white, curdy membrane which can be readily scraped off to reveal an underlying reddened and swollen oropharyngeal mucosa. The physician's diagnosis is thrush, confirmed 2 days later by the laboratory's report of a pure culture of *C. albicans*. What kind of organism causes thrush? D

71. A 2-month-old infant dies and an autopsy is requested. Premortem history included seizures since birth, hydrocephalus, myocarditis, endocarditis, and jaundice. The most striking autopsy finding is the presence of multiple cysts of *Toxoplasma gondii* throughout the body. What kind of organism caused this infant's death? G

72. A 32-year-old sexually active, healthy male donates blood at a local blood drive. Several weeks later he is asked to return to the blood bank and is informed that he has antibodies to HIV. A confirmatory Western blot is positive. What kind of organism has the man developed antibodies against? F

Questions 73 through 76

(A) bunyavirus
(B) *Wuchereria bancrofti*
(C) herpes simplex virus
(D) *Onchocerca volvulus*
(E) *Treponema pallidum*
(F) *Mycobacterium leprae*
(G) *Aspergillus fumigatus*
(H) *Plasmodium vivax*

73. A 54-year-old sexually active male notices a painless, shallow ulceration on his penis. A darkfield examination reveals numerous corkscrew-shaped spirochetes. Which organism is most likely to have caused this ulcer?

74. A 43-year-old Malaysian woman has several hypopigmented nodules on her face that have been slowly enlarging. These nodules have no sensation to touch (hypoesthetic). A biopsy of one of these nodules is remarkable for the presence of numerous acid-fast bacilli. What organism is most likely to have caused these nodules?

75. A 21-year-old sexually active female suddenly develops numerous painful vesicles on her perineum, introtus, and labia. A smear of fluid and cells taken from the base of a vesicle is examined microscopically and is found to contain several multinucleate giant cells with prominent macronucleoli. What organism is most likely to have caused these vesicles?

76. A 56-year-old East Indian develops massive scrotal swelling over a period of several years. A biopsy of the scrotum demonstrates numerous microfilaria in the lymphatics and abundant reactive lymphatic fibrosis. What organism is most likely to have caused this lymphatic obstruction?

Answers and Explanations

1. **(C)** The relationship of the human host and its normal flora is one of a vast number of examples of symbiosis in the animal and plant kingdoms. Symbiosis is the intimate living together of two dissimilar organisms in a mutually beneficial relationship. This evolutionarily conserved relationship is of immense importance, and its delicate balance may be easily disturbed by many factors, such as drug therapy, primary or secondary immunodeficiency, infection, and trauma, with harmful consequences for both symbionts. Commensalism is a relationship between organisms in which one obtains benefits (especially food intake) from the other without benefiting or harming it. A saprophyte lives on dead or decaying organic matter, such as human excreta. Facultative means optional, eg, a facultative pathogen is an organism that is sometimes, but not invariably, pathogenic. A facultative intracellular parasite is one that can survive and reproduce either within or outside of cells. Parasites have a harmful effect on their hosts. Microorganisms of the normal flora (nonparasites) may become parasites in the compromised host and are then called opportunists. *(1:193–197)*

2. **(E)** Gastrointestinal pathogens capable of producing diarrhea in infected human hosts are usually acquired through the ingestion of food or drink which is contaminated by the organisms. The defense mechanisms employed by gut to thwart these invaders include the physical barrier of the mucosa, the acidity of the stomach, the continuous flow of the lumenal contents, secreted mucus and IgA, and competition by commensal organisms. *Klebsiella rhinoscleromatis* infections produce chronic rhinitis, not diarrhea. *(1:219,485)*

3. **(C)** *Mycobacterium leprae*, an acid-fast bacillus, is an obligate intracellular parasite with a strong tropism for macrophages and Schwann cells. It is the cause of Hansen's disease (leprosy), a chronic, indolent infection primarily of skin, peripheral nerves, mucous membranes, and eyes. Leprosy usually begins as a hypopigmented macule (indeterminate leprosy) that gradually progresses to more macules and plaques, which contain granulomas (tuberculoid leprosy) in patients with a cell-mediated immune reaction against the organism. If cell-mediated immunity is lost or becomes weak, the infection becomes much more extensive, and there is less granulomatous reaction (lepromatous leprosy). There is a range of disease severity between the tuberculoid and lepromatous forms (borderline or dimorphous leprosy). The other organisms listed are facultative intracellular parasites. *(2:380–382)*

4. **(E)** The actinobacilli are fastidious gram-negative bacilli and coccobacilli that cause disease in humans and some herbivores. The only species usually associated with human infections is *Actinobacillus actinomycetemcomitans*, which may cause localized purulent granulomas and abscesses, septicemia, endocarditis, and meningitis. It probably is a factor in periodontosis (juvenile periodontitis). Rickettsiae are obligate intracellular parasites of humans and lower animals and are more closely related to bacteria than to viruses. They invade and multiply within endothelial cells, causing vasculitis. *Pseudomonas aeruginosa* can invade extensively both small and large blood vessels in patients with decreased resistance. Another opportunist, *Aspergillus*, also invades blood vessels. *T. pallidum* causes obliterative endarteritis by invading small blood vessels, eg, in skin, liver, bones, central nervous system, and vasa vasorum of the aorta. Infections with organisms that invade blood vessels usually cause proliferative or thrombotic vascular obstruction with ischemic damage or hemorrhage (Table 5–2). *(1:193–212)*

5. **(B)** *Trichuris* has no intermediate host. The eggs are hatched, and the larval forms enter the primary host again. *(2:413)*

6. **(E)** *Y. enterocolitica* causes enterocolitis and mesenteric lymphadenitis, which may range from mild to severe (pseudoappendicitis or pseudo-Crohn's disease). *Y. pseudotuberculosis* also causes acute mesenteric lymphadenitis but is less likely to cause enterocolitis. The I, II, and III serotypes of *Chlamydia trachomatis* cause LGV, a venereal disease characterized by the occurrence (in stages) of genital vesi-

cles, ulcers, lymphadenopathy, and fibrous rectal stricture. *B. suis, B. abortus,* and *B. canis* may colonize the lymphoreticular system and cause an acute or chronic syndrome, with fever, pain, lassitude, lymphadenopathy, hepatosplenomegaly, infarcts, and (infrequently) pneumonia. Cat-scratch disease is an acute, self-limited disease characterized by mild fever and regional lymphadenopathy and probably is caused by an incompletely identified delicate pleomorphic gram-negative bacillus. All of these organisms may cause stellate microabscesses with a granulomatous rim. These may be seen also with some fungal infections and tularemia, but the granulomas in these diseases are more often tuberculoid. Brucellae may cause sarcoid-like granulomas. *(1:205–212)*

7. **(C)** *U. ureolyticum,* a mycoplasma, is a facultative pathogen that causes some cases of nongonococcal urethritis (NGU) but is also commensally present in the urethras of some asymptomatic healthy persons. A more common venereally transmitted cause of NGU (20 to 60% of cases in males and 20% in females) is urethral infection with some serotypes of *Chlamydia trachomatis.* Skin ulcers are not a feature of NGU. Other serotypes of *C. trachomatis* (I, II, and III) cause lymphogranulomas venereum, which usually begins (after a 4- to 21-day incubation) as a small vesicle that quickly evolves into a small ulcer that rapidly heals. The cutaneous lesion is typically painless and evanescent. The initial lesion also may be extracutaneous (rectal, urethral, vaginal, cervical, or oral) and thus may be unrecognized. The primary chancre is the earliest lesion of venereal syphilis and appears after a 2- to 3-week incubation period as a firm papule that superficially erodes to form an indurated, clean-based ulcer that heals spontaneously. It is characterized by obliterative endarteritis and marked plasma cell infiltration. Granuloma inguinale is caused by *Calymmatobacterium granulomatis (donovani),* a tiny, fastidious gram-negative bacillus that causes indolent, gradually progressive cutaneous and mucocutaneous ulcers of the external genitalia, inguinal region, anus, and perianal region. The ulcers are painless or mildly painful and are characterized by proliferation of chronically inflamed granulation tissue and squamous epithelium. *Haemophilus ducreyi* causes an acute venereal disease characterized by ulcers that are chancroid but differ from the primary ulcer of syphilis in that they are not indurated (soft chancre) and are covered by a superficial layer of acute inflammatory exudate. Genital infection with herpes simplex viruses, types 1 and 2, result in multiple, small, grouped vesicles that coalesce into ulcers, especially in moist areas. The virus replicates in the epithelium, causing ballooning degeneration with loss of intercellular bridges (acantholysis), edema, multinucleated cells, and viral inclusions. *(3:944–949)*

8. **(A)** *Staphylococcus aureus* infections characteristically produce acute inflammatory infiltrates, suppuration, and abscess formation. Bacteria that evoke this suppurative pattern of host response possess an ability to resist immediate phagocytosis by neutrophils, monocytes, and macrophages. The initial failure to phagocytize the invading organisms leads to an overabundance of these cellular defenders, producing the associated suppurative pattern. The other listed choices are fungi that produce granulomatous inflammation in sensitized hosts with intact cellular immunity. *(1:210–211)*

9. **(A)** Rapidly progressive glomerulonephritis may occur in association with the five diseases mentioned and also with periarteritis (polyarteritis) nodosa, Wegener's granulomatosis, and essential cryoglobulinemia. Some cases arise without a known antecedent disease (idiopathic). Although the prognosis is poor in all types of rapidly progressive glomerulonephritis, poststreptococcal disease has a better prognosis than the other types, and up to 50% of patients may recover sufficient renal function to avoid chronic dialysis or transplantation. *(3:850–864)*

10. **(B)** The definitive host of the ascarid nematode *Toxocara canis* is the dog and its canine relatives. Many lactating bitches and more than 80% of puppies pass large numbers of infective fertilized eggs in feces for about 6 months after parturition. The fertilized eggs can remain infective for months to years in moist soil. *Toxocara* eggs have been found contaminating 10 to 30% of soil samples taken from public playgrounds and parks in the United States and 24% of soil samples from public places in Britain. A human who ingests infective *T. canis* eggs becomes an accidental host for the larvae. The larvae hatch in the proximal small bowel, penetrate the mucosa, and migrate through the portal circulation to the liver, where they cause granulomatous inflammation. Some migrate on through the systemic circulation to lungs, heart, kidney, central nervous system, and muscles. The larvae do not complete their life cycle. Most infections are mild, but clinically apparent infection generally occurs in one of two patterns, visceral or ocular. The visceral larva migrans syndrome (VLM) is most common in children 1 to 5 years old with geophagous pica and is characterized by fever, malaise, weight loss, marked eosinophilia, hepatomegaly, wheezing, abdominal pain, myalgia, and neurologic signs. The mean age of children with ocular larva migrans (OLM) is 7.5 years (range 2 to 31 years), and a history of pica is unusual. Common signs are failing vision and strabismus. There are three basic lesions: (1) a central granuloma, (2) a peripheral granuloma, which may have elevated retinal folds extending to the disk, and (3) diffuse endophthalmitis or uveitis, sometimes with retinal detach-

ment. The lesions may be mistaken for a retinoblastoma and the eye unnecessarily enucleated. Nematode endophthalmitis was found in 2% of a series of 1000 eyes removed from children under 15 years old and is believed to cause 10% of the cases of uveitis in children (Table 5–3). *(2:414)*

11. **(D)** *Balantidium coli* is a ciliated protozoan. Balantidiasis is associated with abdominal pain, severe diarrhea, malaise, abdominal distention, and vomiting. Humans are infected by ingesting water or food contaminated by animal reservoir feces containing the infective cysts. The excysted organisms invade into the bowel wall to produce the symptoms of the disease. Tetracycline or iodoquinol are effective treatments. *(3:418)*

12. **(B)** Tropical species of mosquitoes in the genera *Culex, Aedes, Anopheles,* and *Mansonia* (family Culicidae, order Diptera, class Insecta, phylum Arthropoda) are the intermediate hosts and vectors of the roundworm (nematode) *W. bancrofti*, a cause of filariasis in humans (the definitive host). When an infected mosquito bites moist skin, the infective larvae in its proboscis creep out, penetrate through the bite, and travel to the lymphatics and lymph nodes, where they mature in a few months into male and female adult worms with tapering ends. The white, threadlike adult worms mate, and the female produces tiny sheathed embryos, microfilariae, that travel from the lymphatic system to the bloodstream, first appearing about a year after the infective bite. The number of microfilariae in the peripheral blood is usually greatest from about 10 PM to 2 AM (nocturnal periodicity), which is the time of peak feeding activity of the mosquito vectors. This is also the optimum time for obtaining blood specimens for diagnostic examination, including centrifuged wet preparations, 5 μm filter preparations, and stained smears. (In the South Pacific, the increase in microfilariae is much smaller and occurs between noon and sunset.) The microfilariae are ingested by mosquitoes taking a blood meal and mature in the mosquito to infective larvae. The larvae are not highly infective, since many fail to penetrate the skin or fail to reach the lymphatics or are injured by the host immune response. The larvae do not multiply in mosquitoes, nor do the adult worms multiply in people. Thus, thousands of bites per person are required to maintain transmission of the disease in a community. *W. bancrofti* filariasis causes lymphatic inflammation and obstruction, which may progress to elephantiasis, especially in the genitalia and lower extremities. The vector of filariasis caused by the nematode *O. volvulus* is the black fly or buffalo gnat of the genus *Simulium*. *O. volvulus* causes subcutaneous swellings and sometimes causes blindness. The flagellate species of the genus *Leishmania* cause visceral leishmaniasis (*L. donovani*), cutaneous leishmaniasis (*L. tropica* and *L. mexicana*), and mucocutaneous leishmaniasis (*L. lutzomyia* and *pschodopygus*). The exclusive vector of malaria is the female *Anopheles* mosquito. *(1:213–220)*

13. **(A)** Mumps is an acute contagious disease caused by a paramyxovirus that is transmitted naturally by respiratory droplets, fomites, or direct contact and enters through the nose or mouth. Although parotitis can be produced in monkeys by injection of mumps virus into the parotid gland or Stenson's duct, the only known natural host is humans. After an incubation period of 2 to 4 weeks, a prodrome of fever, malaise, headache, and anorexia occurs, followed in a day by parotitis, usually bilateral. Most children become infected with the mumps virus and develop lifelong immunity; 80 to 90% of adults over 20 years of age are immune to mumps. More than 50% of cases occur in the 5- to 9-year age group, and 90% occur in children less than 14 years old. Mumps is uncommon in infants less than 1 year old because of placental transfer of maternal mumps antibody. Orchitis is rare before puberty but is the most common extrasalivary manifestation of mumps in postpubertal males, occurring in about 20 to 30% of patients; it is unilateral in about 80% of these. Therefore, mumps rarely causes sterility in males. Mumps may also involve other salivary glands, ovaries, pancreas, and the central nervous system, but sequelae are rare. Mumps virus can be recovered in routine virologic cell culture and causes cytopathic effects, such as intracytoplasmic eosinophilic inclusions and cell fusion. However, inclusions and syncytia are not seen in vivo in infected tissue. Active immunization of all children with live attenuated mumps virus vaccine at age 15 months is recommended. Vaccination produces a noncommunicable subclinical infection followed in more than 95% of vaccinees by protective levels of antibody for at least 10 years. Vaccination is recommended also for adolescent and adult males without a history of mumps. *(3:341–342)*

14. **(D)** *Candida* is by far the most frequent fungus grown from blood cultures. *C. albicans* is the most common isolate, but at least seven other species are known to be pathogenic for humans, including *C. tropicalis, C. pseudotropicalis, C. guilliermondii, C. glabrata, C. krusei, C. paraspilosis,* and *C. stellatoidea*. *C. albicans* is a commensal normally present in the oropharynx, gastrointestinal tract, and vagina. Factors involved in host resistance to *Candida* infection include intact skin and mucosa, neutrophils, circulating and fixed macrophages, eosinophils, lymphocytes, and probably antibodies and complement. *Candida* becomes pathogenic only if the defense mechanisms are compromised. Factors predisposing to *Candida* infection include suppression of inhibitory normal bacterial flora by antibiotic therapy, immunosuppression (human im-

munodeficiency virus infection, steroid therapy, antineoplastic chemotherapy), intravenous drug abuse, skin or mucosal injury (trauma, surgery, chemotherapy, burns), and foreign bodies (intravenous and Foley catheters, prosthetic cardiac valves, ventricular shunt). Candidiasis may involve skin or mucosa (common in diabetes mellitus) or may be disseminated and involve deeper organs. Although aspergillosis is the second most common disseminated mycosis in the compromised patient and hematogenous seeding occurs, blood cultures from patients with aspergillosis rarely are positive. The *Actinomyces* are gram-positive filamentous bacteria that superficially resemble fungi and cause actinomycosis, a chronic suppurative disease. About half of cases are cervicofacial, and about 20% are pulmonary. Lesions spread contiguously, and hematogenous dissemination is very rare. Blood cultures of patients with actinomycosis are negative. Blood cultures may be positive in patients with cryptococcal meningitis, but *Candida* is isolated far more often. *Mucor* is a saprophytic zygomycete that may infect immunocompromised patients with diabetic ketoacidosis, but it is rarely cultured from blood specimens. *(1:213–220)*

15. **(E)** Malaria in humans is caused by species of the genus *Plasmodium: P. falciparum, P. vivax, P. ovale,* and *P. malariae.* All are obligate intracellular protozoa with complex life cycles. Sporozoites injected by an infected female *Anopheles* mosquito penetrate hepatocytes and multiply (primary tissue schizogony) to form merozoites. One *P. falciparum* sporozoite forms up to 40,000 merozoites, whereas sporozoites of the other plasmodia form 2000 to 15,000. Asexual development of merozoites in hepatocytes is called the "pre-erythrocytic cycle." Persistent infection in the liver (exoerythrocytic cycle) may cause periodic relapses of malaria due to *P. vivax* and *P. ovale* for several years. Untreated, nonfatal infections with *P. falciparum* terminate within a year because this organism has no persistent exoerythrocytic cycle. It is very likely that *P. malariae* also has no persistent hepatic infection, but recrudescences may occur for at least 40 years because of latent infection with a small number of circulating parasites (persistent erythrocytic cycle). Because merozoites of *P. falciparum* infect RBCs of all ages, the magnitude of parasitemia (up to 60% of RBCs) is much greater than that of *P. malariae* (which only invades senescent RBCs) and *P. vivax* and *P. ovale* (which only invade reticulocytes and very young RBCs). The level of parasitemia with the last three is usually no more than 1 to 2%. Erythrocytes parasitized by *P. falciparum* develop small electron-dense protrusions (called "knobs") that adhere to vascular endothelium, causing slowed microcirculation with consequent ischemic injury, especially to the cerebrum and kidneys. Although infection with the other plasmodia is rarely fatal, *P. falciparum* malaria is estimated to cause about one million deaths per year in Africa alone. *(3:408–412)*

16. **(A)** Through September 30, 1987, in the United States, 41,770 adult patients with AIDS had been reported to the Centers for Disease Control. No recognized risk factors were reported in only 2059 of these patients (5%). After additional study of these 2059 cases, only 1202 (3%) remain classified as having no identified risk factors. Of these 1202 patients, 596 currently are under investigation, and it is probable that risk factors will be found in a significant proportion. Information was incomplete or unobtainable in 325 of these 1202. After additional information became available, risk factors were not identified for 281 of the AIDS patients. Thus, risk factors were not identified in only a small proportion (3% or less) of adult AIDS patients. Since this proportion has not changed over time, it may be inferred that modes of transmission of HIV have not changed. *(2:227–228)*

17. **(E)** When commercially available test kits licensed by the Food and Drug Administration (FDA) are used by reliable laboratories (such as those inspected by the College of American Pathologists and the American Association of Blood Banks), the specificity and sensitivity of the EIA screening test for anti-HIV are both very high, 99% or greater. This has been established by proficiency testing by the CAP and AABB, studies published in the medical literature, and manufacturers of EIA kits, who have submitted data to the FDA for licensure. *(1:224–226)*

18. **(E)** *N. gonorrhoeae,* a nonencapsulated pyogenic gram-negative diplococcus, attaches to columnar and transitional epithelial cells via surface pili. Strains with fewer pili are less virulent than strains having many pili and tend to cause asymptomatic urethritis or cervicitis. *N. gonorrhoeae* does not attach to squamous epithelial cells. *(3:389–392)*

19. **(A)** *V. cholerae* is a facultatively anaerobic, comma-shaped, gram-negative bacillus with polar flagellation. It does not invade or ulcerate the gut mucosa. It produces a heat-labile protein enterotoxin (choleragen) that has adenosine-diphosphate-ribosyl transferase activity and thus activates the adenylate cyclase of the mucosal cells of the small bowel. This generates increased cyclic adenosine monophosphate (cAMP), causing massive secretion of isotonic fluid in excess of the resorptive capacity of the colon and resulting in severe diarrhea (Table 5–4). *(2:355–357)*

20. **(B)** *C. jejuni* is a motile, nonsporing, comma-shaped, slender microaerophilic rod that is best recovered by culture on selective (antibiotic-containing) media in 5% O_2 and 8 to 10% CO_2. Incubation of pri-

mary plates should be at 42°C to inhibit other fecal bacteria. The reservoir of infection includes poultry, pigs, rabbits, goats, cattle, and dogs. The infection is acquired orally from food, drink, contact with infected animals, or anal–genital–oral sexual activity. *C. jejuni* causes an estimated 2 million cases of diarrhea or dysentery in the United States per year, including 5 to 11% of all cases of diarrhea or dysentery in hospitals. The organism produces enterotoxin, but its clinical significance is not well understood. *C. jejuni* invades the epithelium of the jejunum and ileum, causing hyperemia, edema, acute and chronic inflammatory infiltration, and ulceration. Involvement of the colon produces crypt abscesses and ulcerations. Thus, stools may contain exudate and blood. The incidence is higher in children than adults. After an incubation period of 3 to 5 days, abdominal pain, nausea, headache, and fever occur, along with diarrhea. The disease is usually self-limited, with a 5- to 8-day course, and septicemia and nonenteric infection are uncommon. *C. fetus* (subspecies *fetus* and *intestinalis*) is an opportunistic cause of systemic infection in debilitated patients. *(2:353–357)*

21. **(C)** *Y. enterocolitica* is a facultatively anaerobic, gram-negative rod that causes enterocolitis and mesenteric lymphadenitis. Although endotoxins are present, these have not been shown to have any pathogenic effect on the gut. An enterotoxin is produced in cultures below 30°C but not at 37°C and thus does not appear to be produced in vivo. The pathogenicity appears to be caused by bacterial invasion of the epithelium of the ileum and colon, causing ulceration and inflammation. Refrigeration of culture specimens for 3 weeks at 4°C in phosphate-buffered isotonic saline (with periodic subculture) to enriched media at 22 to 25°C and 37°C) increases the yield, because *Y. enterocolitica* will multiply at this low temperature, and most other fecal organisms are inhibited or killed. The distribution of this pathogen is virtually worldwide, and its reservoirs are extensive, including domestic and wild animals, both sick and healthy, including swine, sheep, cattle, dogs, cats, caged birds, pigeons, deer, rodents, mink, chinchilla, and fish. Transmission to humans is through contaminated food, water, and milk. Person-to-person transmission probably is rare. *(2:357–358)*

22. **(D)** *B. anthracis*, a large, virulent, aerobic, encapsulated, gram-positive rod, produces endospores that resist boiling and disinfectants and persist in soil for years. Infection causes anthrax, primarily a disease of animals, particularly cattle, sheep, horses, goats, and swine. These ingest the spores in soil contaminating the rough vegetation they eat. (Gastrointestinal anthrax is uncommon in humans.) Most human infections result from cutaneous entry of spores from contaminated soil or animal products (hides, carcasses, wool, bone). Within hours to days of entry of spores through a skin scratch, a pruritic red macule appears that soon develops into an edematous papule and then a hemorrhagic vesicle. The vesicle has been called a "malignant pustule," but contains only a few neutrophils, not pus. The vesicle ulcerates, and a small to large black eschar forms. This lesion may heal and no clinical disease results. Alternatively, the ulcer(s) may be followed by severe edema, called "malignant edema," hemorrhagic lymphadenitis, and septicemia. Inhalation of spores, which germinate in the lungs or tracheobronchial lymph nodes, causes hemorrhagic lymphadenitis, mediastinal and pulmonary edema, septicemia, and hemorrhagic bronchopneumonia (woolsorter's disease). *(2:361–362)*

23. **(B)** After larvae of the nematode *O. volvulus* are injected into the skin by an infected *Simulium* blackfly, they migrate to the subcutaneous tissue and mature into filiform adult males and females that may live for years, producing huge numbers of tiny microfilariae. The inflammatory reaction to the adult filariae is successively acute, chronic, and fibrous, forming nodules that eventually may calcify. The serious clinical effects are caused by the microfilariae, which cause dermatitis and eye lesions, including punctate keratitis, pannus formation, corneal fibrosis, iridocyclitis, glaucoma, choroiditis, and optic atrophy. Impaired visual acuity and even river blindness may ensue. Diagnosis is made by finding microfilariae in teased snips or in the anterior chamber of the eye (by slit lamp examination) or by finding adult worms in biopsied nodules. About 30 million people in Africa and about 1 million in Central and South America are infected. *(3:432–433)*

24. **(D)** *Hymenolepis nana* is a tapeworm with humans as both definitive and intermediate hosts. This "dwarf" tapeworm gains entrance to the human intestinal tract when individuals ingest raw foods soiled with infective cysts. Once in the intestine the worm attaches to the mucosa via a scolex mouthpart. The diagnosis may be confirmed by demonstrating the characteristic proglottids in the feces. *(2:420)*

25. **(A)** *A. lumbricoides* is the largest roundworm of humans and infects an estimated 1 billion people worldwide. Fertilized *Ascaris* eggs are passed in the stool and mature to the infective stage in 2 to 3 weeks. When soil contaminated by mature eggs gets on the hands or on raw vegetables and is ingested, larvae hatch in the small intestine, penetrate the mucosa, and migrate in venous blood through the right heart to the lungs. They enter the alveoli, ascend the pulmonary tree, are swallowed, and mature into adult male and female worms in the lumen of the small bowel. In 2 to 3 months, they

begin to produce eggs. Since each female produces up to 200,000 ova per day, ascariasis can be diagnosed by microscopic examination of unconcentrated stool. Since the worm has a short life span of 10 to 24 months and does not multiply in humans, infection is maintained only by ingestion of fertilized eggs. The eggs are resistant to adverse environments and can survive for years in moist soil. Infection and complications are more common in children. Most infestations are asymptomatic and are occasionally recognized because of passage of a worm from the anus, mouth, or nose. Loeffler's syndrome may occur during the pulmonary phase. The most serious complications are obstruction of the intestine, pylorus, common bile duct, or pancreatic duct, volvulus, intussusception, and appendicitis. The worms occur in greatest concentration in the jejunum, but obstruction is most common in the terminal ileum. *(3:439)*

26. **(B)** Influenza A virus causes an acute illness characterized by an 18- to 72-hour incubation period, fever, malaise, myalgia, and sometimes nonexudative pharyngitis and (less often) tracheobronchitis. Pneumonia is uncommon, but the disease predisposes to superimposed bacterial pneumonia. Epidemic and pandemic outbreaks occur often in the winter. The pathogen is an orthomyxovirus with a lipid-rich envelope that has surface proteins (influenzal hemagglutinin, HA), enabling the virus to adsorb to receptors on susceptible respiratory mucosal cells. Mucoproteins (which compete for the receptors) and anti-HA antibodies interfere with viral attachment and infection. Once adsorbed, the virions are transferred into endosomes (cytoplasmic vacuoles), and the envelope fuses with endosome membranes to release the nucleocapsid into the cytosol. The segmented, single-stranded RNA genome dissociates from the capsid proteins and viral replication, assemble, and release by budding allow the infection to spread. The host cell nucleus plays no part in influenza virus replication. Influenza A virus undergoes major phenotypic changes (antigenic shift) associated with pandemic spread of influenza at 10- to 14-year intervals. Interpandemic minor changes (antigenic drift) also occur. There are three major (antigenically distinct) types of influenza virus—A, B, and C. Types B and C usually cause less severe cases of influenza and less serious outbreaks than does type A. *(2:315–316)*

27. **(C)** Polyoma virus (*poly,* many; *oma,* tumor) causes murine adenomas, adenocarcinomas, hemangiomas, fibromas, and fibrosarcomas. In contrast to influenza virus, the polyoma virus is naked (does not have an envelope) and is uncoated (capsid removed) in the host cell nucleus before replication. Polyoma viruses are members of the Papovaviridae family and thus have a circular, double-stranded DNA genome. Members of the Papovaviridae that infect humans are human papillomaviruses, BK virus, which has been isolated from the urine of immunosuppressed renal transplant recipients but does not cause tumors, AS virus, newly described, and JC virus, which causes progressive multifocal leukoencephalopathy (PML), probably by reactivation of a persistent infection. Another polyoma virus, SV40 (simian vacuolating virus) is probably a rare cause of PML. *(2:312–315)*

28. **(D)** HIV, formerly called human T lymphotropic virus III, is a single-stranded RNA retrovirus that has a lipid envelope studded with surface glycoproteins (gp), each of which has two subunits, gp41 (transmembrane gp) and gp120 (surface gp). Human helper T lymphocytes (T4$^+$ cells) and monocytes (macrophages) have a surface antigen called T4 (CD4), which is the receptor for HIV gp120. After HIV gp120 binds specifically to the CD4 receptors, the virion enters the cell. (It has not yet been established whether entry is by direct fusion of the HIV envelope to the cell membrane, by receptor-fusion of the HIV envelope to the cell membrane, or by receptor-mediated endocytosis). Helper T lymphocytes are destroyed by infection with HIV, leading to the severe acquired immunodeficiency syndrome (AIDS). Infected monocytes and macrophages are considerably more refractory to the cytopathic effect of HIV; thus they may serve as a reservoir for persistent HIV infection in the host and also may be the Trojan horse that spreads the infection to the central nervous system, causing encephalopathy. In addition to the CD4 lymphocytes and monocytes, HIV has been found in Langerhans' cells, endothelial cells, astrocytes, oligodendrocytes, microglial cells, and (rarely) neurons. *(3:124–129)*

29. **(A)** The family Paramyxoviridae consists of three genera: *Paramyxovirus* (parainfluenza virus types 1, 2, 3, 4a, 4b, mumps virus, and Newcastle disease virus, and other avian paramycoviruses), *Morbillivirus* (measles, canine distemper, and bovine rinderpest virus), and *Pneumovirus* (respiratory syncytial viruses of humans and cattle and pneumonia virus of mice). Although most other enveloped viruses enter the host cell by receptor-mediated endocytosis, the Parmyxoviridae undergo fusion of the viral envelope with the cell plasma membrane and enter the cytoplasm directly. Adsorption of the virus to the cell surface receptors and envelope–plasma membrane fusion are mediated by viral envelope surface glycoproteins (gp); eg, parainfluenza and mumps viruses have projecting glycoproteins (HN) responsible for adsorption of these viruses, and glycoproteins (Fo) responsible for fusion. Proteolytic cleavage of Fo into two subunits by a host cell enzyme is necessary for fusion and viral penetration. Thus, only cells with the proteolytic enzyme are penetrated and infected. When

the *Paramyxovirus* envelope fuses with the host cell, viral surface proteins become part of the host cell surface, and the cell becomes recognizable as infected and is subject to immune lysis. The Fo gp also is involved in fusion of host cells, spreading by budding of maturing virions from the cell surface. (The lipids of the viral envelope are acquired from the host cell membrane during budding.) The viral HN gp has neuraminidase activity and facilitates release of budding virus. *(2:224–234)*

30. (B)

31. (D)

32. (C)

33. (C)

34. (D)

35. (D)

30 through 35. A large number of mononuclear leukocytes are seen with typhoid fever. Neutrophils predominate in the diarrhea of shigellosis, although (less commonly) some strains of shigella can produce an enterotoxin, resulting in a watery diarrhea without many fecal leukocytes. Salmonellosis and ulcerative colitis cause the appearance of many neutrophils. Ulcerative colitis also may show eosinophils (88% neutrophils, 8% eosinophils). Since little or no inflammatory response is induced by metabolic enterotoxin, inflammatory cells generally are absent in the diarrhea of cholera and infection with enterotoxigenic *E. coli* (Table 5–4). *(1:205–212)*

36. (D) Most patients with AIDS still fall into the categories first observed in 1981. Homosexual and bisexual men constitute the largest group of AIDS patients (73%). *(2:227–228)*

37. (B) A small percentage (1%) of AIDS patients are those with hemophilia who have received multiple units of antihemophilic factor concentrates. *(2:227–228)*

38. (A) Heterosexual men and women who are intravenous drug abusers are the second largest group of people with AIDS (17%) and are becoming an even greater source of new infections. *(2:227–228)*

39. (C) Haitians living in the United States are a small (4%) and decreasing percentage of AIDS patients. Half of these deny homosexual activity and intravenous drug abuse. Thus, a substantial proportion of these could be reclassified as members of the two predominant groups. *(2:227–228)*

40. (D) The anaerobic bacillus, *Clostridium tetani*, is commonly found in the intestinal flora of wild and domesticated animals. The spores produced by these bacteria are deposited out into the environment, especially into the soil, with defecation. Spores enter humans through a traumatic injury. If the wound site becomes anaerobic, the spores germinate and produce a very potent neurologic poison termed "tetanus toxin." This toxin causes uninhibited neural stimulation with resultant tetany, lockjaw, and rigidity of the facial muscles (risus sardonicus). Prolonged spasms of the laryngeal or respiratory muscles can be fatal. Treatment consists of penicillin, tetanus toxoid, immune serum globulin, and the re-establishment of aerobic conditions in the wound. *(3:374–376)*

41. (A) Scarlet fever is an exanthematous disorder associated with acute pharyngitis or tonsilitis caused by erythrogenic strains of *Streptococcus pyogenes*. While infecting the pharynx or tonsil, the organism produces an erythrogenic toxin. This toxin evokes the systemic rash-like reaction which is clinically termed "scarlet fever." The erythematous rash is most abundant over the trunk, inner aspect of the arms and legs, and on the face sparing the mouth. After about a week the rash subsides and the skin begins to scale and desquamate. Prompt antibiotic therapy is necessary during the initial pharyngitis stage to avoid later poststreptococcal sequela, such as glomerulonephritis. *(2:341)*

42. (E) Psuedomembranous colitis is characterized grossly by raised yellowish plaques, measuring between 0.3 and 2.0 cm, cobblestoning the rectosigmoid mucosa. Microscopically the superficial epithelium is eroded and focally covered by a pseudomembrane comprised of fibrin, necrotic debris, and neutrophils. Most individuals with pseudomembranous colitis have been recently treated with antibiotics. This prior antibiotic therapy may alter the normal bowel flora allowing the emergence of *Clostridium difficile*. The organism produces a toxin that damages the colonic mucosa with resultant pseudomembrane formation and usually, diarrhea. The toxin may be detected in the stool of affected individuals, serving as a practical way to confirm the diagnosis. Psuedomembranous colitis is treated with vancomycin, fluids, and electrolyte replacement therapy. *(3:689)*

43. (B) *Clostridium perfringens* is the bacterial organism that most commonly causes gas gangrene. This ubiquitous organism produces a potent myotoxin when grown in anaerobic conditions such as those present in certain contaminated wounds. The myotoxin is a lecithinase which lyses cell membranes causing severe myolysis and hemolysis. Prompt debridement of the wound accompanied by hyperbaric oxygen and antibiotic therapy are critical elements

of treatment. Clinically, the myolysis is fulminating with accompanying crepitus, dusky necrosis, and a foul odor. The combination of gas bubbles (crepitus) and necrosis give rise to the common clinical appellation of "gas gangrene." *(3:373–375)*

44. **(C)** Botulism is usually caused by ingestion of food contaminated by preformed neurotoxins synthesized by *Clostridium botulinum*. Improper home canning, inadequate refrigeration, inadequate smoking, or insufficient curing of foods provides an environment favorable for the bacteria to proliferate, producing a potent neurotoxin. The subsequent ingestion of these foods without sufficient heating results in a symmetric descending paralysis of cranial nerves, limbs, and trunk. Paralysis of respiratory muscles is fatal. Prompt treatment with antitoxin may prove lifesaving. Botulism can be prevented by fully cooking foods, since moderate heating destroys the preformed neurotoxin. *(3:376–377)*

45. **(E)** Epidemic typhus fever is caused by the obligate intracellular organism, *Rickettsia prowazekii*. The organism is transmitted from human to human by body lice (*Pediculus humanus*). After a 1- to 2-week incubation period headache, fever, chills, weakness, and malaise appear. A maculopapular rash soon follows the initial symptoms. Most fatalities in untreated individuals occur in the second or third week after the first symptoms have appeared due to infection of the central nervous system. Microscopically the organisms can be demonstrated in the endothelial cells of the characteristic typhus nodules. *(2:330–332)*

46. **(B)** Rocky Mountain spotted fever is caused by *Rickettsia rickettsii*. The reservoir for this organism is hard-bodied ticks. Ticks transmit the disease to humans when organisms in the ticks' salivary glands are inoculated into bitten individuals. About 1 week after the tick bite, symptoms appear which are characterized by malaise, fever, headache, and myalgia. A rash may then develop as pink macules and later as petechiae. Central nervous system involvement in the second or third week may prove fatal. The organisms may be demonstrated microscopically in infected endothelial cells. Prompt antibiotic therapy is the treatment of choice. *(3:350–351)*

47. **(D)** The chronic suppurative eye disease caused by *C. trachomatis* is one of the leading causes of blindness in the world. The disease is particularly severe in dry sandy regions of the world, where flies and other fomites continually reinfect the conjunctiva. The organism initially evokes a suppurative reaction that later with further reinfection and lack of antibiotic therapy will progress to follicular hypertrophy, conjunctival ulceration, scarring, and finally, blindness. Antibiotics, such as the sulfonamides, readily cure the initial infection. The absence of adequate medical care in many of the world's poorer regions accounts for most of the cases that progress to blindness. *(2:327–328)*

48. **(A)** Human Q fever is caused by the rickettsial organism, *Coxiella burnetii*. This zoonic disease is spread among cattle, sheep, and wild animals by ticks. Humans usually acquire the disease through inhalation of airborne organisms. Slaughterhouse workers, shepherds, cattlemen, and farmhands are most often infected. After a 3-week incubation period, symptoms suddenly develop, characterized by fever, malaise, mayalgias, cough, bradycardia, and hepatosplenomegaly. Most people recover without sequela in about 2 weeks after the beginning of symptoms. Antibiotics speed the recovery. *(2:333)*

49. **(C)** Ornithosis, also termed "psittacosis," is caused by *Chlamydia psittaci*. The organism is transmitted to humans during the inhalation of aerosolized bird excreta. The incubation period varies from 1 to 3 weeks and is followed by the sudden onset of fever, chills, malaise, headache, sore throat, and cough. The most characteristic microscopic finding is interstitial pneumonitis. The mortality rate in individuals not promptly treated with antibiotics ranges from 5 to 40%. *(2:326–327)*

50. **(A)** Chagas' disease is caused by hemoflagellate, *Trypanosoma cruzi*. Cardiac involvement is characteristic with this disease, including acute myocarditis, bundle branch block, interstitial fibrosis, and progressive dilatory cardiac failure. Humans acquire the disease from the bite of "kissing bugs" that inhabit cracks in dilapidated buildings and bite sleeping victims at night. The disease is common from Texas to Argentina. Because of this distribution it is sometimes referred to as "American trypanosomiasis." *(2:407–408)*

51. **(E)** Malaria is a protozoal disease caused by organisms of the *Plasmodium* species. Humans are infected with sporozoites during mosquito bites. The sporozoites travel through the bloodstream to multiply in liver cells. Merozoites are released by the liver and penetrate erythrocytes. Further growth of the parasite in erythrocytes produces both gametocytes and hemolysis. The gametocytes re-enter mosquitoes during a blood meal to complete the infective cycle. *(3:408–412)*

52. **(C)** Lyme disease is a spirochetal disease caused by *Borrelia burgdoferi*. Tick bites transfer the infective agent to humans. Three to four weeks after inoculation a papule develops at the bite site, shortly followed by a ring-like rash that expands outward and lasts from a month to a year. During this expansion phase individuals may complain of

arthritis, myocarditis, or neurologic symptoms. Antibiotics hasten recovery. *(3:358)*

53. **(B)** Amebiasis is a protozoan disease caused by *Entamoeba histolytica*. Infective cysts are found in contaminated water and pass through the stomach to invade the mucosal tissues of the large bowel, especially the cecum. Symptoms may include abdominal pain, nausea, vomiting, and diarrhea. Infrequent, but life-threatening complications, may include bowel perforation or liver abscess formation. The disease is diagnosed by identifying the characteristic cysts and trophozoites in feces. Treatment is via a number of antiprotozoal agents. *(3:414–417)*

54. **(D)** Visceral leishmaniasis (kala-azar) is caused by the protozoan organism, *Leishmania donovani*. Blood-sucking flies transfer the infective promastigotes to humans while biting. The promastigotes invade reticuloendothelial cells, transform into amastigotes, multiply, and are ingested by feeding flies. In the flies the amastigotes transform back into promastigotes, completing the cycle. The involvement of the reticuloendothelial system explains in large part the pathologic features of kala-azar, namely lymphadenopathy, hepatomegaly, hyperplastic bone marrow, and splenomegaly. Treatments include preventative measures, parenteral pentavalent antimonials, and meglumine antimoniate. *(3:406–408)*

55. **(A)** Filariasis, a chronic obstructing fibrosis of the lymph vessels, is caused by the organism, *Wuchereria bancrofti*. The infective form of the organism is transmitted to humans during mosquito bites. Once in the human bloodstream, microfilariae come to rest in lymphatics and mature into adult worms. Immunologic reaction to these adult worms is responsible for the gradual obstructive fibrosis of the lymphatics. Extremities or organs drained by these obstructed lymphatics may later develop pronounced swelling and gigantism, also called "elephantitis." *(1:334)*

56. **(E)** Visceral larva migrans is a disease caused by accidental human infection by animal nematodes parasites, such as the dog roundworm, *Toxocara canis*. The disease typically affects children living with dogs or cats in crowded conditions. Clinical findings include eosinophilia, pneumonitis, and hypergammaglobulinemia. Ocular involvement can lead to retinal detachment. The disease is usually self-limited, and treatment includes diethylcarbamazine or thiabendazole. *(1:886,3:437)*

57. **(D)** Hookworm infestation can be caused by either the Old World hookworm, *Ancylostoma duodenale*, or by the New World hookworm, *Necator americanus*. Both worms live in tropical soils for months as either infective filariform larvae or as free-living rhabdoid larvae and adults. After penetrating the human skin, they circulate into the lungs, migrate to the epiglottis, are swallowed into the stomach, and come to rest in the small intestine where they propagate while feeding on the mucosal villi. Clinically, there is dermatitis, pneumonitis, and iron deficiency anemia. The diagnosis can be confirmed by observing the characteristic eggs shed out into the feces. Treatment is usually with mebendazole. *(3:436)*

58. **(C)** The pork tapeworm is *Taenia solium*. Humans acquire the tapeworm infection through the ingestion of raw or undercooked pork. The encysted larvae excyst in the human intestinal tract, mature into adults, and attach to the intestinal wall via scolex mouthparts. The adults discharge eggs into human feces which may later infect pigs to complete the parasite's life cycle. *(2:420–421)*

59. **(B)** Pinworm infections are caused by the nematode, *Enterobius vermicularis*. Adult worms live in the lower gastrointestinal tract of infected humans. At night the female worms migrate out to the anal skin to lay eggs, resulting in the classical "night itch" associated with the disease. The eggs are readily infective for other household members who accidently ingest them. Numerous effective antihelminths are available to treat infections. Reinfection by dormant eggs in clothing and fomites, however, may necessitate multiple courses of therapy. Rarely the worms infect the fallopian tube or appendix producing salpingitis or appendicitis, respectively. *(2:413)*

60. **(E)** Rhinoviruses are the most common cause of the "common cold." Spread from person to person by aerosol droplets, over 100 different species exist to confound the human immune system. After a brief incubation period of several days, symptoms of nasal stuffiness, runny nose, itchy eyes, sore throat, and mild fever occur. Treatment is symptomatic. The average duration of illness is about a week. *(3:345)*

61. **(A)** Infectious mononucleosis (IM) is caused by the Epstein-Barr virus. In developed nations most symptomatic Epstein-Barr infections occur during adolescence. The clinical features of IM include the triad of fever, sore throat, and lymphadenopathy. In the peripheral blood there is an increased number of circulating atypical lymphocytes. About 2 weeks into the symptomatic phase of the disease, most individuals have developed "heterophile" antibodies which may be detected by laboratory tests to confirm the diagnosis. Over 90% of infected individuals recover without significant sequela. Rarely, splenic rupture, encephalitis, thrombocytopenia,

hemolytic anemia, or meningitis complicate the disease. *(3:338–340)*

62. **(D)** Infection with coxsackievirus type A can produce herpangina, a blistering inflammation of the posterior pharynx, tonsils, and soft palate. The lesions begin as macules, progress to tan papules, and then into vesicles that ulcerate. Myalgia, fever, and malaise may accompany the ulcers. The disease is usually self-limited, resolving without significant sequela in about 2 weeks. *(2:315)*

63. **(B)** Cervical squamous cell dysplasia is strongly linked to prior infection of the cervix by human papillomavirus. Papillomavirus infection at this site usually produces flat condyloma. A small portion of these condylomas fail to resolve and over time display increasing severe degrees of dysplasia. The viral serotypes of 16 and 18 are most likely to initiate these progressive dysplastic changes. *(1:794–795)*

64. **(C)** Rubella virus, the causative agent of German measles, is a togavirus responsible for the "3-day measles." This mild childhood illness is characterized by rash, fever, malaise, and lymphadenopathy. Adult infections of pregnant females may result in fetal malformations. Hence, the public health officials need to test gravid females for immunity to the rubella virus. *(2:318)*

65. **(D)**

66. **(C)**

67. **(B)**

68. **(E)**

69. **(A)**

65 through 69. Many infectious diseases depend on arthropod vectors to carry the transmissible agent to humans. For example, biting fleas and Ixodid ticks spread *Yersinia pestis* (plague) and *Borrelia burgdorferi* (Lyme disease), respectively. The Anopheles mosquito is the vector of malaria. Sleeping sickness is transmitted by the tsetse fly. Smallpox, which has been eradicated, had never been spread by insect vectors, only by human-to-human transmission. *(1:217–219)*

70. **(D)** *Candida albicans* is a fungal organism. It is an opportunistic infectious agent capable of producing disease in individuals with reduced immunity. Infections are commonly seen in the very young, very old, diabetics, after broad spectrum antibiotics, with cancer, with severe burns, with indwelling catheters or prosthetic cardiac valves, and with AIDS. Oral infections, as depicted in the scenario, are termed "thrush" and are frequently seen with insulin-dependent diabetics. *(1:217)*

71. **(G)** *Toxoplasma gondii* is a protozoan organism. Humans are infected by eating undercooked meat contaminated by cat feces containing transmissible cysts. Congenital toxoplasmosis results in severe consequences including brain damage, mental retardation, seizures, deafness, hydrocephalus, encephalitis, and myocarditis. Toxoplasmosis is also commonly seen with AIDS patients. *(2:410–411)*

72. **(E)** The scenario depicts an individual with HIV infection, an obligate intracellular virus. The infective agent is a retrovirus with a central core of RNA, an outer antigenic protein coat, and inner reverse transcriptase enzymes capable of manufacturing DNA templates of the viral RNA for replication. The virus preferentially attaches to CD4 membrane sites of lymphocytes. Parenteral, congenital, and sexual routes account for most infections. *(2:224–229)*

73. **(E)** Syphilis is a venereal disease caused by the spirochetal organism, *Treponema pallidum*. In primary syphilis, as depicted in the scenario, a chancre usually develops on the glans penis of infected males about a week after exposure. Darkfield microscopic examination of fluid expressed from a chancre will demonstrate diagnostic corkscrew-shaped spirochetes. If the organism is not treated with antibiotics at this stage, the infected individual may go on to develop secondary or tertiary syphilis over time. *(2:368–371)*

74. **(F)** Leprosy, also termed "Hansen's disease," is a slowly progressive mycobacterial infection that affects the cooler portions of the body, especially the skin and peripheral nerves. Clinically, the disease is generally divided into tuberculoid and lepromatous varieties. In the tuberculoid variety, granulomatous inflammation is seen microscopically in facial macular lesions. In the lepromatous variant, a foam cell architecture is seen microscopically in the nodular facial lesions. Both types of leprosy contain diagnostic acid-fast mycobacterial organisms. *(2:380–383)*

75. **(C)** The scenario portrays infection with herpes simplex II virus. Most herpetic infections of skin or mucous membranes produce vesicles and ulceration. Examination of the vesicle fluid (Tzanck preparations) will usually demonstrate viral-induced cytopathic changes characterized by multinucleate giant cells containing central large acidophilic intranuclear inclusions. These inclusion bodies contain live and dead viron particles. After the initial vesicular outbreak, the virus retreats to neuroganglia, where it slowly reproduces. Repeated attacks of recurrent vesicles in the anatomic distribu-

tion of the infected nerve characterize the disease over time. *(2:319–320)*

76. **(B)** The scenario portrays a human infection by the microfilarial organism, *Wuchereria bancrofti*. This tropical disease is transmitted from human to human by mosquito bites. Lymphatic filariasis is caused by an inflammatory and fibrous reaction to filarial worms in the lymphatic channels. The gradual development of lymphatic obstruction may produce swelling (elephantisis) of the scrotum, leg, or arm. *(2:417–419)*

REFERENCES

1. Chandrasoma P, Taylor CR: Concise Pathology, Norwalk, Appleton and Lange, 1991
2. Cotran RS, Kumar V, Robbins SL: Robbins Pathologic Basis of Disease, 4th edition, Philadelphia, Saunders, 1989
3. Rubin E, Farber JL: Pathology, Philadelphia, Lippincott, 1988

CHAPTER 6

Genetic, Metabolic, and Environmental Pathology

Forty-six pieces of DNA and protein, called chromosomes, hold the genetic blueprint from which humans are constructed and maintained. The chromosomes are divided into 22 pairs of autosomes and a pair of sex chromosomes. In males, the sex pair is designated XY. In females, the sex chromosomes are XX. The Lyon hypothesis explains the involution of one X chromosome, which leads to formation of the clinically useful Barr body to determine genetic identity in cases of ambiguous secondary sexual differentiation. Hermaphrodites are those rare individuals who possess both ovarian and testicular tissue, regardless of their karyotype or external sexual genitalia. Pseudo-hermaphrodites possess only one type of gonadal tissue and usually have the opposite karyotype or secondary sexual characteristics. Common gross abnormalities of chromosome numbers or composition are shown in Table 6–1.

More subtle abnormalities of chromosomes may affect only one base pair or a short strand of pairs. The damage may affect the individual or remain dormant and be expressed in a later generation. Certain of these genetic disorders have well-understood patterns of inheritance and characteristic clinical symptoms (Table 6–2).

The full maturation of an individual is dependent on appropriate environment and nutrition. Lack of certain nutrients, vitamins, or minerals can be characterized into clinical diseases (Table 6–3). Common chemical substances, termed toxins or poison, can be profoundly harmful (Table 6–4), and environmental conditions, such as heat and radiation, can harm or kill people.

TABLE 6–1. COMMON CHROMOSOMAL ABNORMALITIES

Name	Chromosome Pattern	Clinical Characteristics
Turner's syndrome	45, XO	Webbed neck, short stature, primary amenorrhea, infertility, streak gonads
Klinefelter's syndrome	47, XXY	Eunuchoid habitus with long legs, testicular atrophy, mental retardation, gynecomastia
Down's syndrome	Trisomy 21	Mental retardation, dysplastic ears, epicanthic folds, congenital heart disease
Edward's syndrome	Trisomy 18	Mental retardation, micrognathia, low-set ears, congenital heart disease
Patau's syndrome	Trisomy 13	Mental retardation, microencephaly, microphthalmia, cleft palate, rocker-bottom feet
Cat's cry syndrome	Partial deletion of chromosome 5	Mental retardation, mewing cry, epicanthic folds, microcephaly

TABLE 6-2. INHERITANCE OF GENETIC DISORDERS

Disorder	Inheritance	Molecular Defect	Clinical Features
Galactosemia	Autosomal recessive	Galactose-1 phosphate uridyl transferase	Jaundice, mental retardation, hepatosplenomegaly, cataracts
Alpha,-antitrypsin deficiency	Autosomal recessive	Alpha,-antitrypsin	Emphysema, cirrhosis
Phenylketonuria	Autosomal recessive	Pehnylalanine hydroxylase	Mental retardation
Wilson's disease	Autosomal recessive	Copper excretion	Brain degeneration, cirrhosis (hepatolenticular)
Albinism	Autosomal recessive	Melanin production	Visual impairment, skin cancers
Ochronosis	Autosomal recessive	Homogentisic oxidase	Pigmented cartilage, arthritis
Tay-Sachs disease	Autosomal recessive	Hexosaminidase A	Mental retardation, blindness, cherry red macula
Niemann-Pick disease	Autosomal recessive	Sphingomyelinase	Hepatosplenomegaly, xanthomas, mental retardation, lymphadenopathy
Gauchers' disease	Autosomal recessive	Glucocerebrosidase	Hepatosplenomegaly, bone marrow involvement, mental retardation
Hurler's syndrome (MPS I)	Autosomal recessive	Alpha-L-iduronidase	Hepatosplenomegaly, corneal clouding, dwarfism
Glycogen storage disease (8 types)	Autosomal recessive	Glycogen metabolism	Hepatosplenomegaly, cardiomegaly, skeletal muscle involvement
Glucose-6-phosphate dehydrogenase deficiency	X-linked recessive	Glucose-6-phosphate dehydrogenase	Erythrocyte hemolysis
Fabry's syndrome	X-linked recessive	Trihexosylceramide alpha-galactosidase	Skin, kidney, and neural lesions
Hemophilia	X-linked recessive	Clotting factor VIII or IX	Bleeding
Bruton's agammaglobulinemia	X-linked recessive	Immunoglobulin	Pyogenic infections, autoimmune disorders
Hunter's syndrome	X-linked recessive	L-Iduronosulfate sulfatase	Hepatosplenomegaly, dwarfism, cardiac lesions
Wiskott-Aldrich syndrome	X-linked recessive	Cellular immunity	Loss of cellular immunity, thrombocytopenia, eczema
Duchenne muscular dystrophy	X-linked recessive	Unknown	Muscular weakness, atrophy, and hypertrophy
Achondroplasia	Autosomal dominant	Cartilage cell growth	Short arms and legs
Sickle cell anemia	Autosomal dominant	Hemoglobin	Anemia, autosplenectomy, cirrhosis, gallstones
Huntington;s chorea	Autosomal dominant	Unknown	Cortical and thalamic atrophy, dementia
Polycystic kidney disease	Autosomal dominant	Unknown	Renal and other visceral cysts, renal failure
Thalassemia	Autosomal dominant	Rate of hemoglobin synthesis	Anemia

TABLE 6-3. CLINICAL DEFICIENCY STATES

Substance	Solubility	Deficiency State	Clinical Symptoms
Vitamin A	Lipid	Avitaminosis A	Blindness, xerophthalmia, hyperkeratosis
Vitamin B_1 (thiamine)	Water	Beriberi	Heart failure, Wernicke's psychosis
Vitamin B_2 (riboflavin)	Water	Ariboflavinosis	Cheilosis, glossitis, keratitis, dermatitis
Niacin	Water	Pellagra	Diarrhea, dementia, dermatitis
Vitamin C	Water	Scurvy	Hyperkeratosis, bleeding
Vitamin D	Lipid	Osteomalacia, rickets	Abnormal bone formation
Vitamin K	Lipid	Hypoprothrombinemia	Bleeding
Iron	—	Iron deficiency	Microcytic hypochromic anemia
Total calories and protein	—	Marasmus, kwashiorkor	Edema, depigmentation, fatty liver

TABLE 6-4. HARMFUL CHEMICAL SUBSTANCES

Noxious Substance	Site of Action	Clinical Effects
Carbon monoxide	Hemoglobin	Acute: cherry-red blood, coma, death Chronic: degeneration of basal ganglia
Carbon tetrachloride/chloroform	Microsomes	Hepatic fatty change and necrosis, renal tubular necrosis
Cyanide	Cytochrome oxidase	Systemic asphyxiant, cherry-red blood, bitter almond odor
Mercury	Protein	Mucosal ulcers, renal tubular necrosis, cerebral atrophy
Lead	Blood, brain, bone	Mild anemia with basophilic stippling, encephalopathy, intestinal colic, renal tubular acidosis
Arsenic	Sulfhydryl moieties	Diffuse hemorrhages, coagulation necrosis, thromboses

Questions

DIRECTIONS (Questions 1 through 39): Each of the numbered items or incomplete statements in this section is followed by answers or by completions of the statement. Select the ONE lettered answer or completion that is BEST in each case.

1. Which best determines the genotype of an organism?

    (A) number of microvilli
    (B) deoxyribonucleic acid (DNA) structure
    (C) pinocytosis
    (D) lysosomal content
    (E) rate of metabolism

2. A father and mother are both clinically well heterozygotes for a genetic disease that is expressed only with homozygous recessive, nonsex-linked inheritance. What percentage of their offspring should be affected?

    (A) 0%
    (B) 25%
    (C) 33%
    (D) 50%
    (E) 100%

3. The father is karyotypically normal. The mother is a clinically well heterozygous carrier for an X-linked trait. What percentage of the female offspring also will be carriers?

    (A) 0%
    (B) 25%
    (C) 33%
    (D) 50%
    (E) 100%

4. A Barr body occurs because of

    (A) ribosomes
    (B) endoplasmic reticulum
    (C) Lyon hypothesis
    (D) cytoplasm
    (E) Golgi apparatus

5. How many Barr bodies usually are seen in each cell with Turner's syndrome?

    (A) none
    (B) one
    (C) two
    (D) three
    (E) five or more

6. How many Barr bodies usually are seen in each cell in classic Klinefelter's syndrome?

    (A) none
    (B) one
    (C) two
    (D) three
    (E) four

7. Giemsa and quinacrine dyes are used in chromosome banding to

    (A) accelerate mitosis
    (B) paralyze the centrioles
    (C) stop the cell in metaphase
    (D) identify the karyotype
    (E) repair damaged chromosomes

8. True hermaphroditism is defined as

    (A) ovaries present with male secondary sex characteristics
    (B) absence of any gonadal tissue
    (C) testis present with female secondary sex characteristics
    (D) ambiguous external genitalia
    (E) ovarian and testicular tissue in same organism

9. Expected findings in Turner's syndrome include all of the following EXCEPT

    (A) tall stature
    (B) neck webbing
    (C) primary amenorrhea
    (D) 45,XO karyotype
    (E) streak ovaries

10. The 47,XXY karyotype is called

    (A) normal male
    (B) gonadal dysgenesis
    (C) Turner's syndrome
    (D) normal female
    (E) Klinefelter's syndrome

11. The usual karyotype of Edward's syndrome is

    (A) trisomy 13
    (B) trisomy 18
    (C) trisomy 21
    (D) deletion of short arm of chromosome 5
    (E) normal karyotype

12. Common findings in Down's syndrome include all of the following EXCEPT

    (A) mental retardation
    (B) epicanthic folds
    (C) trisomy 18
    (D) increased incidence of congenital heart disease
    (E) increased incidence of leukemia

13. A 1-year-old infant has a peculiar catlike mewing cry, mental retardation, and congenital heart disease. The abnormal karyotype is

    (A) monosomy 18
    (B) trisomy 18
    (C) trisomy 21
    (D) deletion of short arm of chromosome 5
    (E) monosomy 21

14. An X-linked disorder characterized by lysosomal lack of alpha-galactosidase activity with subsequent accumulation of ceramide trihexoside is

    (A) galactosemia
    (B) Gaucher's disease
    (C) metachromic leukodystrophy
    (D) Fabry's disease
    (E) Wolman's disease

15. Expected findings in Tay-Sachs disease include all of the following EXCEPT

    (A) macular cherry red spot
    (B) death by age 4
    (C) neuronal accumulation of GM2 ganglioside
    (D) deficient sphingomyelinase activity
    (E) mental retardation

16. A 25-year-old man is diagnosed as having an inherited glycogenosis. After heavy exercise, he gets painful cramps, and his urine turns brownish red for a short while. His probable diagnosis is

    (A) type I
    (B) type II
    (C) type IV
    (D) type V
    (E) Pompe's disease

17. With a short-term dose of 15 rad, what effects would be expected?

    (A) death in 2 hours
    (B) minor blood changes, at most
    (C) nausea, vomiting, and 25% mortality rate
    (D) diarrhea, 75% mortality rate
    (E) loss of hair, 50% mortality rate

18. An inherited disorder with abnormality in the rate of hemoglobin's globin chain production is

    (A) Huntington's chorea
    (B) hereditary lymphedema
    (C) spherocytosis
    (D) achondroplasia
    (E) thalassemia

19. An autosomal-dominant inherited disorder with disordered connective tissue, aortic cystic medial necrosis, long extremities, and spider fingers is

    (A) von Willebrand's disease
    (B) Milroy's syndrome
    (C) Alport's syndrome
    (D) Marfan's syndrome
    (E) tuberous sclerosis

20. Identify the FALSE statement about galactosemia

    (A) results from lack of galactose-1-phosphate uridyl transferase activity
    (B) transmitted as autosomal recessive
    (C) jaundice, hepatomegaly, and splenomegaly are common
    (D) mental retardation and cataracts are common
    (E) has low levels of blood galactose

21. The genetic disease characterized by lack of homogentisic oxidase, black-colored urine, and blue-black pigmentation of cartilage is

    (A) albinism
    (B) hypercholesterolemia
    (C) ochronosis
    (D) neurofibromatosis
    (E) von Recklinghausen's disease

22. Which disease is NOT inherited in an X-linked recessive mode?

    (A) hemophilia B
    (B) achondroplasia
    (C) hemophilia A
    (D) Wiskott–Aldrich syndrome
    (E) Bruton's agammaglobulinemia

23. Identify the FALSE statement about sickle cell disease

    (A) abnormal hemoglobin is termed A
    (B) usually caused by point substitution on globin molecule
    (C) homozygotes are most seriously affected
    (D) most common in black populations
    (E) produces chronic hemolytic anemia

24. Which is NOT associated with Niemann–Pick disease?

    (A) accumulation of galactocerebroside
    (B) lysosomal storage disease
    (C) physical and mental retardation
    (D) lipid-laden macrophages
    (E) enlarged spleen, liver, and lymph nodes

25. The pediatric genetic disease characterized by disordered exocrine gland secretion, pancreatic fibrosis, pulmonary bronchiectasis, and meconium ileus is

    (A) cretinism
    (B) erythroblastosis fetalis
    (C) mucoviscidosis
    (D) anencephaly
    (E) newborn respiratory distress syndrome

26. Which is NOT associated with Duchenne type muscular dystrophy?

    (A) first symptoms appear in early childhood
    (B) death usually by age 20
    (C) pseudohypertrophic changes common in lower extremities
    (D) death commonly caused by respiratory or cardiac difficulties
    (E) autosomal dominant inheritance

27. What is the usual mode of inheritance in Wilson's disease?

    (A) sex-linked recessive
    (B) autosomal dominant
    (C) sex-linked dominant
    (D) autosomal recessive
    (E) not an inherited disease

28. All of the following are inherited mucopolysaccharidoses EXCEPT

    (A) Wolman's disease
    (B) Hurler's syndrome
    (C) Morquio's syndrome
    (D) Sanfilippo's syndrome
    (E) Hunter's syndrome

29. An X-linked disorder characterized by absent hypoxanthine-guanine phosphoribosyltransferase activity, self-mutilation, choroeoathetosis, hyperuricemia, and hyperuricosuria is

    (A) Lesch–Nyhan syndrome
    (B) glucose-6-phosphate dehydrogenase (G6PD) deficiency
    (C) pyruvate kinase (PK) deficiency
    (D) Milroy's disease
    (E) Alport's syndrome

30. Common findings in kwashiorkor include all of the following EXCEPT

    (A) hepatomegaly and diarrhea
    (B) diet high in protein, low in carbohydrates
    (C) wasting of extremity muscles, with preserved subcutaneous fat
    (D) depigmentation of skin
    (E) changes in hair color or texture

31. The lipid-soluble vitamin important in mineralization of osteoid is

    (A) vitamin A
    (B) vitamin B
    (C) vitamin C
    (D) vitamin D
    (E) vitamin E

32. Beriberi results from a lack of which water-soluble vitamin?

    (A) vitamin K
    (B) pyridoxine
    (C) niacin
    (D) thiamine
    (E) vitamin B_6

33. Which is NOT true about vitamin K?

    (A) lack predisposes to bleeding
    (B) necessary for synthesis of factor II
    (C) lipid-soluble vitamin
    (D) may be low in diseases with fat malabsorption
    (E) low levels associated with venous thrombosis

34. Niacin deficiency is likely to cause

    (A) scurvy
    (B) pellagra
    (C) pernicious anemia
    (D) hypoprothrombinemia
    (E) ascorbic acid deficiency

35. Iron deficiency usually causes

    (A) macrocytic anemia
    (B) normochromic, normocytic anemia
    (C) megaloblastic anemia
    (D) microcytic, hypochromic anemia
    (E) anemia rarely occurs

36. An unexpected finding in lead poisoning would be

    (A) abdominal pain
    (B) renal tubular acidosis
    (C) polycythemia
    (D) wrist, finger, or foot drop
    (E) encephalopathy

37. A 100 kg healthy man ingests 10 g of sodium cyanide on an empty stomach. The expected result is

    (A) chronic debilitating arthritis
    (B) severe diarrhea
    (C) death within an hour or less
    (D) ataxia for 1 or 2 hours, then gradual improvement
    (E) micronodular cirrhosis

38. Identify the FALSE statement concerning methyl alcohol poisoning

    (A) poisoning can result from ingestion of 20 ml or more
    (B) poisoning can result from inhaled fumes
    (C) metabolic alkalosis occurs with poisoning
    (D) associated with blindness
    (E) can be caused by ingestion of Sterno, paint removers, or solvents

39. Which cell is the MOST radiosensitive?

    (A) ganglion cell
    (B) muscle cell
    (C) mature cartilage cell
    (D) lymphoid cell
    (E) pancreatic epithelial cell

DIRECTIONS (Questions 40 through 91): Each group of items in this section consists of lettered headings followed by a set of numbered words or phrases. For each numbered word or phrase, select the ONE lettered heading that is most closely associated with it. Each lettered heading may be selected once, more than once, or not at all.

Questions 40 through 43

    (A) Down's syndrome
    (B) Edward's syndrome
    (C) Patau's syndrome
    (D) cat's cry syndrome
    (E) Turner's syndrome

40. Deletion of short arm of chromosome 5
41. Trisomy 18
42. Trisomy 21
43. Trisomy 13

Questions 44 through 47

    (A) alpha$_1$-antitrypsin deficiency
    (B) hemophilia
    (C) achondroplasia
    (D) glucose-6-phosphate dehydrogenase (G6PD) deficiency
    (E) albinism

44. Bleeding disorder
45. Emphysema and cirrhosis
46. Dwarfism
47. Erythrocyte hemolysis

Questions 48 through 51

    (A) niacin deficiency
    (B) thiamine deficiency
    (C) protein and total calorie deficiency
    (D) vitamin D deficiency
    (E) iron deficiency

48. Marasmus
49. Beriberi
50. Rickets
51. Pellagra

Questions 52 through 55

    (A) lead poisoning
    (B) cyanide poisoning
    (C) mercury poisoning
    (D) carbon tetrachloride poisoning
    (E) vitamin A poisoning

52. Anemia with basophilic stippling
53. Binds to sulfhydryl groups of proteins
54. Binds to cytochrome oxidase
55. Fatty liver

Questions 56 through 59

    (A) 47,XXY
    (B) 45,XO
    (C) 46,XY
    (D) 46,XX
    (E) 45,YO

56. Normal human male karyotype
57. Normal human female karyotype

58. Klinefelter's syndrome karyotype A

59. Turner's syndrome karyotype B

Questions 60 through 63

(A) Cori's disease
(B) neurofibromatosis
(C) osteogenesis imperfecta
(D) McArdle's disease
(E) Gaucher's disease

60. Autosomal dominant disorder of abnormal collagen synthesis

61. Autosomal dominant disorder with pigmented skin macules and multiple endocrine tumors

62. Hereditary deficiency of glucocerebrosidase

63. Hereditary deficiency of glycogen debrancher enzyme

Questions 64 through 67

(A) Wilson's disease
(B) phenylketonuria
(C) galactosemia
(D) Fabry's syndrome
(E) sickle cell anemia

64. Deficiency of galactose-1-phosphate uridyl transferase

65. Deficiency of phenylalanine hydroxylase

66. Inherited disorder with abnormal hemoglobin molecule

67. Abnormal copper metabolism

Questions 68 through 71

(A) vitamin A
(B) vitamin B_2
(C) vitamin C
(D) vitamin D
(E) vitamin K

68. Lipid-soluble vitamin necessary for the synthesis of clotting factors X and II

69. Deficiency causes scurvy

70. Deficiency is termed "ariboflavinosis"

71. Deficiency state leads to xerophthalmia, night blindness, and follicular hyperplasia

Questions 72 through 75

(A) albinism
(B) iron deficiency
(C) folic acid deficiency
(D) cretinism
(E) von Hippel–Lindau disease

72. Macrocytic anemia

73. Microcytic, hypochromic anemia

74. Autosomal recessive inherited disorder with deficiency of melanin production

75. Autosomal dominant inherited disorder

Questions 76 through 79

(A) heat cramps
(B) smoke inhalation
(C) first-degree burn
(D) third-degree burn
(E) malignant hyperthermia

76. Thermal destruction of the epidermis and adnexal structures

77. Most common cause of fire-related deaths

78. Systemic hyperpyrexia on administration of anesthestics

79. Muscle spasms due to depletion of water and salt

Questions 80 through 83

(A) hypocalcemia
(B) hyponatremia
(C) obesity
(D) bulimia
(E) iodine deficiency

80. Goiter

81. Tetany

82. At least 30% over ideal body weight

83. Eating disorder with binge-and-purge episodes

Questions 84 through 87

(A) cystic fibrosis
(B) ochronosis
(C) muscular dystrophy
(D) hemophilia
(E) female pseudohermaphroditism
(F) male pseudohermaphroditism
(G) Turner's syndrome
(H) Klinefelter's syndrome

84. A 4-year-old male has suffered from progressive weakness of his proximal muscle groups for about 6 months. His serum creatine kinase is markedly elevated. His older brother suffers from the same disorder and is now wheelchair-bound at age 10 and has prominent pseudohypertrophy of his calf muscles. What is the most likely diagnosis?

85. Shortly after birth a white infant is noted to have meconium ileus. Over the next several years the child remains at the lowest tenth percentile for growth and is experiencing malabsorption and repeated respiratory infections. Examination of this child's sweat reveals an elevated sodium and chloride content. What is the most likely diagnosis?

86. A 20-year-old woman is killed in a motor vehicle accident. At autopsy normal female external secondary sexual characteristics are present. However, the gonads are found to be testicular and the decedent's karyotype is 46,XY. What is the most likely diagnosis?

87. A 21-year-old female who has never menstruated is examined by her gynecologist. The patient has a small stature, web neck, poorly developed breasts and widely spaced nipples. No Barr bodies are evident on her buccal smear study. What is the most likely diagnosis?

Questions 88 through 91

(A) lead poisoning
(B) carbon monoxide poisoning
(C) pellagra
(D) scurvy
(E) sickle cell anemia
(F) Wilson's disease
(G) Hunter's syndrome
(H) hemophilia

88. A 4-year-old black female with a long history of microcytic anemia since birth presents to the emergency department complaining of severe left-upper quadrant abdominal pain. Her hemoglobin electrophoresis demonstrates 95% hemoglobin S. What genetic disorder is she most likely to have?

89. A 5-year-old male child presents to the emergency department complaining of knee pain. The child denies any recent trauma to the joint. The joint is distended by unclotted blood. The child's factor VIII is found to be less than 5% of normal. The child's sister is well, but his older brother also has episodes of spontaneous bleeding. What genetic disorder is the child most likely to have?

90. A 19-year-old male has been working on his car in an enclosed garage for about 20 minutes. During this time the car's engine has been running. The man begins to develop an intense headache, nausea, and dizziness. What is the most likely diagnosis?

91. A 43-year-old alcoholic with poor nutritional status is admitted to the hospital. His most serious ailments include dermatitis, diarrhea, and dementia. Which vitamin deficiency disease is he most likely to have acquired?

Answers and Explanations

1. **(B)** The genotype (genetic makeup of an organism) is determined by the molecular structure of its DNA contained in chromosomes. Pinocytosis refers to invaginations of the cell membrane, which is useful in fluid measurement. The lysosomal content, number of microvilli, and rate of metabolism of a cell are in part determined by the cell's genotype but do not themselves direct or define the genotype. They are outward expressions (phenotype) of the DNA structure. *(4:210–212)*

2. **(B)** Half of the offspring will be identical to the parents, that is, heterozygous for the recessive defect but clinically well. One quarter of the offspring will be homozygous normal and clinically well. The remaining offspring, 25% of the total, will be homozygous for the recessive defect and clinically affected. *(4:224)*

3. **(D)** Female offspring receive X chromosomes from the father and mother. The father can contribute only his normal X. The mother can contribute either her normal X or her carrier X. Thus about one half of the female offspring will be carriers. *(4:232–233)*

4. **(C)** According to the Lyon hypothesis, only one X chromatin is genetically active, and the other undergoes heteropyknosis to become the Barr body, inactivation occurs about the 16th day of embryonic life, and inactivation of the same X chromosome persists in all progeny cells. The Barr body is composed mostly of nucleoprotein. *(2:132–133)*

5. **(A)** Turner's syndrome usually has a 45,XO karyotype. According to the Lyon hypothesis, there should be no Barr body (extra X chromosome) in the Turner's cells, since Turner's cells have only one X chromosome. *(4:217–218)*

6. **(B)** Classic Klinefelter's syndrome has a 47,XXY karyotype. According to the Lyon hypothesis, all except one X chromosome will involute and become Barr bodies. The expected number of Barr bodies is then one per cell. *(4:215–217)*

7. **(D)** Giemsa and quinacrine dyes are used to band the chromosomes, allowing enumeration and identification of the karyotype. After staining, colchicine is used to paralyze the centrioles and microtubules, stopping the cell in metaphase. Giemsa and quinacrine stains do not accelerate mitosis or repair damaged chromosomes. *(4:210)*

8. **(E)** True hermaphroditism is defined as an organism possessing both ovarian and testicular tissue. An organism with testicular tissue and female external genitalia is a male pseudohermaphrodite. Female pseudohermaphrodites have ovarian tissue and exhibit male external genitalia. *(2:133–136)*

9. **(A)** Turner's syndrome usually has a 45,XO karyotype, although some people are 46,XX/45,XO mosaic. In the fully expressed syndrome, there are streak ovaries (gonadal dysgenesis), webbed neck, short stature, primary amenorrhea, and congenital heart disease. *(3:48)*

10. **(E)** Klinefelter's syndrome has a male phenotype, sterility, eunochoid body habitus, long legs, and a slight decrease in intelligence. Its karyotype is 47,XXY. Turner's syndrome, also called gonadal dysgenesis, has a karyotype of 45,XO. The normal male and female karyotypes are 46,XY and 46,XX, respectively. *(2:133–134)*

11. **(B)** Edward's syndrome has a karyotype of trisomy 18. Clinical features include mental retardation, cardiac defects, micrognathia, and large occiput. Trisomy 13, trisomy 21, and a deletion of the short arm of chromosome 5 are Patau's syndrome, Down's syndrome, and cat's cry syndrome, respectively. *(2:130)*

12. **(C)** Down's syndrome is caused by a trisomy of chromosome 21. Clinical features include mental retardation, epicanthic folds, horizontal palmar crease, flat facial profile, and muscle hypotonia. The incidence of leukemia and congenital heart disease is increased in Down's syndrome. *(4:214–215)*

13. **(D)** The clinical picture described characterizes cat's cry syndrome, a genetic disorder with a deletion of the short arm of chromosome 5. Infants with monosomies rarely survive birth. Trisomy 18 and trisomy 21 are Edward's syndrome and Down's syndrome, respectively. *(2:132)*

14. **(D)** Fabry's disease is an X-linked recessive disorder caused by lack of alpha-galactosidase activity with lysosomal accumulation of ceramide trihexoside. Affected cells contain doubly refractile lipid material that is lamellated in a myelinlike form by ultrastructural examination. Blue-black pruritic skin eruptions are common with the disease. The other listed diseases have autosomal recessive inheritance. *(3:55)*

15. **(D)** Tay-Sachs disease is a glycolipid storage disease caused by absent hexosaminidase A activity. Neurons accumulate GM2 ganglioside with resultant mental retardation, deafness, blindness, and death by age 4. The macular cherry red spot is an expected clinical finding. Deficient sphingomyelinase activity is seen in Niemann–Pick disease. *(2:145–146)*

16. **(D)** Of the listed choices, only type V, McArdle's disease, is compatible with a normal life span. The defect in McArdle's disease, muscle phosphorylase, causes skeletal muscle damage, with resultant pain and myoglobinuria after heavy exercise. All of the other glycogenoses listed usually are fatal in early childhood. *(2:151–153)*

17. **(B)** A short-term dose of 15 rad would be expected to produce minor blood changes, if anything. Higher short-term doses, up to about 200 rad, are necessary to produce a mortality rate of about 20%. Over 800 rad, there is a 100% mortality rate. *(3:249–251)*

18. **(E)** Thalassemia is an autosomal dominant inherited disorder characterized by an abnormal rate of globin chain production. All of the other choices are autosomal dominant inherited disorders but have no direct effect on the rate of globin synthesis. *(2:670–676)*

19. **(D)** Marfan's syndrome is a genetic disorder of connective tissue. Aortic cystic medial necrosis is a characteristic lesion and results in a propensity for thoracic dissecting aneurysms. Other features of the disorder include autosomal dominant inheritance, long slender extremities, and long fingers. *(2:138–139)*

20. **(E)** Galactosemia is a genetic disorder with autosomal recessive inheritance characterized by absent galactose-1-phosphate uridyl transferase activity. This blocked metabolic pathway causes high blood galactose levels and galactosuria. Common findings in the disease are mental retardation, cataracts, jaundice, and hepatosplenomegaly. *(2:532–533)*

21. **(C)** Ochronosis is an autosomal recessive disorder characterized by the lack of homogenitisic oxidase, black-colored urine, and pigmentation of the cartilage. The pigmented cartilage is more susceptible to osteoarthropathy. The other choices have genetic modes of transmission but lack the clinical findings seen in ochronosis. *(2:143–144)*

22. **(B)** X-linked recessive inheritance has a genetic abnormality carried on the X chromosome. Because of this, the disease usually is apparent only in about half of the male offspring of clinically unaffected heterozygote carrier females. Unaffected males do not transmit the disease. The hemophilias are both X-linked, bleeding disorders. Bruton's agammaglobulinemia and Wiskott–Aldrich syndrome are both X-linked immunodeficiency disorders. Achondroplasia, or dwarfism, is an autosomal dominant affliction. *(3:58–60)*

23. **(A)** Sickle cell disease is a genetic disease caused by an inherited abnormal hemoglobin. The most common form in North America, the S form, is caused by a point substitution on the beta-globulin molecule. Normal hemoglobin molecules are termed "A." Sickle hemoglobin is termed "S." Homozygotes are most severely affected with anemia. Vasoocclusive complications and chronic infections hallmark the disease. The S hemoglobin is most common in black populations. *(2:666–670)*

24. **(A)** Niemann–Pick disease is a lysosomal storage disease caused by reduced or absent sphingomyelinase activity. Sphingomyelin accumulates within lysosomes of the reticuloendothelial cells and macrophages of the spleen, liver, and lymph nodes, causing clinical enlargement as well as physical and mental retardation. An accumulation of galactocerebroside is seen in Krabbe's disease, alternatively called globoid cell leukodystrophy. *(2:146–148)*

25. **(C)** Mucoviscidosis, also called "cystic fibrosis," is characterized by disordered exocrine gland secretion, pancreatic fibrosis, and chronic bronchiectasis. The other disorders, cretinism, newborn respiratory distress syndrome, anencephaly, and erythroblastosis fetalis are pediatric diseases resulting from lack of thyroxine, lack of surfactant, lack of cranial development, and maternal red blood cell alloantibodies, respectively. *(4:225–226)*

26. **(E)** Duchenne type of muscular dystrophy is an X-linked recessive disorder usually limited to males. Pelvifemoral muscle weakness usually first appears in early childhood. Later in the disease, the

shoulder, arms, and trunk are involved. Pseudohypertrophic changes are distinctive of this dystrophy. Death by age 20 usually results from respiratory failure, pulmonary infections, or cardiac disorders. *(4:1401–1403)*

27. **(D)** Wilson's disease, also called "hepatolenticular degeneration," is a genetic abnormality of copper metabolism. The usual mode of inheritance is autosomal dominant. The clinical picture is one of cirrhosis, cerebellar and basal ganglia degeneration, and a pigmented ring in the cornea (Kayser-Fleischer ring). Treatment with penicillamine has markedly improved the prognosis for this disorder. *(2:461,956–957)*

28. **(A)** The mucopolysaccharidoses are inherited disorders of mucopolysaccharide metabolism. Lack of degradative enzymes results in lysosomal accumulation of mucopolysaccharides. Eventually, the excessive retained mucopolysaccharides result in cell injury and death. Of the listed choices, only Wolman's disease is not a mucopolysaccharidoses. The defect in Wolman's disease is lack of acid esterase enzymatic activity, leading to accumulation of triglyceride and cholesterol esters in the liver, spleen, adrenal gland, and kidney of affected individuals. *(2:149–151)*

29. **(A)** Lesch–Nyhan syndrome has absent hypoxanthine-guanine phosphoribosyltransferase activity with resultant hyperuricemia, hyperuricosuria, and uric acid renal calculi. The major clinical features of the disease are neurologic self-mutilation, mental retardation, spastic movements, and choreoathetosis. Deficiencies of G6PD and PK are X-linked chronic hemolytic anemias. Milroy's disease (hereditary lymphedema) and Alport's syndrome (nephropathy, deafness) are autosomal dominant disorders. *(3:59)*

30. **(B)** Kwashiorkor is a nutritional imbalance caused by inadequate protein consumption with adequate or high carbohydrate intake. It usually follows weaning when children are switched to a calorically adequate grain diet with limited quantities of nutritionally poor protein. The clinical picture includes hair changes, skin depigmentation, hepatomegaly, diarrhea, and muscle wasting. Subcutaneous fat usually is preserved. *(2:437–438)*

31. **(D)** Vitamin D is important for the proper mineralization of newly made osteoid. Vitamin D is a steroid-based molecule and is lipid-soluble. Other lipid-soluble vitamins include vitamins A, E, and K. All of the B vitamins are water-soluble. *(1:156–164)*

32. **(D)** Beriberi is caused by a lack of dietary thiamine. The disease consists of high output heart failure, complicating infections, serous effusions, acute pulmonary edema, and hepatic congestion. Niacin deficiency, pellagra, has skin and mucous membrane lesions. Pyridoxine, also called "vitamin B_6," deficiency has a variable clinical appearance. Vitamin K is a fat-soluble vitamin necessary to synthesize certain coagulation proteins. *(4:319–321)*

33. **(E)** Vitamin K is a lipid-soluble vitamin necessary for the synthesis of blood clotting factors II, VII, X, and XI. Lack of vitamin K predisposes to bleeding and can be seen in fat malabsorption diseases, such as chronic pancreatitis and obstructive jaundice. Venous thromboses are less likely to occur with low levels of vitamin K. *(1:159–160)*

34. **(B)** Niacin is an active component in many oxidation–reduction reactions in the body through nicotinamide-adenine dinucleotide (NAD) and NAD phosphate intermediaries. The niacin deficiency state is termed "pellagra" and is associated with dermatitis, dementia, and diarrhea. Scurvy, pernicious anemia, and hypoprothrombinemia are associated with low levels of vitamin C (ascorbic acid), vitamin B_{12}, and vitamin K, respectively. *(1:156–164)*

35. **(D)** Iron is an important constituent of hemoglobin, and iron deficiency can lead to anemia. The anemia produces red blood cells that are microcytic and hypochromic. *(1:164)*

36. **(C)** Lead poisoning usually has mild anemia not polycythemia. Accompanying the anemia is basophilic stippling of the erythrocytes. Other common clinical features in lead poisoning include abdominal colic and pain, encephalopathy, gingival lead lines, renal tubular acidosis, and finger, wrist, or foot drop. *(3:205–208)*

37. **(C)** Ingestion of less than 0.1 g of the inorganic salt of cyanide usually is rapidly fatal. A 10-g dose is massive; death would occur within 10 to 20 minutes. In acute cyanide poisoning, the cyanide binds to cytochrome oxidase to produce asphyxiation. The blood is cherry red color and has a pungent bitter almond shell. *(4:296–297)*

38. **(C)** Methyl alcohol is found in solvents, Sterno, and paint remover. As little as 20 ml of ingested methyl alcohol can be toxic. Poisoning also occurs if fumes are inhaled for a prolonged time, particularly in unventilated rooms. A marked anion gap metabolic acidosis develops. The principal sites of body damage are the brain and retina. Blindness is a common sequela. *(3:197–198)*

39. **(D)** Cells with high radiosensitivity (the ability to be easily damaged by radiation), include lymphoid cells, hematopoietic cells, germ cells, and intestinal

epithelium. In general, the higher the mitotic rate of the tissue, the more likely that the tissue will be damaged by radiation. *(3:256–258)*

40. (D)

41. (B)

42. (A)

43. (C)

40 through 43. All of the syndromes have chromosomal aberrations. Down's syndrome, Edward's syndrome, and Patau's syndrome are trisomies of chromosomes 21, 18, and 13, respectively. Cat's cry syndrome (cri du chat) has a deletion of the short arm of chromosome 5. *(2:130)*

44. (B)

45. (A)

46. (C)

47. (D)

44 through 47. All of the listed conditions are inherited. The mode of inheritance is X-linked recessive in hemophilia and G6PD deficiency. Achondroplasia is an autosomal dominant disorder. The cirrhosis and emphysema seen in alpha$_1$-antitrypsin deficiency is inherited in an autosomal recessive mode. *(1:239)*

48. (C)

49. (B)

50. (D)

51. (A)

48 through 51. Deficiencies of the B vitamins, niacin and thiamine, cause pellagra and beriberi, respectively. Lack of protein and total calories is called "marasmus" and is characterized by severe weight loss, edema, depigmentation, and diarrhea. Vitamin D deficiency results in poor mineralization of osteoid and is rickets in infants and children. In adults, the deficient state is osteomalacia. *(1:156–164)*

52. (A)

53. (C)

54. (B)

55. (D)

52 through 55. Lead poisoning is characterized by anemia, erythrocytic basophilic stippling, encephalopathy, renal tubular acidosis, and colic. Cyanide poisons by binding to cytochrome oxidase and asphyxiating all the cells of the body. Mercury damages cells by binding to sulfhydryl protein groups. The kidney is a major site of damage. Carbon tetrachloride poisoning is characterized by hepatic fatty change and necrosis. *(3:205–208)*

56. (C)

57. (D)

58. (A)

59. (B)

56 through 59. The normal human male and female karyotypes are 46,XY and 46,XX, respectively. Klinefelter's syndrome has a 47,XXY karotype and is characterized by tall eunuchoid habitus, female distribution of hair, small penis, gynecomastia, and infertility. Turner's syndrome has a 45,XO or 45,XO/46,XX mosaic karyotype and is characterized by short stature, web neck, lymphedema, immature nipple development, primary amenorrhea, streak gonads, skeletal abnormalities, and congenital heart disease. *(1:235–236)*

60. (C)

61. (B)

62. (E)

63. (A)

60 through 63. Osteogenesis imperfecta is a genetic disorder with abnormal collagen production. There is a defect in the synthesis of type I collagen, the major (90%) matrix constituent of bone. The mode of inheritance is autosomal dominant. Affected individuals suffer from extreme bone fragility, multiple fractures, dental imperfections, and blue sclera. Neurofibromatosis is an autosomal dominant disorder characterized by numerous pigmented skin lesions, multiple neural tumors, Lisch nodules, and a tendency for reduced intelligence. Gaucher's disease is an autosomal recessive lysosomal storage disorder in which there is an intracellular accumulation of glucocerebroside due to the genetic lack of glucocerebrosidase enzyme. Clinical features include hepatosplenomegaly, progressive central nervous system degeneration, and skeletal lesions. Cori's disease is an autosomal recessive disorder of glycogen metabolism due to the absence of the debrancher enzyme. There is accumulation of massive quantities of glycogen throughout the body with

64. (C)

65. (B)

66. (E)

67. (A)

64 through 67. Galactosemia is an autosomal recessive disorder which is most often due to the genetic lack of the enzyme galactose-1-phosphate uridyl transferase. Infants are normal at birth. But, shortly after ingesting galactose containing foods, such as human or bovine milk, there is a marked elevation of galactose levels in serum and urine with subsequent jaundice, vomiting, hepatomegaly, liver failure, neurologic damage, and cataracts unless a galactose-free diet is maintained. Phenylketonuria is an autosomal recessive disease due to an absence of the enzyme phenylalanine hydroxylase. There is hyperphenylalaninemia and increased urinary excretion of its phenylketone metabolites. Clinically, progressive mental retardation is observed unless a phenylalanine-free diet is maintained. Sickle cell disease is an inherited hemoglobinopathy in which there is abnormal beta globin chain production. The abnormal hemoglobin spontaneously deforms the erythrocytes into sickle- and leaf-shaped structures when deoxygenized. These deformed red blood cells hemolyse or clog the smaller blood vessels causing ischemia. Wilson's disease, hepatolenticular degeneration, is an autosomal recessive disorder of copper metabolism characterized by marked accumulation of copper in the brain, liver, and eye. There are usually very low levels of the copper transport protein, ceruloplasmin. *(2:530–533,633–670,956–957)*

68. (E)

69. (C)

70. (B)

71. (A)

68 through 71. The lipid-soluble vitamin K is necessary for the synthesis of blood clotting factors II, VII, IX, and X in the liver. The resultant abnormality of blood clotting is seen clinically as easy bruising, hematuria, or melena. Scurvy is caused by a deficiency of the water-soluble vitamin C. Scurvy is characterized by abnormal collagen maturation, bleeding gums, abnormal wound healing, and abnormal bone growth. Ariboflavinosis, a lack of vitamin B_2, is associated with fissuring of the lips (cheilosis), fissuring at the angles of the mouth (angular stomatitis), tongue atrophy, and corneal vascular opacities. A lack of the lipid-soluble vitamin A can produce night blindness (nyctalopia), conjunctival dryness (xerophthalmia), corneal opacities, corneal ulcerations, and follicular deratosis. *(1:156–162)*

72. (C)

73. (B)

74. (A)

75. (E)

72 through 75. Macrocytic anemia is usually seen with a deficiency of folic acid. Folic acid is a necessary cofactor for the synthesis of nucleic acids. Folic acid is most plentiful in raw green and yellow vegetables. Iron deficiency produces a microcytic, hypochromic anemia. Chronic blood loss is the most frequent cause of iron deficiency. Albinism is a recessive autosomal disorder due to an inherited lack of effective melanin production. The lack of melanin predisposes these individuals to the early development of actinic-induced skin cancers. Von Hippel–Lindau disease is an autosomal dominant disorder in which there is an increased incidence of hemangioblastomas, angiomas, adenomas, pheochromocytomas, cysts, and carcinomas in various organs throughout the body. A genetic alteration has recently been mapped to chromosome 3. *(2:140, 143,455,459–461)*

76. (D)

77. (B)

78. (E)

79. (A)

76 through 79. Thermal burns are divided into three categories by the depth of tissue destruction. First-degree burns are defined as the thermal loss of only the epidermis. Burns that destroy the epidermis and the superficial dermis, but spare the underlying adnexal structures are termed second-degree. Third-degree burns involve the loss of the epidermis, dermis, and adnexal structures. Smoke inhalation is the most common cause of fire-related deaths. In a house fire, for example, most people die of hypoxia while breathing smokey air with little remaining oxygen and abundant carbon monoxide. Only after the individual expires of asphyxia does most thermal burning of the body occur. Malignant hyperthermia is a genetic disorder characterized by the development of marked hyperpyrexia during administration of anesthetics. Widespread skeletal muscle necrosis occurs with resultant myoglobinemia, myoglobinuria, and acute renal failure. Exercising in hot, humid weather encourages the loss of water and salt predisposing an individual to develop muscle cramps. These spasms of the voluntary muscles can be prevented and treated by salt and water replacement *(1:169–172)*

80. **(E)**

81. **(A)**

82. **(C)**

83. **(D)**

80 through 83. Goiter, a diffuse enlargement of the thyroid gland, is usually seen with iodine deficiency. Iodine is a necessary element in the synthesis of thyroid hormones. One of the body's responses to the lack of this hormone is to encourage hyperplasia of the thyroid gland. Tetany, an involuntary twitching or contracting of muscles, is seen with hypocalcemia. Insufficient parathyroid hormone is the most common cause of hypocalcemia. Obesity is usually defined as a weight at least 30% in excess of ideal body weight. Obese individuals are at increased risk for heart disease, stroke, hypertension, and some forms of cancer. Bulimia is an eating disorder characterized by episodic overeating usually followed by induced vomiting. Bulimics may sustain esophageal tears, aspiration pneumonia, cardiac arrhythmias, acid erosion of their teeth, and occasionally, death. *(1:28,848–849)*

84. **(C)** Duchenne muscular dystrophy is an X-linked recessive, inherited disorder characterized by progressive muscle weakness. The weakness is usually first detected at age 3 or 4 and begins in the proximal muscle groups, such as the shoulder, trunk, or pelvis. There is a persistent elevation of the serum creatine kinase enzyme throughout the disease. This elevated enzymatic marker is also useful in identifying the heterozygous carrier state. By age 10 most victims are wheelchair-bound. Pseudohypertrophy of the calf muscles due to fatty replacement of diseased muscle is a characteristic finding in the later stages of the disease. Death usually results from muscular respiratory insufficiency. *(4:1401–1403)*

85. **(A)** Cystic fibrosis is an inherited disorder affecting exocrine gland secretion throughout the body. The enigmatic genetic alteration is present at the long arm of chromosome 7. Meconium ileus may occur in utero or shortly after brith heralding the onset of the disorder. More commonly, however, the disorder is first diagnosed in 2- or 3-year-old infants who have had repeated pulmonary infections, malabsorption, a retarded growth rate, and poor development. Analysis of sweat reveals the characteristic elevation of both sodium and chloride. Many individuals with cystic fibrosis now live into their mid-20s. Death is usually due to infectious complications. *(2:533–536)*

86. **(F)** The scenario describes male pseudohermaphroditism, a phenotypic female with male karyotype. Unless these individuals are serendipitously studied for karyotype, primary amenorrhea, infertility, or develop tumors in their abdominal testes, most will live their lives as normal, albeit sterile, females. The disorder is usually inherited in an X-linked manner. The corresponding biochemical defect is an inability of cells to respond to androgenic hormones. In utero the lack of androgenic action leads to incomplete descent of the testes and subsequent formation of normal female external genitalia, including a vagina. The uterus, however, is not formed so that primary amenorrhea and sterility result. Chromosomal analysis is diagnostic revealing a male karyotype. The intraabdominal gonads are testes and this cryptorchidism predisposes to the development of testicular malignancies. *(1:250–251)*

87. **(G)** The karyotype of Turner's syndrome is usually 45,XO. A few individuals are 45,XO/46,XX mosaics. Turner's syndrome may include the following features: webbed neck, short stature, primary amenorrhea, widely spaced nipples, coarctation of the aorta, wide carrying angle of the arms, poor breast development, rudimentary or streak gonads, lymphedema, hypoplasia of the nails, abnormal teeth, high arched palate, craniofacial abnormalities, metatarsal and metacarpal deformations, and multiple pigmented nevi. *(2:217–218)*

88. **(E)** Sickle cell disease is a hereditary hemoglobinopathy in which an aberrant beta hemoglobin chain is made due to an inherited point mutation in the genetic code. This mutation results in the substitution of the amino acid valine for glutamic acid in the sixth position of the beta chain. Upon deoxygenation this abnormal hemoglobin spontaneously polymerizes in the erythrocyte deforming the cell into a sickle- or leaf-like shape. The sickled erythrocytes hemolyze and occlude small blood vessels. The vascular occlusion may result in ischemic tissue destruction. Most homozygous infants do not develop profound anemia and ischemic sequela until 5 or 6 months after birth due to the protective effect of residual fetal hemoglobin. The common clinical features of sickle cell disease in patients older than 6 months usually include anemia, hyperbilirubinemia, chronic infections, painful vascular occlusive events, and later in the progression of the disease, splenic autoinfarction. Heterozygotes are clinically well and derive a mild protective effect against malarial erythrocytic infection. *(2:666–670)*

89. **(H)** Hemophilia A is an X-linked disorder in which the activity of blood clotting factor VIII is insufficient for normal hemostasis. These individuals suffer from spontaneous hemorrhages, particularly into the joints. Exsanguination from unexpected trauma or surgical procedures is not unheard of. Replacement therapy with factor VIII concentrates is helpful for temporary correction of the bleeding diathesis in individuals who have not developed inhibitor antibodies. The transfusion of factor VIII concentrates do, however, carry a risk of hepatitis and AIDS transmission. *(2:698)*

90. **(B)** Carbon monoxide poisons by binding irreversibly to hemoglobin with resultant systemic asphyxiation. This colorless, odorless gas is readily formed by incomplete combustion, such as in automobile engines powered by fossil fuel derivatives. Hypoxia is first noted as headache, nausea, and vomiting with a 20% to 30% saturation of hemoglobin. Unconsciousness and death are likely at concentrations above 60% saturation. Chronic low-dose poisoning may result in cystic necrosis of the brain. *(2:495)*

91. **(C)** The scenario depicts an individual with pellagra, a deficiency of niacin. Pellagra usually has a constellation of symptoms termed "the three Ds"—dermatitis, diarrhea, and dementia. The dermatitis affects the sun-exposed skin which becomes darker because of increased melanin pigmentation and redder because of increased vascularity. There are atrophic mucous membrane changes throughout the gastrointestinal tract with resultant diarrhea. The dementia occurs due to degeneration of neurons in the cerebral cortex. Niacin is required for the synthesis of nicotinamide adenine dinucleotide, a cofactor active in many oxidation reduction reactions in the cell. *(1:163)*

REFERENCES

1. Chandrasoma P, Taylor CR: Concise Pathology, Norwalk, Appleton and Lange, 1991.
2. Cotran RS, Kumar V, Robbins SL: Robbins Pathologic Basis of Disease, 4th edition, Philadelphia, Saunders, 1989
3. Kissane JM (ed): Anderson's Pathology, 9th edition, St. Louis, Mosby, 1990
4. Rubin E, Farber JL: Pathology, Philadelphia, Lippincott, 1988

CHAPTER 7

Neoplasia and Abnormalities of Growth

Our first priority is to recognize that cancer is only a name given to one part of the collective processes of tissue disorganization, that it has no one external cause, that many external and internal agencies predispose to its development, that it is cell mediated but generally arises without any specific, once-for-all, genetic origin and that, though it may regress or become benign, its tendency is to progress irregularly in several of its growth characteristics.
—Sir David Smithers (1971)

Neoplasia: An abnormal mass of tissue, the growth of which exceeds and is uncoordinated with that of the normal tissues and persists in the same excessive manner after cessation of the stimuli which evolve the change.
—R.A. Willis

The biologic and clinically important subject of neoplasia should be seen in the perspective of abnormal growth and cellular reproduction. This is particularly seen in the concept of the role of genes and gene products—the control of cellular proliferation and growth.

BASIC FACTS AND DEFINITIONS

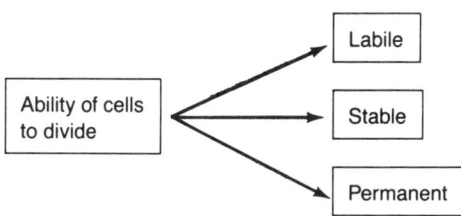

The various types of growth abnormalities are summarized in Table 7–1 and further defined in Table 7–2. The normal ability of cells to divide is based on whether they are labile, stable, or permanent.

TABLE 7–1. ABNORMALITIES IN GROWTH

Alteration in Number of Cells	Alteration in Size of Individual Cells	Alteration in Cell Composition and Maturation
Aplasia	Agenesis	Metaplasia
Hypoplasia	Atrophy	Dysplasia
Hyperplasia	Hypertrophy	Neoplasia

Two of the most important distinctions in cell proliferation are between hyperplasia and neoplasia (Table 7–3) and benign vs malignant neoplasia (Table 7–4).

Various types of carcinogenic agents identified in human cancer can be seen in Table 7–5. The older concepts of initiation and promotion in chemical carcinogenesis, the multiple hit theory of physical and chemical carcinogenesis, virus oncogenesis, hereditary and acquired carcinogenic chromosomal abnormalities, and their relationship with growth factors and control mechanisms are summarized schematically in Figures 7–1 and 7–2. Carcinogenesis can therefore be regarded as an interference in the normal gene regulation of growth.

In Table 7–6 some of the mechanisms of increased oncogene activation are summarized. Suppressor genes,

TABLE 7–2. DEFINITIONS

Terminology	Definition
Aplasia	Lack of normal cellular proliferation with resultant absence of tissue, eg, aplastic anemia
Hypoplasia	Decrease in mass of tissue or organ due to decrease in normal cellular proliferation resulting in decrease before tissue or organ reaches normal mature size
Hyperplasia	Increase in mass of tissue or organ because of cellular increase beyond normal range
Agenesis	Congenital lack of tissue or organ owing to total lack of cells concerned
Atrophy	Acquired decrease in mass of tissue or organ because of decrease in size of cellular components after full maturity has been achieved
Hypertrophy	Acquired increase in mass of tissue or organ owing to increase in size of cellular components
Metaplasia	Acquired change of tissue or organ because of change of one adult cell type to a different adult cell type
Dysplasia	Abnormal sequence of changes in maturation or development of cell type in a tissue or organ
Neoplasia	Formation of new growth by abnormal cell proliferation

TABLE 7-3. ESSENTIAL DIFFERENCE BETWEEN HYPERPLASIA AND NEOPLASIA

Neoplasia	Hyperplasia
Spontaneous or abnormal proliferative response to a stimulus (often unknown type)	A proliferative cellular response to an overstimulation of a normal type
Often not proportional to the stimulus, and proceeds	Proliferation proportional to the stimulus
Unabated in the absence of continuation of stimulus	Ceases on cessation of the stimulus

Note: There are circumstances when the two conditions are superimposed and difficult to separate

TABLE 7-4. ESSENTIAL DIFFERENCES BETWEEN BENIGN AND MALIGNANT NEOPLASIAS

Benign	Malignant
Noninvasive by groups of cells or individual cells	Invasive
Encapsulated	Nonencapsulated
Highly differentiated, closely resembling normal cells of origin	Well differentiated or poorly differentiated
Mitoses rare	Mitoses relatively frequent
Slowly growing	More rapidly growing
Nonmetastatic to distant sites	Metastatic to distant sites

often referred to as anti-oncogenes, have been shown in some neoplasms to have a control effect and are related to prognosis. Some examples in human cancer are shown in Table 7-7. It is important to be able to classify the different types of human neoplasms and this is summarized in detail in Table 7-8.

The effects that neoplasms can produce clinically is best understood by the awareness of their mode of spread (Fig 7-3 and Table 7-9) and the various products of tumor expression, which can be exploited diagnostically (Table 7-10). The response of the body to growing neoplasm via the policing immune system is summarized in Table 7-11. The major effects of tumors in terms of their clinical presentation are summarized in Table 7-12. It is important to be aware of the different incidence and death rate for cancer not only in the United States (Table 7-13) but the geographic differences and epidemiology aspect of cancer (Table 7-14).

TABLE 7-5. SUMMARY OF CARCINOGENIC AGENTS IN HUMAN TUMORS

Chemical	Physical	Viral	Genetic Chromosomal	Hormonal
Polycyclic Hydrocarbons	Radiation	HTLV-1	Retinoblastoma (Chromosome 13)	Androgen Estrogen
Tobacco	Ultraviolet Light	HIV	Wilms' tumor (Chromosome 11)	D.E.S.
Asbestos		Papilloma Viruses	Burkitt's lymphoma (Chromosome 14)	? Prolactin
Aflatoxins		Herpes II	Chronic myeloid leukemia (Chromosome 22)	
Aromatic Amines		E.B. Virus	Acute myeloid leukemia	
Nitrosamines		Hepatitis B	Acute lymphoblastic leukemia	
Heavy metals		Molluscum Contagiosum	Neurofibromatosis	
Arsenic		Cytomegalovirus	Multiple endocrine adenomatosis	
Vinyl chloride			Familial polyposis coli	
Chemotherapy drugs			Nevoid basal cell carcinoma syndrome	

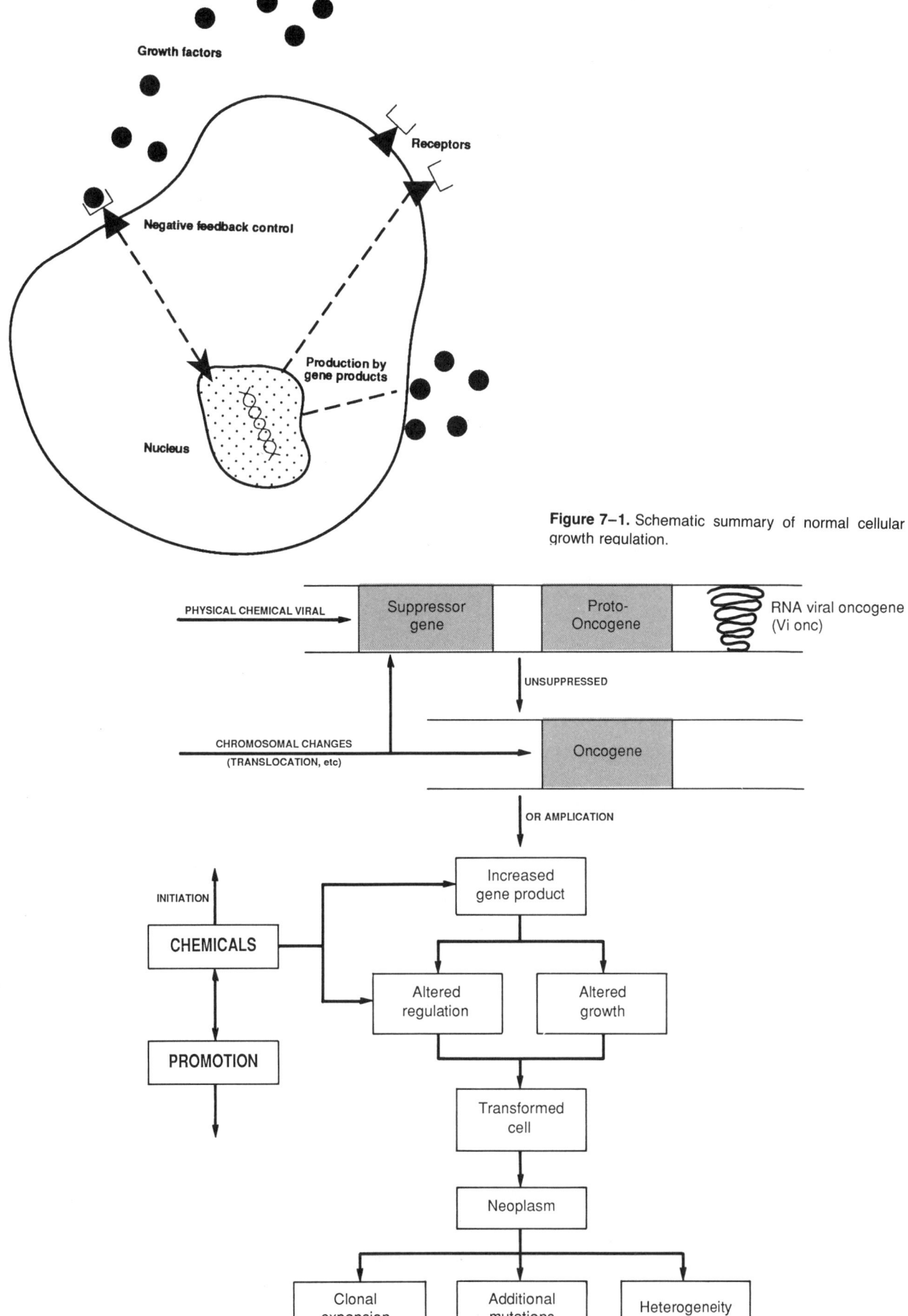

Figure 7-1. Schematic summary of normal cellular growth regulation.

Figure 7-2. Carcinogenesis is a unifying concept.

TABLE 7-6. EXAMPLES OF POTENTIAL MECHANISMS OF ONCOGENE EXPRESSION

Genetic Alteration	Oncogene Activity	Associated Tumors
Mutation	Recombinant oncogenes	B cell lymphomas
	Insertional activation	Colon carcinoma (K-ras, C-src)
		Myelodysplasic syndromes (K-ras)
Amplification	Increase expression of oncogenes	Neuroblastoma (N-myc)
		Small cell carcinoma of lung (C-myc)
		Breast carcinoma (C-erb)
Decrease	Suppressor genes (anti-oncogenes)	
Deletion	Suppressor genes (anti-oncogenes)	

TABLE 7-7. EXAMPLES OF HUMAN CANCER IN WHICH SUPPRESSOR GENES (ANTI-ONCOGENES) HAVE BEEN RELATED TO PROGNOSIS

- Neuroblastoma
- Renal cell carcinoma
- Colon carcinoma
- Gliomas
- Wilms' tumor
- Bladder carcinoma
- Breast carcinoma
- Retinoblastoma
- Small cell carcinoma of lung
- Osteogenic sarcoma
- Meningioma

TABLE 7-8. CLASSIFICATION OF TUMORS

Tissue or Cell of Origin	Benign	Malignant
Epithelial		
Ectodermal		
Endodermal		
Squamous	Squamous papilloma	Squamous cell carcinoma (epidermoid carcinoma)
Transitional	Transitional cell papilloma	Transitional cell carcinoma
Glandular	Adenoma	Adenocarcinoma (columnar cell mucous secretion, etc.)
	Adenomatous polyp	
	Cystadenoma	
Basal cell	Basal cell papilloma	Basal cell carcinoma (locally malignant)
Melanocyte[a]	Nevus	Malignant melanoma
	Junctional	
	Compound	
	Intradermal	
Connective Tissue		
** Mesodermal**		
Fibrous tissue	Fibroma	Fibrosarcoma
	Dermatofibroma	Dermatofibrosarcoma
	Myxofibroma	Myxofibrosarcoma
Nerve sheath	Neurofibroma	Neurofibrosarcoma
Adipose tissue	Lipoma	Liposarcoma
Smooth muscle	Leiomyoma	Leiomyosarcoma
Skeletal muscle	Rhabdomyoma	Rhabdomyosarcoma
Cartilage	Chondroma	Chondrosarcoma
Bone	Osteoma	Osteogenic sarcoma
Blood vessel	Hemangioma	Hemagiosarcoma

(continued)

TABLE 7–8. CLASSIFICATION OF TUMORS (continued)

Tissue or Cell of Origin	Benign	Malignant
Embryonic cells		
Retinoblasts		Retinoblastoma
Neuroblasts (ganglion)		Neuroblastoma
Kidney		Nephroblastoma (Wilms' tumor)
Liver		Hepatoblastoma
Pancreas		Pancreatic blastoma
Notochord		Chordoma
Enamel organ		Ameloblastoma (adamantinoma)
Rathke's pouch		Craniopharyngioma
Medulloblast (cerebellum)		Medulloblastoma
Mixed Cell Type	Benign teratoma	Malignant teratoma
Miscellaneous		
Kidney	Renal cell adenoma	Renal cell carcinoma (hypernephroma)
Liver parenchyma		Hepatocellular carcinoma (hepatoma)
Placenta (trophoblasts)	Hydatidiform mole	Choriocarcinoma
Lymphatics	Lymphangioma	Lymphangiosarcoma
Mesothelium	Mesothelioma (benign) (?)	Malignant mesothelioma (Wilms' tumor)
Hematopoietic and Reticuloendothelial		
Lymphatic tissue	Lymphoma (?)	Malignant lymphoma
Lymphocytes		Lymphatic leukemia
Granulocytes		Myeloid leukemia
Monocytes		Monocytic leukemia
Platelets		Megarkaryocytic leukemia
Plasma cells	Plasmacytoma	Multiple myeloma
Red cell precursors	Some forms of polycythemia rubro vera	Erythroderma (DiGuglielmo's disease)
Nervous System		
Glial cells (astrocytes)		Glioblastoma multiforme
Ependymal cells		Ependymoma
Meduloblasts		Medulloblastoma
Choroid plexus		Papilloma of choroid plexus
Pineal gland		Pinealoma
Schwann cells		Schwannoma (neuroadenoma)
Testis		Seminoma
		Teratoma
Ovary		Dysgerminoma
	Granulosa/thecoma	
	Serous cystadenoma	Serous cystadenocarcinoma
	Mucinous cystadenoma	Mucinous cystadenocarcinoma
		Papillary cystadenocarcinoma
		Solid undifferentiated carcinoma
	Brenner tumor	
		Arrhenoblastoma
		Endodermal sinus tumor
	Benign cystic teratoma	Solid malignant teratoma (choriocarcinoma)

^aOften considered under a separate heading. Since the melanocyte is derived from neural crest and resides in an epithelial location, it is included in this classification as part of epithelial tumors.

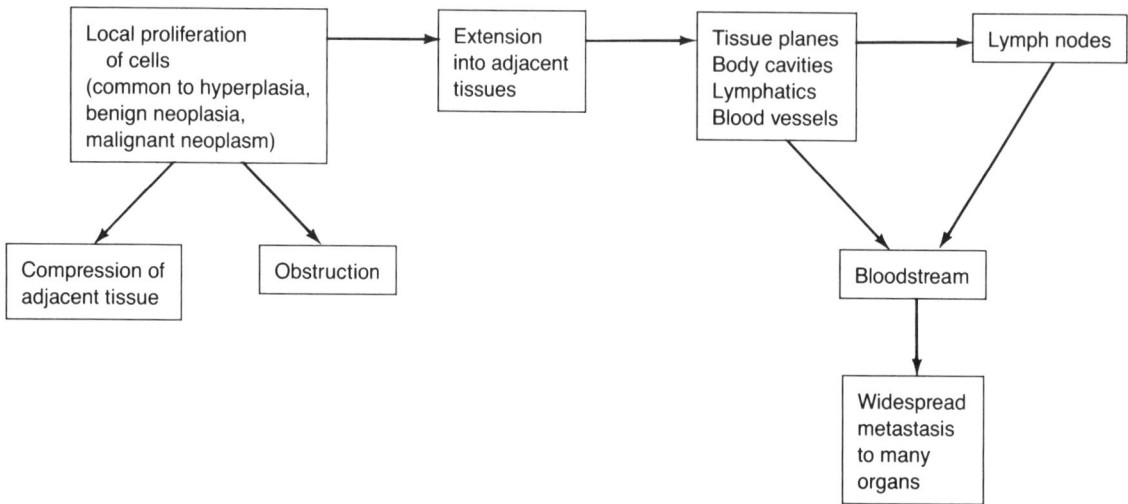

Figure 7–1. Sequential pathways in tumor growth or spread.

TABLE 7–9. IMPORTANT MODES OF TUMOR SPREAD WITH COMMON EXAMPLES

Mode of Spread	Example
Local spread or invasion	Most common malignant tumors Basal cell carcinoma almost exclusively
Coelomic cavities	Many types of primary epthelial tumors, such as carcinoma of stomach, ovary, and lung Many secondary (metastatic) tumors, such as carcinoma of breast
Cerebrospinal fluid	Primary brain tumors involve the meninges Metastatic carcinomas and malignant melanoma
Lymphatic spread to lymph nodes	Particular epithelial tumors (carcinomas), very occasional mesodermal tumors (sarcomas)
Bloodstream spread	Particularly mesodermal tumors—sarcomas and, in later stages of spread, carcinomas

TABLE 7–10. SOME EXAMPLES OF TUMOR PRODUCTS AND MARKERS OF IDENTIFICATION

Carcinoembryonic antigen (CEA)	Carcinomas and breast, colon, stomach, pancreas, and lung
Alphafetoprotein (AFP)	Hepatocellular carcinoma, some germ cell neoplasms
Human chorionic gonadotrophin (HCG)	Trophoblastic tumors and some germ cell tumors
Prostatic specific antigen (PSA)	Prostatic carcinoma
Prostatic acid phosphatase	Prostatic carcinoma
Catecholamines	Pheochromocytoma or neuroblastoma
Calcitonin	Medullar carcinoma (C-cell) of thyroid
Serotonin on 5HIAA	Carcinoid tumors
Neurone specific Enolase	Small cell carcinoma of lung neuroblastoma
Glycoprotein complex	
CA-125	Ovarian carcinoma
CA 19-9	Colonic and pancreatic carcinoma
CA 15-3	Breast carcinoma

TABLE 7-11. EXPRESSION OF IMMUNOLOGICAL REACTION IN PATIENTS WITH CANCER

Immune surveillance and spontaneous regression

Lymphocytic/monocyte and plasma cell influence in early cancer

Antitumor antibodies   < against live tumor cells
                              < against tumor products

Immune complexes contact tumor antigens   <serum tissue

In-vitro cell mediator immune reaction < Cytotoxic B and T cells
                                          T-cell - surveillance
                                          NKCL - NK cells
                                                  - macrophages

Response to various forms of immunotherapy (*often limited*)

TABLE 7-13. RELATIVE INCIDENCE OF SELECTED CANCERS IN THE UNITED STATES

Rank	Male	Female
1.	Prostate	Breast
2.	Lung	Colon/Rectum
3.	Colon/Rectum	Lung
4.	Urinary	Uterus
5.	Leukemia/Lymphoma	Leukemia/Lymphoma
6.	Oral	Ovary
7.	Skin (excluding melanoma)	Skin (excluding melanoma)
8.	Pancreas	Pancreas

TABLE 7-12. EXAMPLES OF MAJOR EFFECTS OF TUMORS

Obstruction or compression	Hyperplasia of prostate with urinary obstruction Benign neoplasia of bronchus, bowel, or base of brain Malignant tumors of bronchus, bowel, etc.
Ulceration	Skin tumors, benign or malignant, especially basal cell rodent ulcer, carcinoma of stomach, colon carcinoma
Infection	Any tumor of skin with surface ulceration or tumor of bronchial tree of gastrointestinal tract or bladder Lymphomas and leukemias in which immune suppression may occur
Anemia	Effect of blood loss from ulcerated tumor, effects of bone marrow replacement by tumor cells Unknown mechanisms
Cachexia	Extremely variable and complex, seen in a variety of metastatic tumors or obstructive tumors, such as esophageal carcinoma
Effects of products of tumors	Hormones: thyroid, adrenal, catecholamine, protein by appropriate neoplasms of these tissues Inappropriate hormone production, ie, antidiuretic hormone by bronchogenic carcinoma

TABLE 7–14. AGE-ADJUSTED CANCER DEATH RATES IN 50 COUNTRIES

	Highest Ranks		Lowest Ranks		USA (Rank)	
	Male	*Female*	*Male*	*Female*	*Male*	*Female*
All cancers	Hungary Czechoslovakia Belgium	Denmark Scotland Hungary	Peru (50th)	Peru (50th)	26th	20th
Lung	Scotland Belgium Holland	Scotland HongKong United States	Peru (50th)	Peru (50th)	12th	3rd
Colon/Rectum	Czechoslovakia Denmark Austria	New Zealand Denmark Hungary	Peru (50th)	Peru (50th)	22nd	20th
Prostate	Martinique Switzerland Norway		HongKong (50th)		23rd	
Breast		England Malta Denmark		Peru (50th)		16th
Leukemia	Luxenburg Iceland Hungary	Kuwait Luxenburg Denmark	Surinam (50th)	Surinam (50th)	6th	11th
Stomach	Costa Rica Japan Former Soviet Union	Former Soviet Union Costa Rica Ecuador	United States (50th)	United States (50th)	50th	50th

Questions

DIRECTIONS (Questions 1 through 50): Each of the numbered items or incomplete statements in this section is followed by answers or by completions of the statement. Select the ONE lettered answer or completion that is BEST in each case.

1. Which of the following is NOT a neoplasm of epithelial origin?

    (A) carcinoma of the esophagus
    (B) carcinoma of the stomach
    (C) rhabdomyosarcoma
    (D) basal cell carcinoma
    (E) laryngeal papilloma

2. A biopsy of the liver shows tumor nodules composed of mucus-secreting adenocarcinoma. The most likely site of origin outside the liver is

    (A) cerebellum
    (B) prostate
    (C) bladder
    (D) colon
    (E) anal canal

3. Which of the following characteristics is NOT typical of a sarcoma?

    (A) pleomorphism
    (B) blood vessel invasion
    (C) lymphatic invasion
    (D) mesodermal origin
    (E) metastases to distant sites

4. The process described as angioneogenesis is

    (A) invasion of blood vessels by tumor cells
    (B) blood-borne spread of tumor cells
    (C) a tumor arising from primitive blood-forming tissue
    (D) the ingrowth of new blood vessels into a growing tumor
    (E) the central necrosis seen in rapidly growing tumors due to outgrowing of the blood supply

5. Which of the following tumors is LEAST associated with hormone dependence?

    (A) carcinoma of the prostate
    (B) carcinoma of the breast in females
    (C) carcinoma of the thyroid
    (D) carcinoma of the colon
    (E) carcinoma of the endometrium

6. A keloid is

    (A) a protruding tumorlike scar
    (B) the outcome of most infected wounds
    (C) a form of early granulation tissue
    (D) a benign tumor of melanocytic origin
    (E) a granuloma in response to mycobacteria

7. A tumor composed of tissues representing all three embryologic germ layers is called

    (A) adenocarcinoma
    (B) carcinosarcoma
    (C) mixed mesodermal tumor
    (D) teratoma
    (E) papillary adenocarcinoma

8. A biopsy shows what appears to be an abnormal amount and arrangement of normal tissue that is appropriate or normal for the area in which the tissue arises. This is best described as

    (A) teratoma
    (B) mixed tumor
    (C) hamartoma
    (D) embryonal tumor
    (E) carcinosarcoma

9. Which of the following best describes the phenomenon of epithelial dysplasia?

    (A) an increase in thickness of the epithelium because of increased number of cells
    (B) a decrease in thickness of the epithelium owing to decrease in number of dividing cells
    (C) an irregular proliferation and maturation of cells throughout the layers of the epithelium
    (D) an increase in thickness of the epithelium owing to enlargement of the component cells
    (E) absence of epithelium because of lack of cell proliferation

10. Which of the following is the LEAST correct statement?

    (A) the incidence of malignancy tends to increase with age
    (B) carcinoma of the breast is more frequent in males than in females
    (C) hormones may inhibit or promote tumor growth
    (D) certain tumors characteristically appear in certain age groups
    (E) carcinoma of the breast is more frequent in females than in males

11. Which of the following is NOT a neoplasm of mesenchymal origin?

    (A) papilloma
    (B) hemangioma
    (C) lipoma
    (D) rhabdomyoma
    (E) leiomyoma

12. The pathologic condition in which one type of adult tissue is replaced by another is termed

    (A) dysplasia
    (B) anaplasia
    (C) metaplasia
    (D) aplasia
    (E) hypoplasia

13. The single most important feature of malignancy is

    (A) cellular pleomorphism
    (B) numerous mitotic figures
    (C) metastases
    (D) lymphocytic infiltration at the edges of the tumor
    (E) plasma cell infiltration at the edges of the tumor

14. Decrease in size of a previously normal-sized and normally developed organ is called

    (A) aplasia
    (B) hypoplasia
    (C) atrophy
    (D) metaplasia
    (E) agenesis

15. A tumor composed of columnar epithelium arranged in glandular configuration with nests of cells invading into adjacent normal tissue is best described as

    (A) adenomatous polyp
    (B) adenomatous hyperplasia
    (C) adenomyosis
    (D) adenocarcinoma
    (E) carcinosarcoma

16. Multiple nodules are discovered in the gastric mucosa and small intestinal mucosa. The cells composing the nodules are pleomorphic and contain fine granules of brownish pigment. The most likely source of this tumor is

    (A) gastric carcinoma
    (B) small intestinal adenocarcinoma
    (C) hepatocellular carcinoma
    (D) malignant melanoma
    (E) adrenal cell carcinoma

17. The most common cause of death from cancer in women in the United States is

    (A) carcinoma of the urinary bladder
    (B) carcinoma of the liver
    (C) carcinoma of the cervix of uterus
    (D) carcinoma of the breast
    (E) carcinoma of the ovary

18. The most common form of cancer seen in most black African countries is

    (A) carcinoma of the colon
    (B) carcinoma of the cervix and uterus
    (C) carcinoma of the breast
    (D) carcinoma of the lung
    (E) carcinoma of the pancreas

19. Which of the following tumors has been associated most strongly with a possible viral etiology?

    (A) leiomyoma of the uterus
    (B) carcinoma of the lung
    (C) carcinoma of the esophagus
    (D) Burkitt's lymphoma
    (E) histiocytic lymphoma

20. Which of the following tumors has been most clearly associated with production of carcinoembryonic antigen (CEA)?

    (A) carcinoma of the esophagus
    (B) malignant lymphoma
    (C) carcinoma of the colon
    (D) testicular seminoma
    (E) testicular teratoma

21. Which of the following characteristics is NOT typical of benign neoplasms?

    (A) encapsulation
    (B) low mitotic index
    (C) blood vessel invasion
    (D) slow growth
    (E) well differentiated

22. An increase in tissue associated with an increase in the number of cells composing the tissue is best described as

    (A) aplasia
    (B) agenesis
    (C) hypertrophy
    (D) hyperplasia
    (E) metaplasia

23. The etiology of bronchogenic carcinoma is most clearly associated with

    (A) genetic abnormalities in patients
    (B) familial tendency
    (C) cigarette smoking
    (D) respiratory viruses
    (E) emphysema

24. Workers in the aniline dye industry are most prone to which of the following tumors?

    (A) carcinoma of the lung
    (B) carcinoma of the stomach
    (C) squamous cell carcinoma of the skin
    (D) basal cell carcinoma of the skin
    (E) carcinoma of the urinary bladder

25. Exposure to sunlight is most closely associated with

    (A) carcinoma of the lung
    (B) basal cell carcinoma of the skin in blacks
    (C) squamous cell carcinoma of the skin in blacks
    (D) malignant melanoma of the skin in whites
    (E) intraocular malignant melanoma in blacks

26. Which term is most likely to fit the description of the uterus during pregnancy?

    (A) hyperplasia
    (B) hypertrophy
    (C) aplasia
    (D) agenesis
    (E) dysplasia

27. Which of the following best describes postmenopausal small uterus?

    (A) hyperplasia
    (B) hypertrophy
    (C) aplasia
    (D) agenesis
    (E) atrophy

28. Which term most closely describes lack of development in a lobe of the lung in a newborn infant?

    (A) hyperplasia
    (B) hypertrophy
    (C) aplasia
    (D) agenesis
    (E) atrophy

29. A localized thickness of the buccal mucosa resulting from an increase in the number of epithelial cells is

    (A) hyperplasia
    (B) hypertrophy
    (C) aplasia
    (D) agenesis
    (E) dysplasia

30. Which of the following tumors is most associated with ingestion of aflatoxins?

    (A) carcinoma of the cervix
    (B) carcinoma of the endometrium
    (C) carcinoma of the urinary bladder
    (D) hepatocellular carcinoma (hepatoma)
    (E) carcinoma of the stomach

31. Which of the following is most associated with industrial exposure to naphthalenes and related products?

    (A) carcinoma of the cervix
    (B) carcinoma of the stomach
    (C) carcinoma of the endometrium
    (D) carcinoma of the urinary bladder
    (E) hepatocellular carcinoma (hepatoma)

Questions 32 through 35. Refer to Figures 7–4 and 7–5.

32. The gross appearance (Fig 7–4) is best described as

    (A) an ulcer
    (B) an adenoma
    (C) an inflamed polyp
    (D) a papilloma
    (E) a sarcoma

33. The high-power view (Fig 7–5) enables the epithelium to be recognized as

    (A) columnar epithelium
    (B) stratified squamous epithelium
    (C) transitional cell epithelium
    (D) mesothelium
    (E) smooth muscle

34. On the basis of the appearance, the lesion is best classified as

    (A) sweat gland adenoma
    (B) transitional cell carcinoma
    (C) squamous papilloma
    (D) squamous cell carcinoma (poorly differentiated)
    (E) leiomyosarcoma

132   7: Neoplasia and Abnormalities of Growth

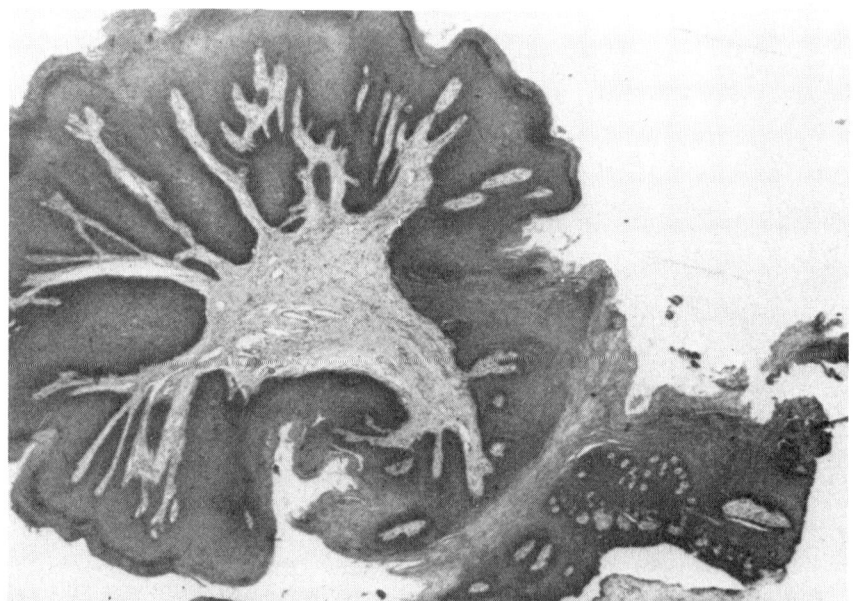

Figure 7–4. Low-power photomicrograph of a skin lesion removed from the shoulder of a 40-year-old white male.

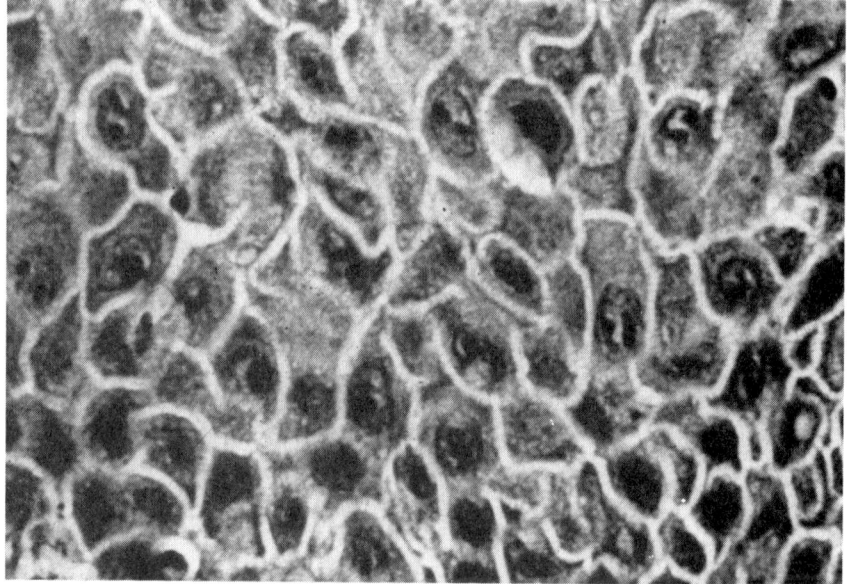

Figure 7–5. High-power photomicrograph of a section taken from the lesion depicted in Figure 7–4.

35. After complete excision of the lesion, the most likely sequela would be

(A) metastatic spread to regional lymph nodes
(B) metastatic spread to lungs via the bloodstream
(C) recurrence of the lesion locally
(D) none of the above
(E) all of the above

Questions 36 through 38. Refer to Figure 7–6.

36. The photomicrograph demonstrates

(A) malignant spindle cells
(B) malignant epithelial cells
(C) ferruginous (asbestos) bodies
(D) acid-fast bacilli
(E) Curschmann's spirals

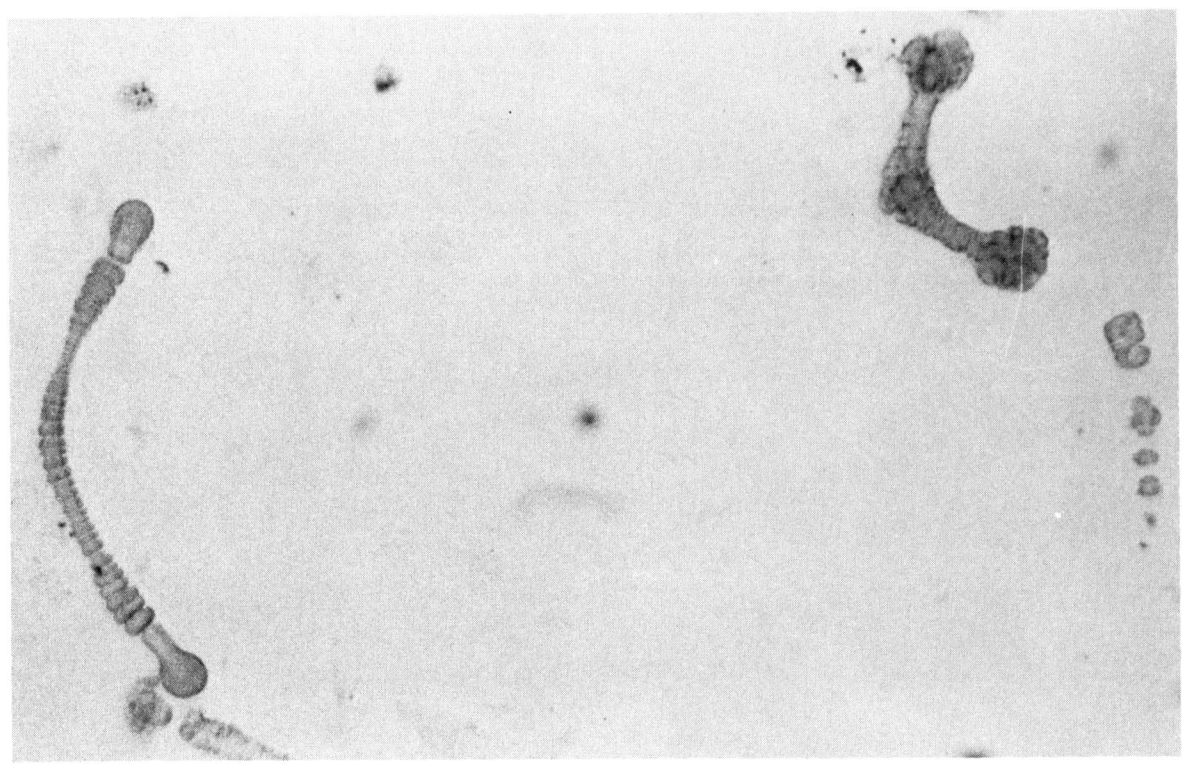

Figure 7-6. A 60-year-old male has dyspnea and bilateral pulmonary infiltrates. Sputum examination shows features seen in the photomicrograph.

37. Additional history useful in assessing this patient includes

    (A) excessive smoking
    (B) asthma
    (C) exposure to tuberculosis
    (D) occupation
    (E) none of the above

38. The patient also is more likely to have or develop

    (A) mesothelioma of pleura
    (B) history of other allergies
    (C) metastatic tumor deposits in lymphatics of the lung
    (D) tuberculous pneumonia
    (E) status asthmaticus

Questions 39 and 40. Refer to Figure 7-7.

39. The photomicrograph shows

    (A) normal cervical squamous epithelium
    (B) transitional epithelium
    (C) chronic cervicitis
    (D) squamous carcinoma in situ (intraepithelial carcinoma)
    (E) invasive squamous carcinoma

40. The chance that this patient has metastatic carcinoma in the inguinal lymph nodes is

    (A) 0%
    (B) 10%
    (C) 30%
    (D) 50%
    (E) 100%

Questions 41 and 42. Refer to Figure 7-8.

41. The photomicrograph demonstrates

    (A) normal squamous epithelium to the right and squamous epithelium showing dysplasia to the left
    (B) normal squamous epithelium to the left and squamous epithelium showing dysplasia to the right
    (C) variants of cervical squamous epithelium
    (D) normal squamous epithelium to the left and metaplastic epithelium to the right
    (E) squamous metaplasia of epithelium at left and malignant squamous epithelium at right

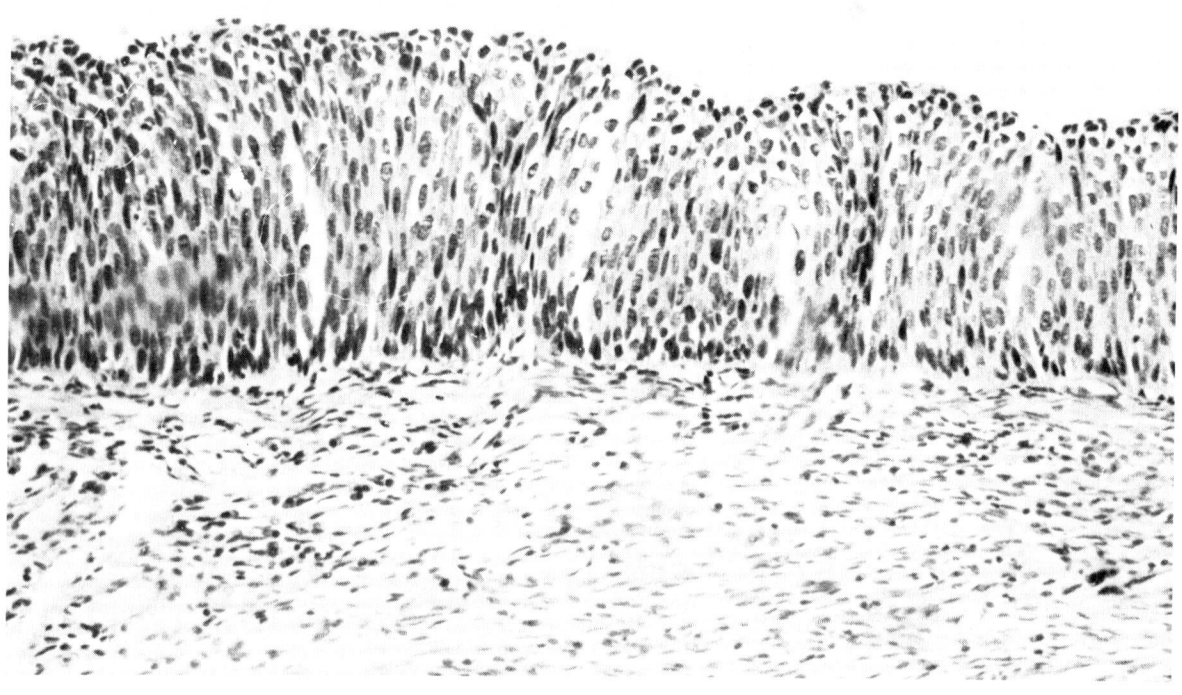

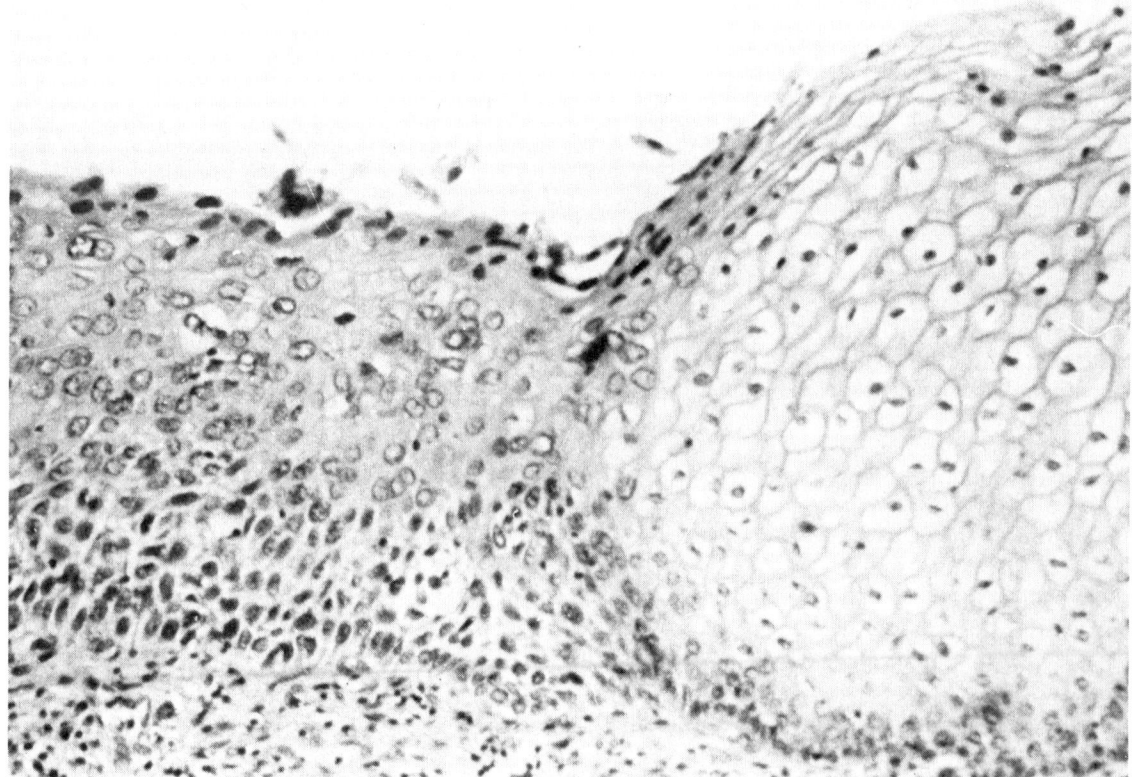

Figure 7–8. Photomicrograph of a section taken from a biopsy of the cervix performed after a Papanicolaou smear that contained abnormal cells.

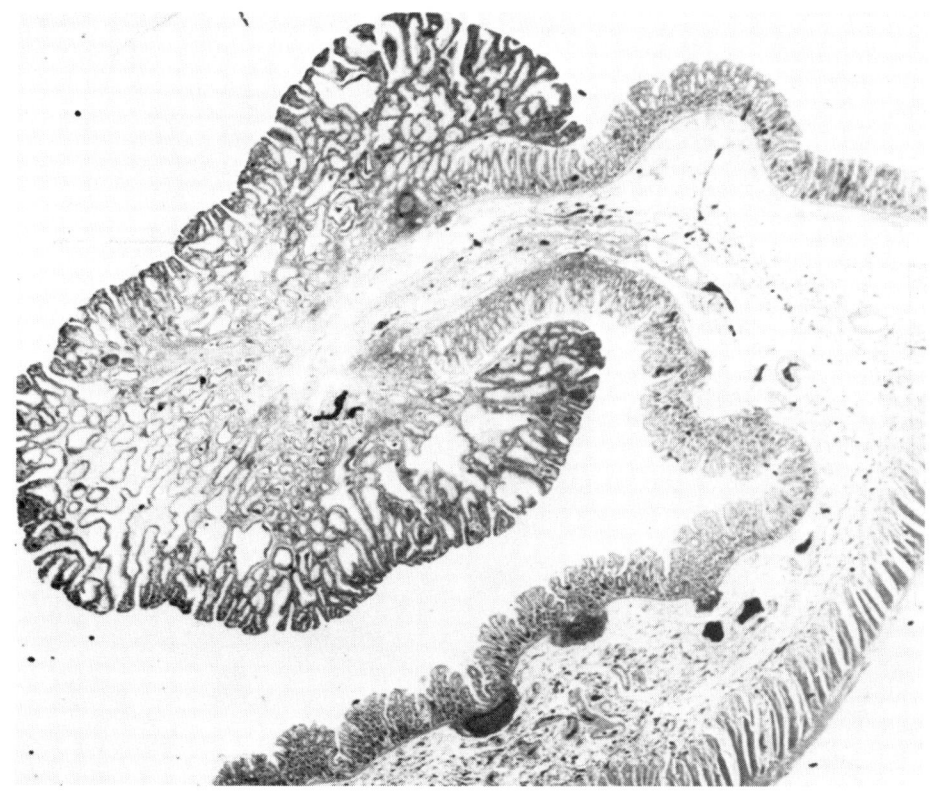

Figure 7-9. Low-power photomicrograph of a segment of large intestine.

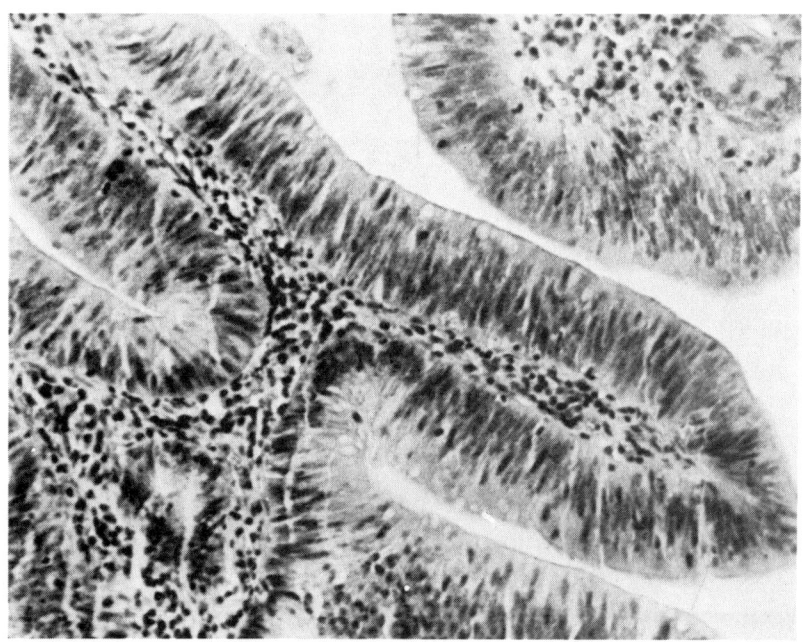

Figure 7-10. High-power view of the lesion shown in Figure 7-9.

42. The lesion depicted may

    (A) regress
    (B) remain unchanged
    (C) develop into carcinoma
    (D) all of the above
    (E) none of the above

Questions 43 through 46. Refer to Figures 7–9 and 7–10.

43. The low-power appearance (Fig 7–9) is best described as

    (A) diverticulum
    (B) pseudopolyposis
    (C) sessile polyp
    (D) pedunculated polyp
    (E) annular constriction

44. The high-power appearance (Fig 7–10) is best described as

    (A) well-differentiated adenocarcinoma
    (B) poorly differentiated adenocarcinoma
    (C) inflammatory polyp
    (D) adenomatous polyp
    (E) metaplasia

45. The ultimate outcome of the lesion is

    (A) metastasis via the lymphatics
    (B) blood-borne tumor spread to the liver
    (C) both of the above
    (D) neither of the above
    (E) no further growth after removal

46. The best assessment of prognosis based on these findings alone is

    (A) poor
    (B) moderate
    (C) excellent
    (D) impossible to determine
    (E) dependent on patient's age

Questions 47 through 50. Refer to Figure 7–11.

47. The lesion is most likely

    (A) inflammatory
    (B) ischemic
    (C) infectious
    (D) neoplastic
    (E) immunologic

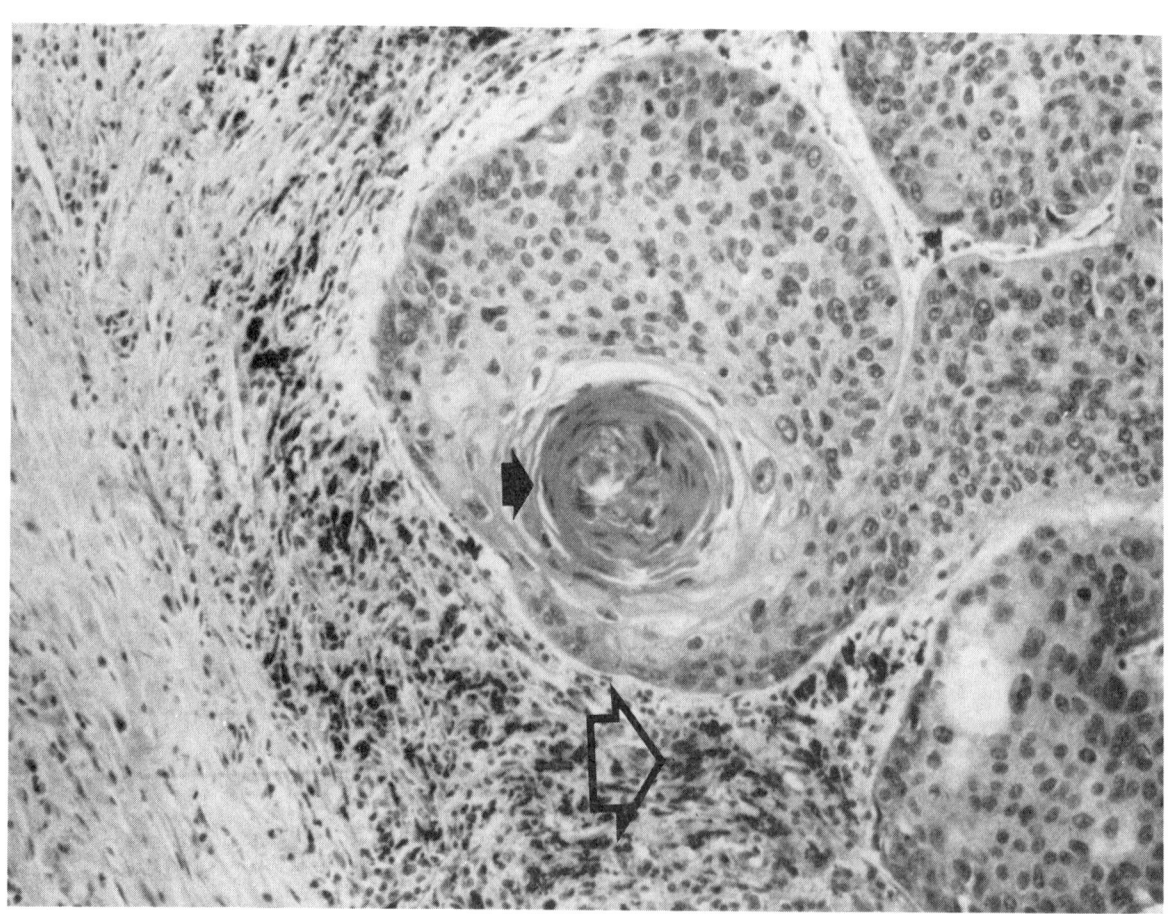

Figure 7–11. Histologic section of a lesion removed from a 60-year-old male.

48. The lesion is most likely

    (A) tuberculous pneumonia
    (B) healing pulmonary infarction
    (C) Wegener's granulomatosis
    (D) bronchogenic carcinoma
    (E) centrilobular emphysema

49. The small solid arrow points to

    (A) a Langhans' giant cell
    (B) coagulated bronchial epithelium
    (C) fibrinoid necrosis of a pulmonary artery
    (D) a squamous pearl
    (E) a psammoma body, or calcospherite

50. The large open arrow points to

    (A) degenerating elastic fibers
    (B) epithelioid cells
    (C) polymorphonuclear leukocytes
    (D) anthrocotic pigment
    (E) pores of Kohn

DIRECTIONS (Questions 51 through 110): Each group of items in this section consists of lettered headings followed by a set of numbered words or phrases. For each numbered word or phrase, select the ONE lettered heading that is most closely associated with it. Each lettered heading may be selected once, more than once, or not at all.

Questions 51 through 53

    (A) malignant neoplasm
    (B) benign neoplasm
    (C) hyperplasia
    (D) aplasia
    (E) teratoma

51. Adenoma B

52. Lack of red cell precursors in bone marrow D

53. Liposarcoma A

Questions 54 and 55

    (A) carcinoma
    (B) sarcoma
    (C) adenoma
    (D) papilloma
    (E) teratoma

54. A benign tumor of epithelial origin attached to the normal epithelium by a stalk D

55. A malignant tumor of mesodermal origin B

Questions 56 through 61

    (A) a tumor that predominantly metastasizes via the bloodstream
    (B) a lymph node filled with tumor composed of abnormal epidermoid cells
    (C) a Krukenberg tumor
    (D) a tumor that produces alpha-fetoprotein (AFP)
    (E) cells that produce human chorionic gonadotropin (HCG)

56. Choriocarcinoma E

57. Secondary carcinoma of the stomach in ovaries C

58. Hepatocellular carcinoma D

59. Osteogenic sarcoma A

60. Bronchogenic carcinoma B

61. Fibrosarcoma A

Questions 62 through 64

    (A) neuroblastoma
    (B) malignant fibrous histiocytoma
    (C) bronchogenic carcinoma
    (D) squamous cell carcinoma
    (E) adenocarcinoma

62. Cells of origin thought to be derived from fetal neural crest A

63. More common in childhood than in adult life A

64. The adrenal is the most common site A

Questions 65 and 66

    (A) stage I
    (B) stage II
    (C) stage III
    (D) stage IV
    (E) insufficient data to stage completely

65. Breast carcinoma, T1, N0, M0 A

66. Colon carcinoma, T3, N2, M1 D

Questions 67 and 68

    (A) papillary thyroid carcinoma
    (B) mammary fibroadenoma
    (C) pleural mesothelioma
    (D) gastric adenocarcinoma
    (E) liver cell carcinoma

67. A tumor associated with asbestos exposure in a non-smoker C

68. A tumor associated with hepatitis B virus carrier state E

Questions 69 through 72

(A) hyperplasia (hypertrophy)
(B) dysplasia
(C) atrophy
(D) aplasia
(E) metaplasia

69. Increase in the thickness of the cardiac left ventricle with essential hypertension   A ?

70. Cellular change seen with cervical intracellular neoplasia (CIN), grade II   B

71. Congenital absence of a pulmonary lobe or segment   D ?

72. Squamous epithelium found in the bronchial mucosal of a smoker   E

Questions 73 and 74

(A) prostate specific antigen
(B) calcitonin
(C) catecholamines
(D) CA 19-9
(E) CA 15-3

73. Most likely product of a medullary carcinoma of thyroid   B

74. Most likely product of a pheochromocytoma   C

Questions 75 through 78

(A) lipoma
(B) osteogenic sarcoma
(C) rhabdomyosarcoma
(D) renal cell carcinoma
(E) liposarcoma

75. Malignant tumor of adipocytes   E

76. Benign tumor of adipocytes   A

77. Production of osteoid by malignant cells   B

78. Myosin may be detected with monoclonal antibodies   C

Questions 79 through 82

(A) adenoma
(B) adenocarcinoma
(C) chondroma
(D) chondrosarcoma
(E) leiomyoma

79. Benign neoplasm of smooth muscle cells   E

80. Malignant neoplasm arising from glandular cells   B

81. Benign neoplasm arising from glandular cells   A

82. Benign neoplasm arising from cartilage cells   C

Questions 83 through 86

(A) gastric adenocarcinoma
(B) cervical squamous cell carcinoma
(C) colonic adenocarcinoma
(D) cutaneous basal cell carcinoma
(E) appendiceal adenocarcinoma

83. More frequently seen in Western populations with high-fat, low-fiber diets   C

84. More frequently seen in African women   B

85. More frequently seen in whites who have extensive actinic dermatitis   D

86. More frequently seen in Japanese and Russian populations   A

Questions 87 through 90

(A) Epstein-Barr virus
(B) hepatitis B virus
(C) mumps virus
(D) human immunodeficiency virus
(E) human papilloma virus

87. Carcinoma of the cervix   E

88. Hepatocellular carcinoma   B

89. Burkitt's lymphoma   A

90. Kaposi's sarcoma   D

Questions 91 through 94

(A) undescended testicle
(B) tuberous sclerosis
(C) ulcerative colitis
(D) Paget's disease of the bone
(E) xeroderma pigmentosum

91. Increased incidence of cutaneous neoplasms   E

92. Increased incidence of colonic adenocarcinoma   C

93. Increased incidence of seminoma   A

94. Increased incidence of osteosarcoma   D

Questions 95 through 98

(A) hepatic angiosarcoma
(B) liver cell carcinoma
(C) vaginal adenosis
(D) mammary phylloides tumor
(E) oral carcinoma

95. Ingestion of aflatoxins B

96. Chewing betel nuts and leaves E

97. Maternal antepartum administration of diethylstilbesterol C

98. Vinyl chloride exposure A

Questions 99 through 102

  (A) neuron stimulating factor
  (B) monoclonal immunoglobulin
  (C) corticosteroids
  (D) prostate-specific antigen
  (E) erythropoietin

99. Renal cell carcinoma E

100. Prostatic adenocarcinoma D

101. Multiple myeloma B

102. Adrenal cortical adenoma C

Questions 103 through 106

  (A) malignant melanoma
  (B) malignant mesothelioma
  (C) adenocarcinoma
  (D) squamous cell carcinoma
  (E) transitional cell carcinoma
  (F) lymphoblastic leukemia
  (G) Hodgkin's disease
  (H) fibrosarcoma

103. A 62-year-old man who has been smoking two packs of cigarettes a day for the past 35 years is found to have a 2.5 cm solitary nodule in the left upper lobe of his lung. A fine needle aspiration biopsy reveals abundant malignant cells with intercellular bridges, intracellular keratin production, and keratin pearl formation. No glandular structures are evident. What is the most likely diagnosis? D

104. A 32-year-old woman is seen by her family physician because of an enlarging pigmented skin lesion on her back that now measures about 2 × 1.5 cm. It is variegated by hues of brown, black, and pink. The central portion of the lesion is raised and beginning to ulcerate. A biopsy shows nests of atypical melanocytes scattered up through the epidermis and invading down into the dermis. What is the most likely diagnosis? A

105. A 6-year-old child with Down's syndrome is noted to have recent onset of bleeding gums and pallor. At the doctor's office the child's white blood cell count is found to be markedly elevated due to a monomorphic population of immature lymphoid cells. A bone marrow biopsy reveals almost complete replacement of the medullary space by similar appearing blast cells. What is the most likely diagnosis? F

106. A 67-year-old postmenopausal woman has been feeling excessively tired for about 2 months. Her lab work is remarkable for a microcytic anemia and an elevated CEA. A barium enema x-ray study reveals an "applecore" mass lesion in the right colon. A biopsy of this area demonstrates malignant gland-forming epithelial cells. What is the most likely diagnosis? C

Questions 107 through 110

  (A) adenocarcinoma
  (B) lymphoma
  (C) adenoma
  (D) hemangioma
  (E) transitional cell carcinoma
  (F) insulinoma
  (G) malignant astrocytoma
  (H) chronic myelogeneous leukemia

107. A 45-year-old male has had a slowly growing reddish nodule on his forearm for about 2 years. He finally decides to have a surgeon remove it. Microscopically the nodule is composed of benign varying sized blood vessels. What is the most likely diagnosis? D

108. A 51-year-old female is found to have an elevated white blood cell count on her annual physical. The elevated count is due to an increased number of myelocytes, metamyelocytes, and band neutrophils. A chromosomal analysis of these myeloid cells reveals the presence of a Philadelphia chromosome. What is the most likely diagnosis? H

109. A retired rubber worker notices that his urine is occasionally brownish or reddish in color. At the doctor's office this tinctorial abnormality is found to be hematuria. His bladder is examined via cystoscopy and a biopsy of a large ulcerating tumor is obtained. The lesion is composed of malignant transitional cells. What is the most likely diagnosis? E

110. A 41-year-old woman has a seizure while at work and is taken to the hospital. On examination she denies ever having had seizures before. A CAT scan of the brain demonstrates a large poorly circumscribed, focally necrotic tumor in the frontal and parietal lobes. A biopsy of this area contains malignant astrocytes. What is the most likely diagnosis? G

Answers and Explanations

1. **(C)** This is a question of terminology (Table 7–8). The terms "carcinoma" and "papilloma" are used to denote neoplasms that are of epithelial origin. Rhabdomyosarcoma is a tumor as designated by *sarcoma* (of mesodermal origin) and the prefix *rhabdo* (of striated muscle origin). *(1:270–274)*

2. **(D)** This is a practical problem often faced by pathologists and clinicians when patients have symptoms of metastasis before the primary site is discovered. All primary tumors, with the exception of those of the cerebellum, can produce metastasis to the liver, but the colon is by far the most common site and often produces a mucus-secreting adenocarcinoma arising from the glandular epithelium. *(2:900–902)*

3. **(C)** Although sarcomas may occasionally spread via the lymphatic invasion route, with very few exceptions they tend either to remain locally invasive or to spread by the bloodstream. This probably is related to the fact that they are of mesodermal original (Tables 7–8 and 7–9) and often have large vascular spaces that readily connect with the vasculature of normal surrounding tissues, hence, their ability to spread more rapidly by that route. Pleomorphism or a variation in size and shape and appearance of the nuclei and the cell in general is relatively characteristic of these neoplasms. *(4:197; 5:151–153)*

4. **(D)** As the name implies, angioneogenesis is the formation of new blood vessels. It has been shown that these often are of host origin, growing into the tumor and stimulated by the release from the tumor of substances designated angiogenesis factors. *(1:305)*

5. **(D)** There is little direct evidence to suggest that colonic carcinoma is directly under hormonal influence. All of the others may be altered by treatment or manipulation, such as ablation of estrogen-producing tissues in carcinoma of the breast or castration and administration of estrogen in carcinoma of the prostate. In the thyroid, the cancer actually may produce thyroid hormone and be destroyed by uptake of radiolabeled iodine by the functioning tumor cells. Not all of the cancer cells in prostate, breast, or thyroid, however, are hormone dependent. This depends on the presence of estrogen or progesterone receptors in breast cancer, the production of hormone receptors in prostate cancer, and the actual production of a functioning hormone in carcinoma of the thyroid. *(1:291–292)*

6. **(A)** Keloid is an overexuberant production of collagen bundles, usually following a wound that may be trivial. It often is a tumorlike mass but is not neoplastic in the true sense of the word in that the phenomenon is self-limiting and does not progress or spread or metastasize as do other forms of neoplastic growth. The formation of keloid often is a racially determined condition, and blacks have a high propensity for producing such scarring, with gross distortion, particularly in response to burns. *(5:89–90)*

7. **(D)** Teratoma, which may be benign or malignant, is the only tumor type in which all three germ cell layers are represented. All the others contain one or two cell types. Teratomas typically are seen in the ovaries or testis but also occur in other sites, such as the mediastinum and retroperitoneum. *(2:241)*

8. **(C)** Hamartoma is a conglomeration of tissues that are normal to the area but haphazardly arranged in an abnormal fashion. All of the neoplasias listed contain a mixture of different cell types, but only in the hamartoma are the cells normal to that particular area. These are best regarded as developmental anomalies rather than true neoplasms, and they are never malignant and, therefore, do not metastasize. *(2:241–243)*

9. **(C)** This is a question of definition of the different types of cell growth (Tables 7–1 and 7–2). As described, dysplasia is an abnormal sequence of changes in maturation or development of cell types in a tissue or organ. It is best seen in the cervix of the uterus, where normally an ordered regular maturation of basal cells results in flattened squamous epithelium at the surface. In dysplasia, nucleated

cells appear throughout the layers even at the surface and can be shared and thus recognized in cytologic preparations. Dysplasia can, therefore, occur in any epithelium where maturation produces a series of layers. Dysplasia, in company with dyscrasia and dystrophy, is often used in describing tissues with other perversions of cell growth. All are self-limiting and distinct from neoplasia. *(4:173)*

10. **(B)** It is true that incidence of malignancy tends to increase with age. It also is true that hormones may inhibit or promote tumor growth. Certain tumors characteristically appear in certain age groups. Carcinoma of the breast, however, is more frequent in the female than the male, and cancer of the male breast, although it does occur, is particularly rare. *(1:266–293)*

11. **(A)** Hemangioma, lipoma, rhabdomyoma, and leiomyoma are tumors of mesenchymal mesodermal origin (Table 7–8), whereas papilloma is a tumor arising from epithelium, ectoderm, or endoderm and is a benign epithelial tumor usually producing an exophytic growth on a stalk (see Question 6). *(1:266–274)*

12. **(C)** Metaplasia is defined as an acquired change of tissue or organ resulting from change in one adult cell type to a different adult cell type (Table 7–2). All of the other terms describe various forms of cellular proliferation or lack of proliferation, but only metaplasia implies a change from one established adult type to another. An example is squamous metaplasia of the bronchus, in which the normal stratified squamous epithelium replaces the normal columnar cell epithelium. Similar changes are seen in the uterine cervix, in which columnar epithelium sometimes replaces the squamous epithelium at the squamocolumnar junction. *(4:173)*

13. **(C)** Cellular pleomorphism, numerous mitotic figures, lymphocyte infiltration at the edge of the tumor, and plasma cell infiltration at the edge of the tumor are features common to all forms of malignancy and may even be seen in some benign tumors. However, as shown in Table 7–4, metastasis, ie, spread of the tumor beyond the normal site widely in the body, is a feature characteristic of only truly malignant tumors. *(2:243–249)*

14. **(C)** The definitions of the various types of cellular proliferations or abnormalities of cell proliferation and development are shown in Table 7–2. A decrease in the size of a previously normal-sized and developed organ is defined as atrophy. It is an acquired decrease in the size of cellular components after full maturation has been achieved. This is in contradistinction to agenesis, where the tissue or organ may never reach the normal adult size because of lack of tissue components. Examples are disuse atrophy of muscles that have become denervated or atrophy of the uterus in the postmenopausal period. *(2:30–33; 4–173)*

15. **(D)** The term or prefix *adeno* implies a tumor of glandular epithelial origin. However, adenomatous polyp simply implies growth that is limited and does not exhibit the changes described here of invasion into the adjacent tissue (Table 7–8). Adenomyosis is the appearance of glandular elements in the myometrium, and a carcinosarcoma, although containing invasive and glandular components, also has a sarcomatous element, as its name suggests. The best example, therefore, is an adenocarcinoma in which all of the features described are present. *(1:266–274)*

16. **(D)** A malignant tumor that produces multiple nodules and, therefore, metastatic spread in a structure, such as the gastric mucosa and small intestine, is a relatively rare phenomenon. Added to this, the presence of fine granules of brownish pigment would fit the description of melanin, and, therefore, malignant melanoma, a malignant tumor rising from the melanocytes of the skin, fits this description best. Malignant melanoma is one of the few tumors to metastasize to the stomach and small intestine. It is often pigmented because of the production of melanin, although sometimes the tumor is so undifferentiated as to no longer produce melanin (so-called amelanotic melanoma). *(4:202–207)*

17. **(D)** It is estimated that in 1991, 44,000 women in the United States died of breast carcinoma, and the age-corrected death rate per 100,000 of the population was 27.4 for breast cancer. *(1:274–279)*

18. **(B)** The incidence of cancer differs considerably both in its crude incident rate and in its death rate in underdeveloped countries, particularly in black African countries as compared to white races in the United States and Europe. Carcinoma of the lung, colon, breast, and pancreas tend to be major neoplasms in Western developed countries and are relatively uncommon in Africa. Carcinoma of the uterine cervix, however, is one of the most frequent malignancies in African countries. It has been suggested that this is associated with early and frequent sexual activity. Recent data related this antecedent to herpes virus infections. *(3:116–118)*

19. **(D)** There has been a great deal of investigation of the possible etiologic role of viruses, which has established the oncogene and oncovirus theories. A number of tumors have come under suspicion, including some forms of cancer of the uterine cervix and possibly some lymphomas. Burkitt's lymphoma is associated with the Epstein-Barr virus and was described first in young African children. There is

no direct evidence that leiomyoma of the uterus, carcinoma of the lung, and carcinoma of the esophagus have viral etiologies. This is another example of the fact that malignancy may occur morphologically in different forms and may have different pathways of etiology and that chemical carcinogenesis, hereditary factors, viruses, and other factors may interact at different levels and have more or less strong associations in a specific type of tumor. *(1:289–291)*

20. **(C)** CEA is a form of glycoprotein. It usually is expressed by cells of the fetal intestine. Although it is produced in some form by a variety of tumors and some nonneoplastic conditions, it is most typically seen in carcinoma of the colon. Its very consistent appearance in carcinoma of the colon has led to its use not only diagnostically but in following up patients after surgery to determine if recurrence or metastasis has occurred. Some of the other tumors listed, particularly testicular teratomas and seminomas, may produce similar by-products that are unrelated to CEA. *(1:312)*

21. **(C)** As seen in Table 7–4, benign tumors tend to be encapsulated and slowly growing. Therefore, they have a low mitotic index; ie, at any time, particularly when sections are taken of the fixed tissue at death of the tumor, few mitoses are seen. In this respect, they appear closely similar to their normal tissue counterparts and tend to be well differentiated. All of these factors, however, are variable. The inability to invade in single cells or groups of cells and not to produce metastasis via the blood vessels and lymphatics is a particularly important distinction between benign and malignant. *(2:243–249)*

22. **(D)** The term "hyperplasia" (Tables 7–2 and 7–3) is an increase in mass of tissue or organ because of cellular increase beyond the normal range. The terms "aplasia," "agenesis," "hypertrophy," and "metaplasia" clearly are different and usually are easily distinguishable. *(2:30–35)*

23. **(C)** The relationship between cigarette smoking and lung cancer is probably one of the most convincing associations between a social habit and a prevalent form of neoplasia. Although there may be other factors, including the role of such substances as asbestos and even viruses, cigarette smoking is clearly and unequivocally shown to be a major carcinogenic event in this very important tumor. *(3:87–88)*

24. **(E)** The increased incidence of bladder cancer among aniline dye workers was one of the earliest industrial cancers recognized before the turn of the century and was thought to be caused by naphthylamines and related amines, including benzene. There is a complex relationship between the enzyme beta-glucuronidase and the release of 2-amino-l-naphthol in the bladder. This is further exaggerated by cigarette smoking, which increases the carcinogenic effect by interfering with betaglucuronidase production. *(3:82–84)*

25. **(D)** Production of malignant melanoma of the skin in the white races, particularly those of Celtic origin, in such countries as Australia and New Zealand and parts of the Untied States, eg, Texas, Arizona, and New Mexico, has a clear, direct relationship with ultraviolet light. Carcinoma of the lung has no such relationship with sunlight, and the skin of blacks is particularly immune to the effect of ultraviolet light in production of both basal cell and squamous cell carcinoma. Intraocular malignant melanoma is an extremely rare tumor in blacks and is unrelated to sunlight as far as can be determined. *(3:132–134)*

26. **(B)** Table 7–2 shows that hyperplasia is an increase in the size of an organ or tissue resulting from increase in cell proliferation, whereas hypertrophy is an increase in size of an organ resulting from increase in size of the cells. This is what happens in the uterus during pregnancy. Dysplasia may occur in the uterine cervix but is not related to pregnancy per se. *(4:173)*

27. **(E)** The postmenopausal small uterus results from a decrease in the size of the component cells (atrophy) (Table 7–2). It is the opposite of the answer to Question 26. *(4:173)*

28. **(D)** Lack of development of the lobe of the lung in a newborn fits the term "agenesis," which is a congenital lack of tissue or organ resulting from total lack of cells. Although aplasia may share certain features, it is often an acquired rather than a congenital lack of development and is seen also in adults. *(5:201)*

29. **(A)** Hyperplasia is an increase in mature tissue or organs resulting from increase in cell number beyond the normal range (Tables 7–2 and 7–3). A localized thickness of the buccal mucosa resulting from increased numbers of epithelial cells fits this description. This is not hypertrophy, since the cells do not necessarily increase in size and there are more cells than normal. Dysplasia may often accompany hyperplasia in some situations, but the two may be separate entities, as in this case. *(2:30–35)*

30. **(D)** Aflatoxins produced by certain fungi may contaminate food and have been shown to produce changes in the liver in humans and in other ani-

mals, including the turkey. It is closely associated with hepatocellular carcinoma, particularly in parts of Africa. *(3:34–38)*

31. **(D)** Industrial exposure to naphthalene, as seen in aniline dye workers (see Question 24), is associated with an increased incidence of urinary bladder carcinoma caused by by-products of naphthalene and their concentration in the urine. It is another form of chemical carcinogenesis that has been well established and proven. *(2:271–273)*

32. **(D)** The low-power photomicrograph (Fig 7–4) shows a papillary tumor on a stalk that is well circumscribed with what appears to be a central core of connective tissue and an epithelial covering. The high-power photomicrograph (Fig 7–5) shows the cells to be of squamous type with intercellular bridges and the pavement type epithelium characteristic of squamous epithelium. The tumor is, therefore, a papilloma (Table 7–8). Because the cells of origin are clearly squamous in type and it is well differentiated, the tumor is referred to as a well-differentiated benign squamous cell papilloma. *(4:173)*

33. **(B)** *(4:173)*

34. **(C)** After complete excision of this lesion, the most likely predictable sequence would be that nothing further would occur, since the benign tumor has been completely excised. Therefore, by definition, it would not spread to regional lymph nodes or to the bloodstream and should not occur locally unless tissue was left behind. The prognosis is good with such a lesion if it is adequately treated. *(4:173–196)*

35. **(D)** *(4:173–196)*

36. **(C)**

37. **(D)**

38. **(A)**

36 through 38. The association between mesothelioma, which is a malignant tumor of the pleura, and asbestos exposure over many years has now been well established. It is reasonably well established that there is an increased incidence of cancer arising from the bronchial epithelium, so-called bronchogenic carcinoma. The characteristic asbestos bodies are demonstrated clearly (Fig 7–6) in the photomicrograph, and the other features are clearly distinguishable. Although excessive smoking may add to the problem, this is not particularly the case in mesothelioma, although it would be in lung cancer. *(2:479–483)*

39. **(D)**

40. **(A)**

39 and 40. The photomicrograph (Fig 7–7) shows epithelium from the ectocervix in which there is total disorganization of the cells, with nucleated cells appearing throughout the layers and with the cells showing marked pleomorphism and irregularity in the size and shape of the nuclei. This is the picture of carcinoma in situ or a malignant process still confined to the epithelial layer, with no evidence of invasion of the underlying tissue. If the area of the cervix is completely removed at this stage, there is no further likelihood of malignant spread. *(2:1141–1145)*

41. **(A)**

42. **(D)**

41 and 42. The photomicrograph from the cervix (Fig 7–8) shows normal squamous epithelium to the right and squamous epithelium showing severe dysplasia to the left. The distinction between the severe dysplasia seen in this photomicrograph and that in Figure 7–7 may be difficult to determine in some instances, but there is still an attempt at regular layering of the cells even though there are nucleated cells shedding at the surface. If this is the situation, the lesion may under some circumstances regress, may remain unchanged for periods of time, or may develop into a true in situ or even invasive malignancy. It is for this reason that such severe dysplasia is regarded as potentially malignant. *(2:1141–1145)*

43. **(D)**

44. **(D)**

45. **(D)**

46. **(C)**

43 through 46. The low-power photomicrograph (Fig 7–9) shows a pedunculated structure composed of glandular spaces on a stalk that is connected to epithelium characteristic of the large intestine. The high-power photomicrograph (Fig 7–10) shows the epithelium to be well differentiated, similar to that seen in the normal bowel but disorganized in the fashion of a glandular tumor. There is no evidence of invasion of the stalk by groups or clumps of cells; therefore, this represents a benign tumor of glandular type, ie, an adenoma (Table 7–8). Because of its pedunculated nature, it is described as an adenomatous polyp. These lesions are extremely common throughout the large bowel and can produce malignant change with subsequent invasion. In this instance, there is no such evidence, and, therefore, the prognosis is excellent. This is similar to that seen in Questions 32 through 35, where the pedunculated lesion of the skin was removed completely with no residual area of tumor, resulting in cure. *(4:2–5)*

47. (D)

48. (D)

49. (D)

50. (D)

47 through 50. The photomicrograph (Fig 7–11) clearly shows a neoplastic process. There are sheets and clumps of cells that do not have a normal appearance of any tissue. The tumor is composed of cells of an epithelial type, and the center shows an area of keratohyalin, which is characteristic of squamous cell carcinoma or a carcinoma arising from squamous cell epithelium. There is, adjacent to the tumor, black pigment characteristic of anthracotic pigment, which often is seen in the lungs of city dwellers and in those who smoke cigarettes. Although the anthracotic pigment is not related directly to cigarette smoking, it is a clue to the site of the tumor. The tumor is, therefore, a squamous cell carcinoma arising in the lung and is a characteristic of bronchogenic carcinoma. *(4:228–233)*

51. (B)

52. (D)

53. (A)

51 through 53. These definitions are described in Table 7–8. An adenoma is defined as a benign neoplasm that is growing locally and is well circumscribed and very similar in appearance to the cells from which it arose. The term "adenoma" usually applies to a particular benign neoplasm of glandular origin. The lack of production of red cell precursors in bone marrow is a description of aplasia; often this results in a disease known as "aplastic anemia," in which the red cells are no longer replenished from the stem cell pool and severe anemia results. There are many other reasons why red cells are not replaced or are actually destroyed, but in this situation, it is a lack of production of the precursors. A liposarcoma is a sarcoma or malignant neoplasm of mesodermal or mesenchymal origin, the prefix *lipo* meaning "of fat cells." This is a particularly rare form of malignant tumor arising from the adipose tissue. *(1:270–274)*

54. (D)

55. (B)

54 and 55. The benign tumor of epithelial origin attached to the normal epithelium by a stalk is a papilloma (Table 7–8). If the epithelium is of glandular type, it can be referred to as a "papillary adenoma," which is a combination of these descriptions. A malignant tumor of mesodermal origin, by definition, is a sarcoma. The prefix determines the cell of origin, eg, *lipo*sarcoma, *fibro*sarcoma, and *osteo*sarcoma. *(1:270–274)*

56. (E)

57. (C)

58. (D)

59. (A)

60. (B)

61. (A)

56 through 61. A choriocarcinoma is a malignant neoplasm of trophoblastic origin that, although it may predominantly metastasize via the bloodstream, most characteristically produces HCG, as does the normal trophoblast. A secondary carcinoma of the stomach in the ovaries, the Krukenberg tumor, is a metastatic tumor that originates in other sites than the stomach, although that is the most classic, and metastasizes to the ovaries either via the bloodstream or via the peritoneal cavity or both. A hepatocellular carcinoma is one of the tumors that secretes AFP, a substance normally seen only in fetal life and the fetal equivalent of albumin. Other tumors, such as teratomas and testicular tumors, may also produce AFP. Osteogenic sarcoma is a malignant neoplasm of mesodermal origin (Table 7–8) and arises from cells of the osteoblast type in bone. It is a highly malignant tumor usually seen in young people, with a second peak at an older age. It characteristically metastasizes via the bloodstream, although there have been rarer occasions when lymph nodes have been involved in some forms of osteogenic sarcoma. Bronchogenic carcinoma, however, a tumor of epithelial origin arising in the lungs and characteristic of epithelial tumors, tends to go via the lymphatic rather than the bloodstream, although it can eventually be widely disseminated through the bloodstream after traversing the lymphatics and the lymph nodes. A fibrosarcoma is a malignant neoplasm of mesodermal origin from fibroblastic tissue and is characteristically metastasized via the bloodstream through thin-walled blood vessels often closely associated with the tumor. Very occasionally, a fibrosarcoma may metastasize primarily via the lymphatics (Table 7–9). *(1:270–274; 4:197)*

62. (A)

63. (A)

64. (A)

62 through 64. Neuroblastoma is a malignant neoplasm thought to arise from primitive neural crest cells. It is a tumor of infancy and early childhood, most commonly occurring in the adrenal gland. Most patients have an enlarging abdominal mass. Examination of the urine reveals elevated levels of the neuroendocrine metabolites, metanephrine, and vanillylmandelic acid. Hematogenous metastases occur early in the disease. The karyotypic abnormalities associated with neuroblastoma include partial deletion of the short arm of chromosome 1 and amplification of the oncogene N-myc. Treatment is a combination of surgery, chemotherapy, and radiation. The prognosis depends on the age of the patient, stage of disease, histology of the tumor cells, and oncogene status. *(1:873–875)*

65. (A)

66. (D)

65 and 66. The TNM staging system is a useful method to quickly enumerate the extent of malignant disease, categorize patients for therapy, and predict prognosis. The T icon represents the size of the primary tumor, with T1 being the smallest sized tumor, and T2 through T4 designating increasingly larger tumor sizes. The N icon is for the nodal status. N0 indicates no known nodal metastases. N1 through N3 indicate increasing, more distant lymph node involvement. The absence or presence of distant non-nodal metastases is designated by M0 or M1, respectively. The stage of disease is determined by plugging the appropriate T, N, and M numbers into a site- or organ-specific staging formula. For example, a stage I breast carcinoma is T1, N0, M0. Whereas a stage II breast carcinoma is T1, N1, M0; or T2, N0, M0; or T2, N1, M0; or T3, N0, M0. The prognosis decreases with each increasing stage. The 5-year survival for stages I, II, II, and IV breast cancers are 85%, 66%, 41%, and 10%, respectively. *(1:829,623; 2:901–902,1200)*

67. (C)

67 and 68. Asbestos is strongly associated with an increased risk of subsequently developing malignant mesothelioma. Asbestos is a fiber-shaped silicate found in nature occurring in crocidolite, chrysotile, and amosite forms. Inhaled fibers are deposited in the alveolar spaces and phagocytized by macrophages. Eventually interstitial pulmonary fibrosis may result. Ferruginous bodies are iron-coated asbestos fibers and may be seen microscopically. Pleural thickening and mesothelioma occur not only in individuals who work with asbestos, such as shipbuilders, but also in their family members who are exposed to the worker's asbestos-soiled clothes. The hepatitis B viral carrier state is associated with an increased risk of developing hepatoma (liver cell carcinoma). Preceding the emergence of the cancer there is antecedent cirrhosis and liver cell dysplasia. Hepatoma is most common in Africa and the Far East in geographic areas with a high prevalence of the hepatitis B carrier individuals. *(1:544–545,658–659)*

69. (A)

70. (B)

71. (D)

72. (E)

69 through 72. A number of terms exist (Tables 7–1 and 7–2) to define alterations either in the number of cells, the size of individual cells, the composition of cells, or the maturation of cells. Hyperplasia is the increase in size of individual cells. Left ventricular hypertrophy due to essential hypertension is a common physiologic example. Dysplasia is a preneoplasic abnormality of maturation associated with nuclear hyperchromatism and enlargement. Aplasia is the absence of normal cellular proliferation or populations. It can involve a few cells, a complete developmental line of cells, a portion of an organ, or an entire organ. Metaplasia is the acquired change of one adult cell type into another adult cell type. Usually metaplasia is a protective alteration since the metaplastic cells are frequently more resistant to the inciting physiologic or environmental stresses. *(2:30–35)*

73. (B)

74. (C)

73 and 74. The products synthesized by certain benign and malignant tumors can be used as markers of identification for diagnosis and as an aid in detecting tumors at an earlier stage (Table 7–10). Medullary carcinoma arises from the parafollicular C cells of the thyroid. These cells manufacture and secrete the hormone calcitonin. Medullary carcinomas either secrete increased serum levels of calcitonin, or calcitonin molecules can be demonstrated in these tumor cells with special techniques. Pheochromocytomas are neoplasms of the adrenal medulla. They characteristically produce increased levels of catecholamines and their metabolites. *(5:1141–1144,1154–1156)*

75. (E)

76. (A)

77. (B)

78. (C)

75 through 78. Liposarcoma is a malignant tumor composed of fat-forming cells. These malignant tumors of adipocytes occur most commonly in the retroperitoneum, mesentery, and soft tissues of middle-aged and elderly individuals. A lipoma is a benign tumor of adipocytes. It is seen most often in the hypodermis of middle-aged and elderly individuals. Osteogenic sarcoma is a malignant tumor of bone-forming cells. Osteoid production is a characteristic feature. Rhabdomyosarcoma is a malignant tumor of skeletal muscle cells. Myosin can be demonstrated immunohistochemically in most of these tumors. Osteogenic sarcoma and rhabdomyosarcoma are most commonly encountered in children and young adults. The nomenclature for tumors is detailed in Table 7–8. *(5:143–146)*

79. (E)

80. (B)

81. (A)

82. (C)

79 through 82. The nomenclature of tumors can be complex (Table 7–8). In general, benign tumors are named by combining the cell type with the suffix *oma*. For example, a benign tumor of chondrocytes (cartilage cells) is called a "chondroma," and a benign tumor of leiomyocytes (smooth muscle cells) is called a "leiomyoma." Malignant epithelial tumors are generally named by adding the cell type to the suffix *carcinoma*. For example, a malignant tumor of glandular cells (adenocytes) is called an "adenocarcinoma." Malignant tumors of mesenchymal cells are usually named by adding the suffix *sarcoma* to the cell type. For example, a malignant tumor of chondrocytes is termed a "chondrosarcoma." *(2:240–243)*

83. (C)

84. (B)

85. (D)

86. (A)

83 through 86. Colonic carcinoma occurs most commonly in Western populations with high-fat, low-fiber diets. A low residual diet slows colonic transit times perhaps exposing the bowel epithelium to carcinogenic fatty substances for prolonged periods of time. African female populations have a high incidence of cervical squamous cell carcinoma for a number of reasons: lack of pap smear screening, high prevalence of viral promotors, and early age of first sexual activity. Basal cell carcinomas of the skin occur much more frequently in individuals with extensive actinic dermatitis. Gastric adenocarcinoma is most common in Japan and the former Soviet Union, and relatively rare in North American populations (Table 7–14). The reason for this disparity is not known. *(1:274–279; 2:897–902)*

87. (E)

88. (B)

89. (A)

90. (D)

87 through 90. Close viral associations are seen with several types of human cancers. Dysplasias and carcinoma of the cervix are strongly associated with genital infection of the human papilloma virus, particularly subtypes 16, 18, 31, and 33. Hepatocellular carcinoma is seen with hepatitis B virus carrier states. Dysplasia and cirrhosis may precede the development of liver cell carcinoma. Burkitt's lymphoma of the African type is strongly associated with Epstein-Barr viral infections. Epstein-Barr virus infection is also related to the subsequent development of nasopharyngeal carcinomas. Kaposi's sarcoma is seen most frequently in individuals with AIDS due to human immunodeficiency virus infection. *(1:290)*

91. (E)

92. (C)

93. (A)

94. (D)

91 through 94. A number of clinical conditions and disorders predispose to the later emergence of neoplasms. Xeroderma pigmentosum, for example, is a genetic disorder which lacks the usual DNA cellular repair mechanisms for mitigating against actinic damage. As a result these individuals develop multiple skin cancers at an early age. Ulcerative colitis is another disorder associated with subsequent neoplastic transformation. In this disease there is chronic ulcerative inflammation of the large intestine, epithelial dysplasia, and a significantly increased risk of colonic adenocarcinoma. Undescended testes are associated with sterility and an increased risk of germ-cell tumors such as seminoma. Individuals with Paget's disease of the bone have an increased incidence of subsequent osteosarcoma. *(1:295–298)*

95. **(B)**

96. **(E)**

97. **(C)**

98. **(A)**

95 through 98. A number of chemical substances are related to tumorous development. Aflatoxin, a fungal metabolite, can contaminate improperly stored food, particularly grains and peanuts. The ingested aflatoxin is oxidized in the liver and exerts its carcinogenic effect by binding to quanine. Chewing betel leaves and nuts is likely to produce oral carcinomas. This practice correlates with Sri Lanka's and parts of India's high incidence of oral tumors. The maternal antepartum administration of diethylstibesterol produces an increased risk of subsequent vaginal adenosis and vaginal clear cell carcinoma in their female offspring. These tumors usually do not make their appearance until the daughters are at least age 20. Vinyl chloride workers are at increased risk to develop angiosarcomas of the liver. *(1:284–288)*

99. **(E)**

100. **(D)**

101. **(B)**

102. **(C)**

99 through 102. Renal cell carcinoma may secrete erythropoietin, a hormonal red cell growth factor. Erythrocytosis and polycythemia may occur. Prostate adenocarcinoma may secrete prostate-specific antigen and prostatic acid phosphatase. Early detection of localized disease may be achieved by measuring the serum levels of these markers. Multiple myeloma is a malignancy of plasma cells. The malignant plasma cells may secrete intact whole immunoglobulin molecules, free light chains, or rarely, free heavy chains. The immunoglobulins may be observed in the serum, urine, or both serum and urine. Adrenal cortical carcinomas may retain their native cell's ability to secrete corticosteroid products. These products may be measured in the serum or the metabolites may be detected in the urine. *(1:300–301)*

103. **(D)** Squamous cell carcinoma of the lung is seen most commonly in cigarette smokers. Squamous metaplasia and squamous cell dysplasia usually precede the development of an overt malignancy. The microscopic appearance of the tumor is varied, depending on the grade of the tumor. Usually multicell keratin pearl formation, intercellular bridges (prickles), or intracellular keratin production must be observed histologically to definitively diagnose the squamous cell type. Other associated features include sheetlike architecture, enlarged hyperchromic nuclei, and eosinophilic cytoplasm. Early lesions may be cured by surgery. However, the overall prognosis of lung carcinoma is dismal since the 5-year survival is only 8%. *(1:550–556)*

104. **(A)** Melanoma is a malignant neoplasm of melanocytes. Most melanomas arise in basal layers of the epidermis and remain confined to the epidermis in a radial growth phase for some time. Later in the tumor's development it will grow down into the dermis (vertical growth phase) and gain access to the lymphatics. Clinically most melanomas display a variegated brown, tan, pink, or black appearance. Irregular edges, enlargement, and central nodular ulceration may also be noticed. The microscopic appearance is characterized by nests of cells and single cells with eccentric nuclei, prominent macronucleoli, and cytoplasmic melanin pigment. The prognosis of melanoma is related to its depth of invasion measured by either the Clark's level or Breslow's thickness. Deeply invading tumors and thicker tumors are associated with a poor prognosis. *(1:895–896)*

105. **(F)** Down's syndrome is caused by a trisomy of chromosome 21. Prominent epicanthal folds, mental retardation, congenital cardiovascular abnormalities, oblique palpebral fissures, increased susceptibility to infections, hyperflexibility, muscle hypotonia, dysplastic ears, and infertility characterize the syndrome. Individuals with Down's syndrome have a 20-fold increased risk of developing lymphoblastic leukemia during childhood. *(2:129–132)*

106. **(C)** Adenocarcinoma is the most common type of malignancy arising in the large intestine. Iron deficiency microcytic, hypochromic anemia, may be the presenting symptom due to bleeding from tumorous ulceration. Alternatively, the tumor may be suspected by detection of occult fecal blood tests, bowel obstruction, or through the development of hepatic enlargement due to metastases. The gross appearance of the tumors is usually polypoid or ulcerating. Many ulcerating tumors involve the full circumference of the bowel and appear radiographically as an "applecore" lesion. The microscopic appearance is that of gland-forming malignant cells. Usually mucin production is prominent. The prognosis is related to the stage of the disease. TMN and modified Duke's staging protocols are clinically useful to predict an individual's prognosis. *(1:620–623)*

107. **(D)** Hemangiomas are benign tumors composed of blood vessels. They occur in the dermis of all age groups, although they are most common in infancy and childhood. Those tumors forming large vessels may be termed "cavernous hemangiomas." Those formed by small blood vessels are called "capillary hemangiomas." Most hemangiomas are removed for diagnostic or cosmetic reasons. Rarely, rupture of an intravisceral hemangioma can be fatal. The malignant counterpart, angiosarcoma, is distinguished by the anaplasia its endothelial cells demonstrate, invasiveness, and ability to metastasize. *(2:587–592)*

108. **(H)** Chronic myelogenous leukemia is a myeloproliferative disease of middle age with a slight male predominance. Common clinical features include splenomegaly, hepatomegaly, anemia, fatigability, easy bruising, and bleeding. Examination of the peripheral blood reveals an increased number of myeloid white blood cells, mostly segmented neutrophils, band neutrophils, metamyelocytes, and myelocytes. The bone marrow displays trilineage hyperplasia. The Philadelphia chromosome is present in about 90% of cases. This karyotypic abnormality consists of a translocation of a portion of the long arm from chromosome 22 to chromosome 9. *(5:1069–1071)*

109. **(E)** Malignant tumors composed of bladder transitional epithelium are termed "transitional cell carcinomas." They are commonly associated with employment in the dye, rubber, paint, and chemical industries due to exposure to occupational carcinogens. The most frequent initial complaint is that of gross hematuria. The tumors are divided histologically into three grades, with grade I tumors being the most (well) differentiated and grade III tumors being the least (poorly) differentiated. The prognosis and treatment is determined by the stage of disease at initial presentation. *(5:905–907)*

110. **(G)** Malignant tumors composed of astrocytes are called "malignant astrocytomas." These tumors occur most frequently in middle-aged and elderly adults. The heralding clinical event may be a seizure. Malignant astrocytomas are characterized microscopically by proliferations of atypical astrocytes with anaplasia and increased mitoses. Those tumors that, in addition, demonstrate glomeruloid endothelial hyperplasia, extreme astrocytic pleomorphism, and palisading of tumor cells next to necrotic foci are termed "glioblastoma multiforme." Malignant astrocytoma and glioblastoma multiforme have a dismal prognosis, with most affected individuals dying within a year of diagnosis. *(5:1469–1471)*

REFERENCES

1. Chandrasoma P, Taylor CR: Concise Pathology, Norwalk, Appleton and Lange, 1991
2. Cotran RS, Kumar V, Robbins SL: Robbins Pathologic Basis of Disease, 4th edition, Philadelphia, Saunders, 1989
3. Hutt MSR, Burkitt DP: The Geography of Non-Infectious Diseases, New York, Oxford University Press, 1986
4. Lewis MG, Rowden G: Histopathology, A Step by Step Approach, Boston, Little, Brown, 1984
5. Rubin E, Farber JL: Pathology, Philadelphia, Lippincott, 1988.

CHAPTER 8

Photographic Exercises
Questions

DIRECTIONS: Each of the numbered items or incomplete statements in this section is followed by answers or by completions of the statement. Select the ONE lettered answer or completion that is BEST in each case.

Questions 1 through 5. Refer to Figure 8–1.

1. Which of the following statements most accurately describes Figure 8–1?

    (A) hyperplasia of the epithelial lining
    (B) loss of continuity of the epithelial surface
    (C) neoplastic transformation of the epithelium
    (D) metaplastic transformation of the epithelium
    (E) atrophic changes of the epithelium

2. Which of the following is the most appropriate diagnostic statement for the illustrated condition?

    (A) hypertrophic gastritis
    (B) peptic ulcer
    (C) gastric carcinoma
    (D) intestinal metaplasia of gastric mucosa
    (E) congenital gastric atrophy

3. The most likely etiology is

    (A) ingestion of carcinogens in the diet
    (B) the result of megaloblastic anemia
    (C) associated with overproduction of acid and pepsin
    (D) an inherited enzyme deficiency
    (E) a viral organism

4. Which type of tissue alteration does this condition illustrate?

    (A) gummatous inflammation
    (B) tuberculous inflammation
    (C) ulcerative inflammation
    (D) fat necrosis
    (E) granulomatous inflammation

5. What is the most likely complication of the illustrated condition?

    (A) gastric leiomyomatosis
    (B) hypertension
    (C) atrophic gastritis
    (D) pernicious anemia
    (E) hemorrhage

Questions 6 through 9. Refer to Figures 8–2 and 8–3.

6. Which of the following processes best describes the pathologic changes illustrated in Figures 8–2 and 8–3?

    (A) chronic nongranulomatous inflammation
    (B) chronic granulomatous inflammation
    (C) acute suppurative inflammation
    (D) peptic ulceration
    (E) hyperplasia

7. Which is the most probable outcome if untreated?

    (A) malignant transformation
    (B) complete resolution
    (C) ischemic necrosis with perforation
    (D) spontaneous healing and repair
    (E) atrophy

8. Characteristic morphologic findings include all of the following EXCEPT

    (A) neutrophils
    (B) luminal suppurative debris
    (C) edema and vascular congestion
    (D) acute inflammation
    (E) malignant mucin-producing cells

9. Which statement about this pathologic process is true?

    (A) usually resolves without treatment
    (B) always is associated with a carcinoid tumor
    (C) may be associated with obstruction by a fecalith
    (D) more frequently seen in underdeveloped rather than developed societies
    (E) never seen in elderly individuals

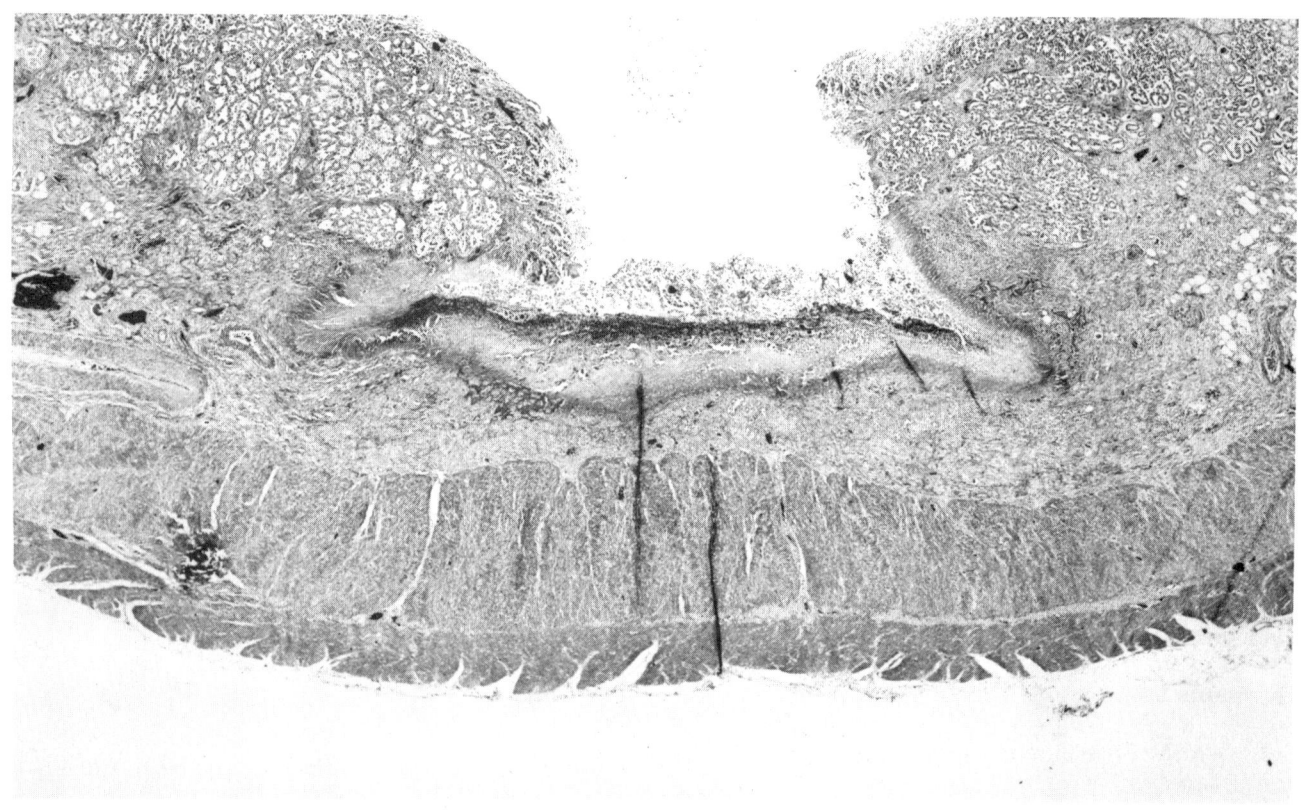

Figure 8–1. Low-power photomicrograph of a lesion in the stomach.

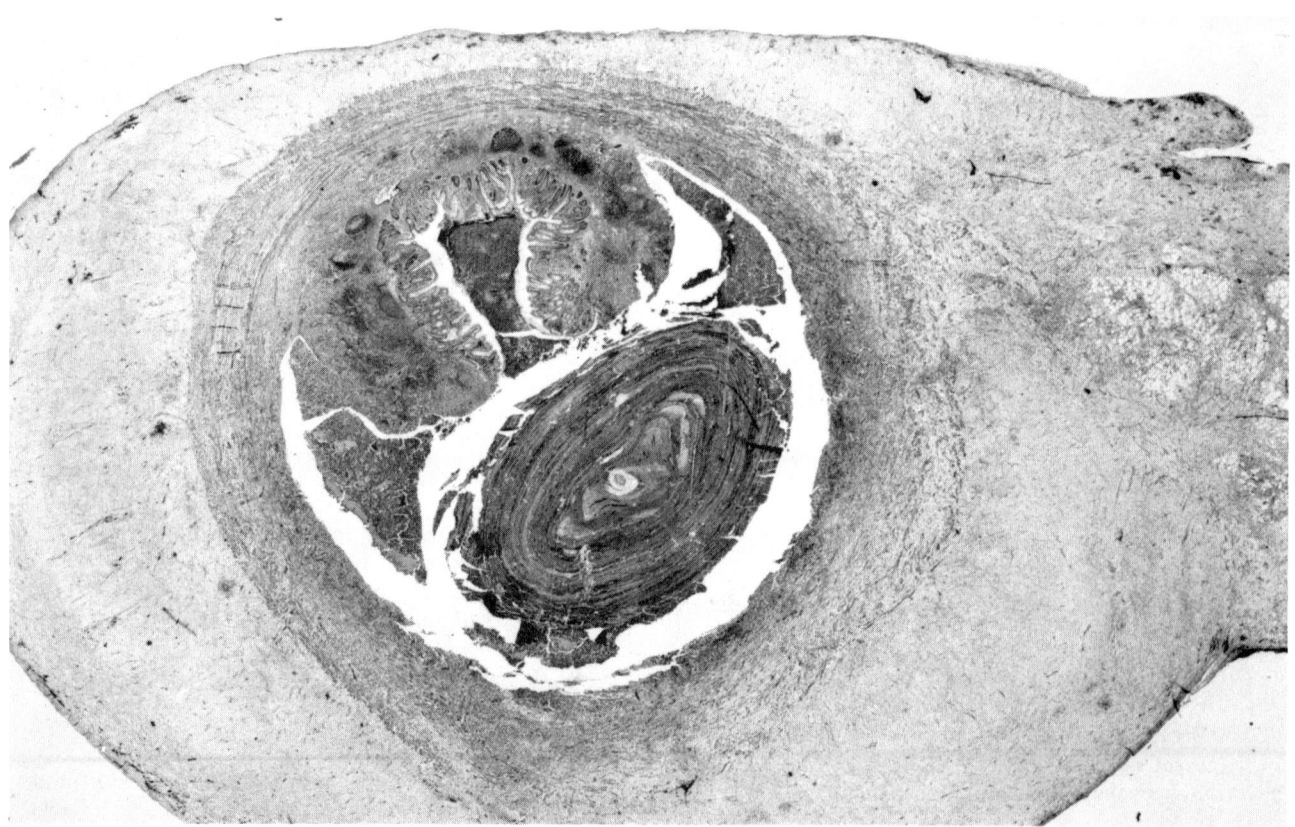

Figure 8–2. Low-power photomicrograph of a transverse section of appendix.

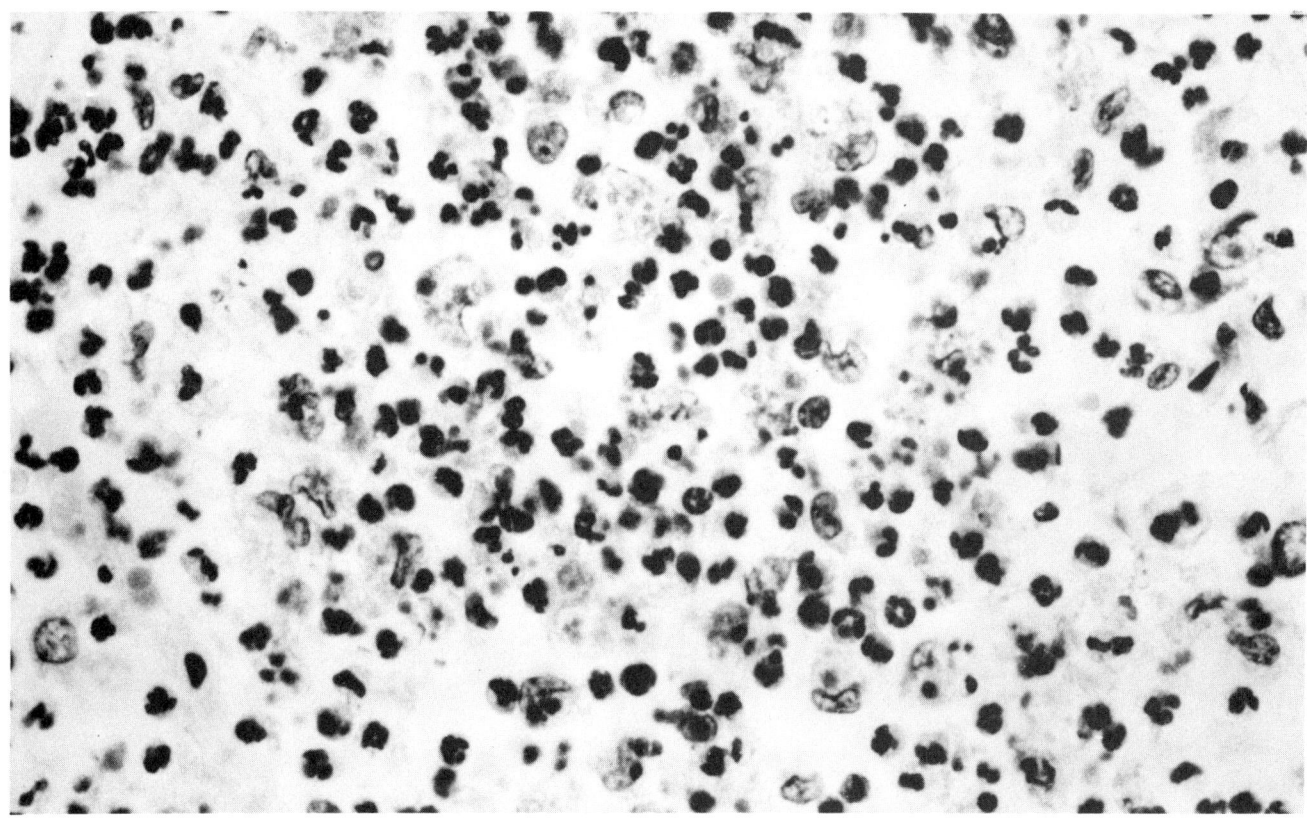

Figure 8–3. High-power photomicrograph of a transverse section of appendix.

Questions 10 through 13. Refer to Figures 8–4 and 8–5.

10. Which of the following is the most appropriate description?

    (A) diffuse interstitial pneumonia
    (B) lobar pneumonia
    (C) lobular (broncho) pneumonia
    (D) chronic granulomatous disease
    (E) pulmonary fibrosis

11. Which of the following is the most likely cause?

    (A) adenovirus
    (B) *Streptococcus pneumoniae* (pneumococcus)
    (C) *Escherichia coli*
    (D) *Mycobacterium tuberculosis* (tubercle bacillus)
    (E) asbestos particles

12. The characteristic microscopic feature seen in the acute phase of this process is

    (A) multinucleate giant cells
    (B) fibrin and neutrophils in the alveoli
    (C) lymphocytic inflammation
    (D) fibrocytes and granulation tissue
    (E) granulomatous inflammation

13. The most likely sequela is

    (A) malignant nodal metastasis
    (B) calcification
    (C) gangrene
    (D) complete resolution
    (E) dense fibrosis and scar formation

Questions 14 through 17. Refer to Figures 8–6 and 8–7.

14. Which of the following is the most appropriate description?

    (A) diffuse interstitial pneumonia
    (B) lobar pneumonia
    (C) lobular (broncho) pneumonia
    (D) chronic granulomatous disease
    (E) pulmonary fibrosis

15. Which of the following is the most likely cause?

    (A) adenovirus
    (B) pneumococcus *Streptococcus pneumoniae* (pneumococcus)
    (C) *Escherichia coli*
    (D) *Mycobacterium tuberculosis* (tubercle bacillus)
    (E) asbestos particles

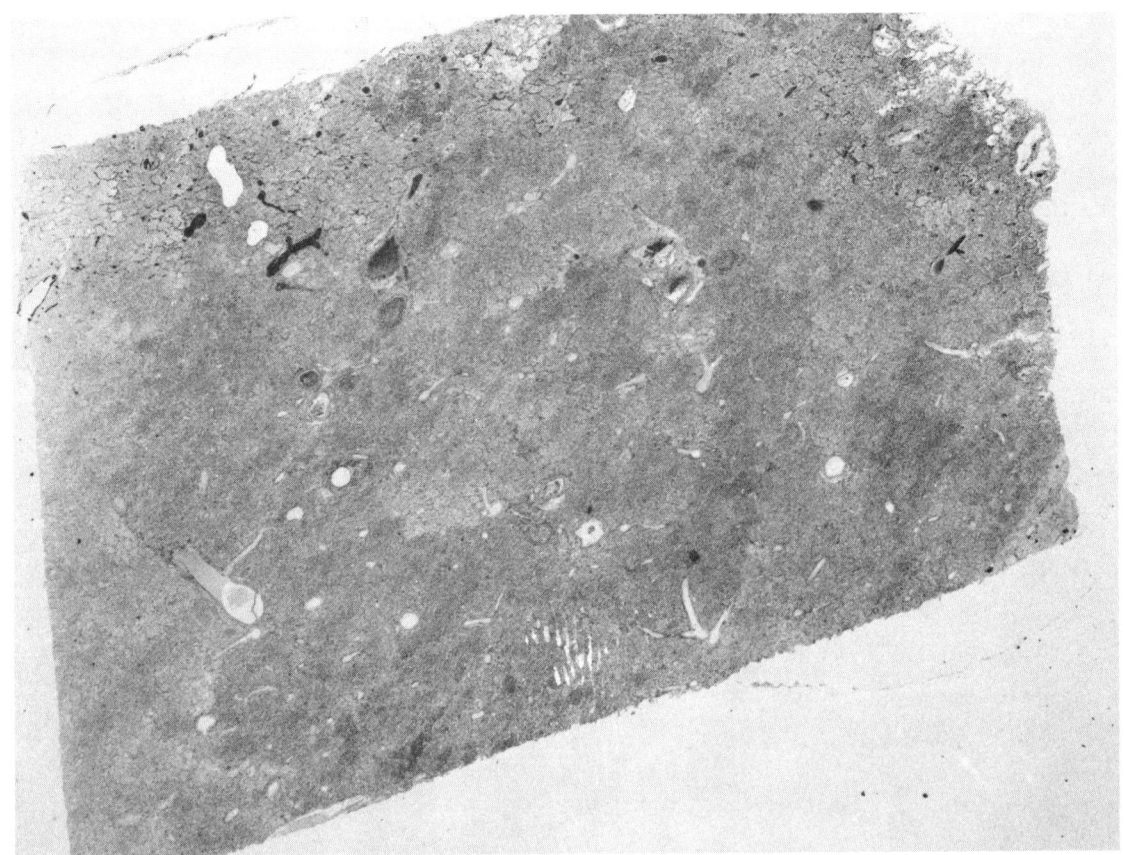

Figures 8–4 and 8–5. Low-power and high-power photomicrographs of an inflammatory process in the lung.

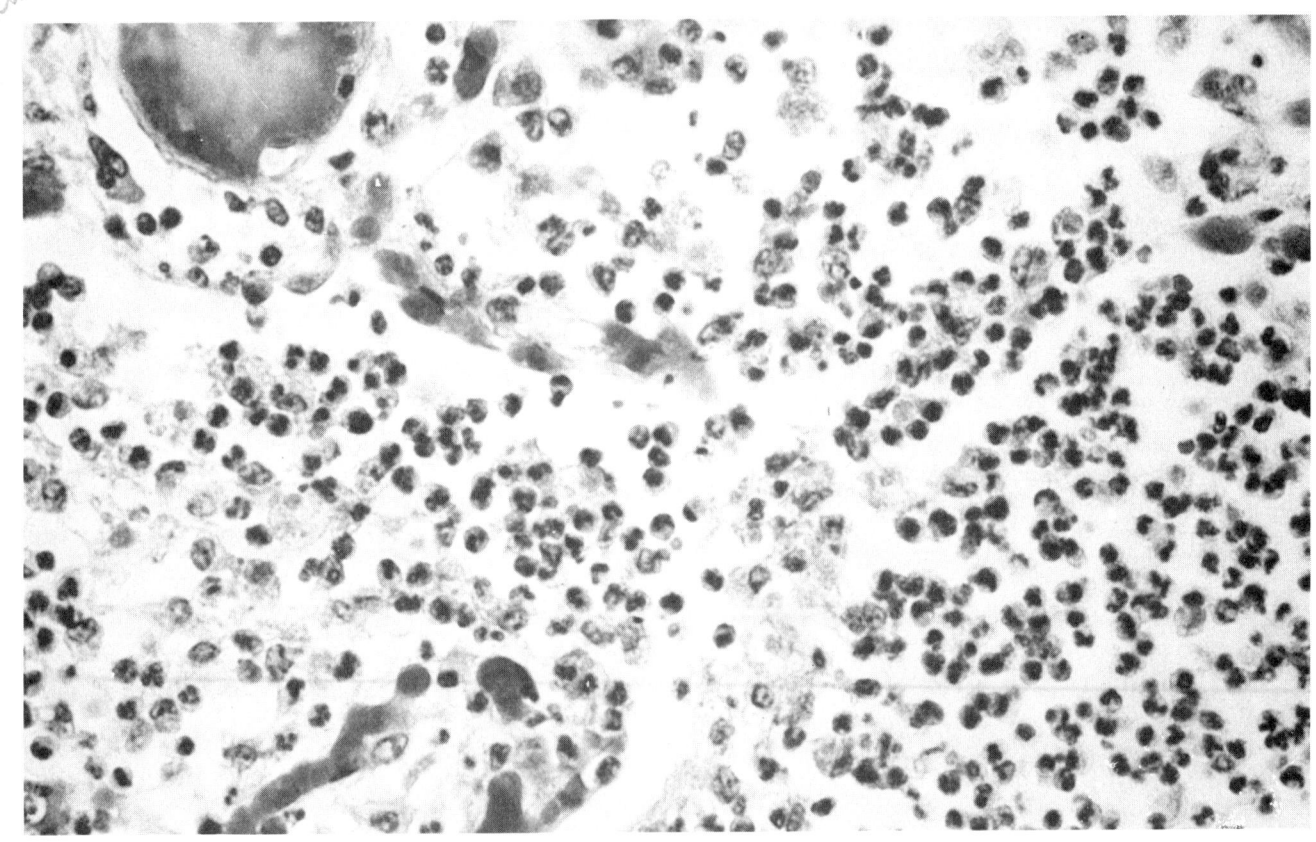

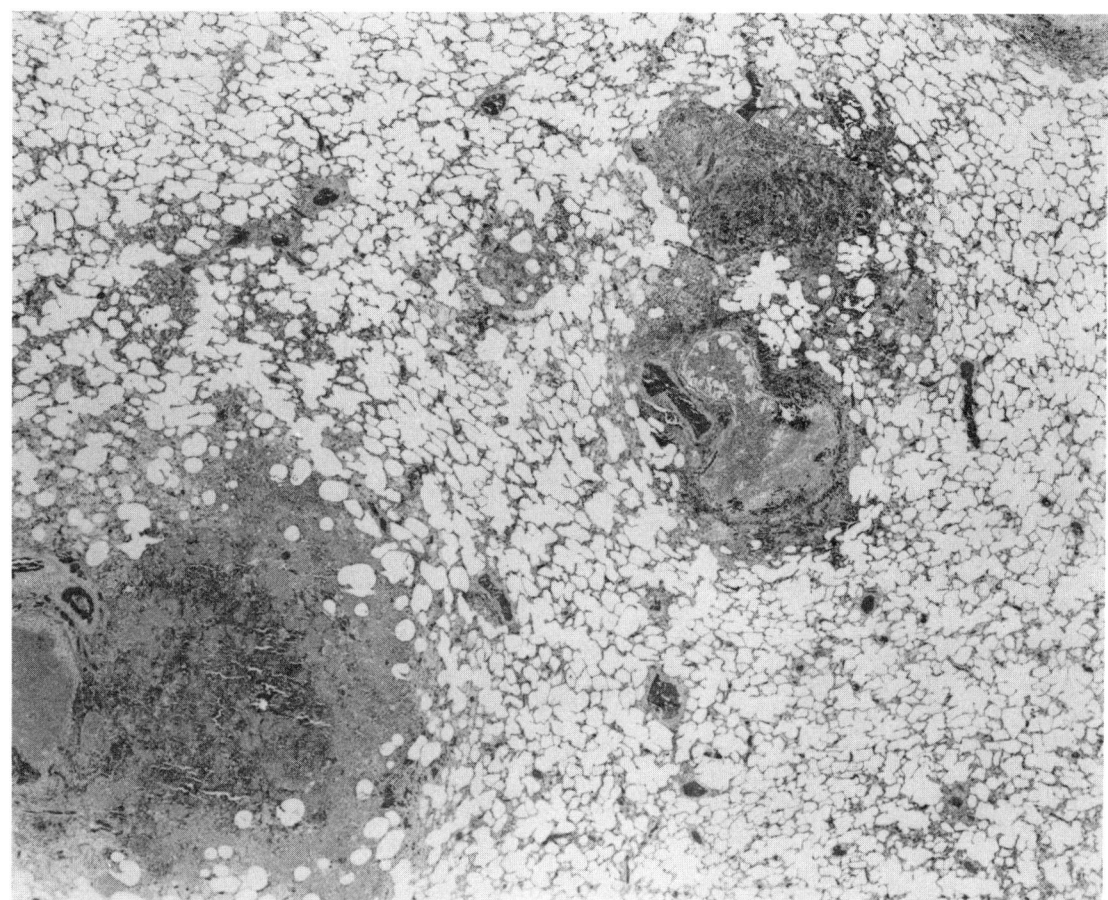

Lobular (Broncho) pneumonia

Figures 8–6 and 8–7. Photomicrographs of lung.

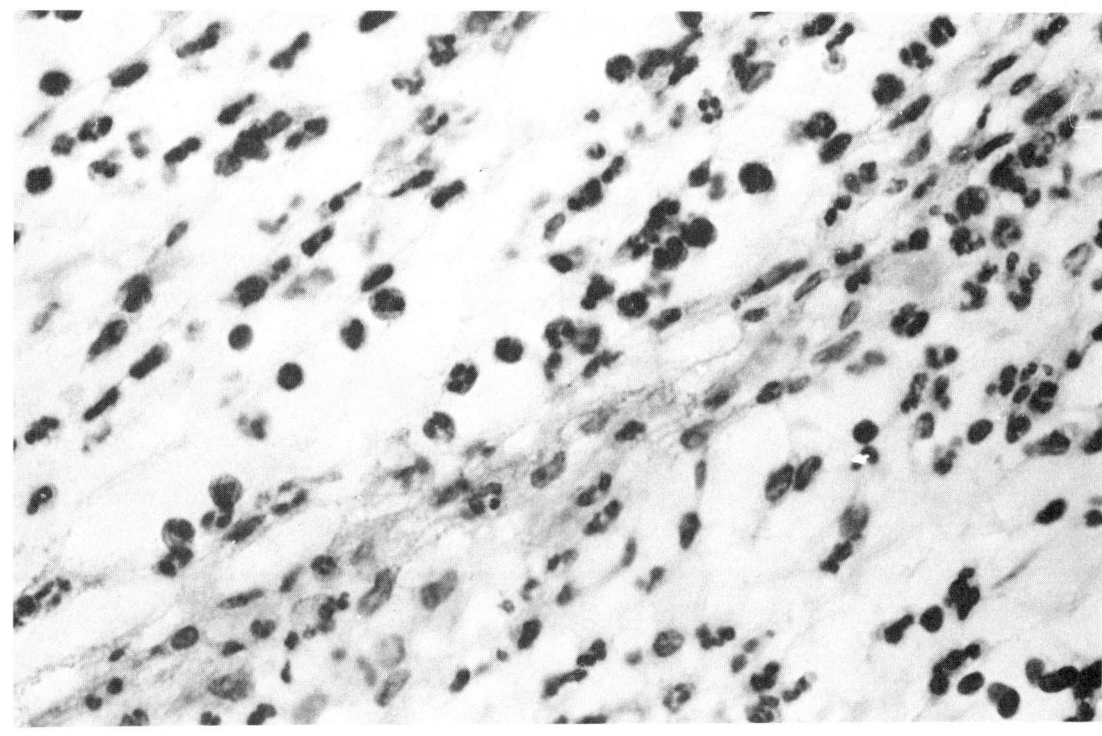

16. The characteristic microscopic feature of this process is

    (A) malignant gland-forming cells
    (B) ferruginous bodies
    (C) peribronchial and bronchial neutrophilic inflammation
    (D) giant cell granulomas
    (E) malignant squamous cells

17. Which is most likely outcome of the process?

    (A) pancreatitis
    (B) complete resolution with no residual abnormalities
    (C) widespread calcification
    (D) partial resolution with some permanent damage to bronchi and bronchioles
    (E) gangrene

Questions 18 through 21. Refer to Figures 8–8 and 8–9.

18. Which is the most appropriate description of Figures 8–8 and 8–9?

    (A) diffuse interstitial pneumonia
    (B) lobar pneumonia
    (C) lobular (broncho) pneumonia
    (D) abscesses
    (E) chronic granulomatous disease

19. Which is the most likely causative agent?

    (A) adenoviruses
    (B) *Mycobacterium tuberculosis* (tubercle bacillus)
    (C) mixed aerobic and anaerobic pyogenic bacteria
    (D) asbestos particles
    (E) *Mycoplasma pneumoniae*

20. What is the most likely predisposing event?

    (A) inhalation of asbestos material
    (B) aspiration of infected material into the respiratory tract or septicemia
    (C) opportunistic infection with *Mycoplasma pneumoniae*
    (D) pneumoconiosis
    (E) idiopathic pulmonary fibrosis

21. Which of the following events is LEAST likely to occur?

    (A) empyema
    (B) brain abscess
    (C) focal scar formation
    (D) complete resolution
    (E) abscess formation in the pleural cavity

Questions 22 through 25. Refer to Figures 8–10 and 8–11.

22. The process demonstrated is

    (A) postmortem blood clot
    (B) thrombotic occlusion
    (C) acute inflammation
    (D) chronic inflammation
    (E) tumor embolus

23. The most probable outcome of this process is

    (A) acute suppurative inflammation
    (B) chronic granulomatous inflammation
    (C) metastatic spread of tumor cells
    (D) infarction of tissue distal to the obstruction
    (E) dissolution and disappearance of the blood clot

24. The extent and final outcome of this process depends on all of the following EXCEPT

    (A) degree of occlusion
    (B) whether the vessel is an end-artery type
    (C) state of collateral circulation
    (D) osmolality
    (E) state of tissue oxygenation before occlusion

25. Predisposing factors include all of the following EXCEPT

    (A) thrombocytopenia
    (B) damage to intima of vessel wall
    (C) alterations of blood flow
    (D) hypercoagulable state
    (E) stasis of blood

Questions 26 through 29. Refer to Figures 8–12 and 8–13.

26. The pathologic process is best described as

    (A) hyperplasia of the epithelium
    (B) granulomatous inflammation
    (C) malignant neoplasm
    (D) benign neoplasm
    (E) acute suppurative inflammation

27. The microscopic picture would suggest

    (A) ulcerative colitis
    (B) Crohn's disease of the colon
    (C) adenocarcinoma of the colon
    (D) adenomatous polyp of the colon
    (E) amebic dysentery

28. Which is LEAST likely to occur if this process is left untreated?

    (A) resolution with healing
    (B) ulceration
    (C) metastases
    (D) hemorrhage
    (E) obstruction

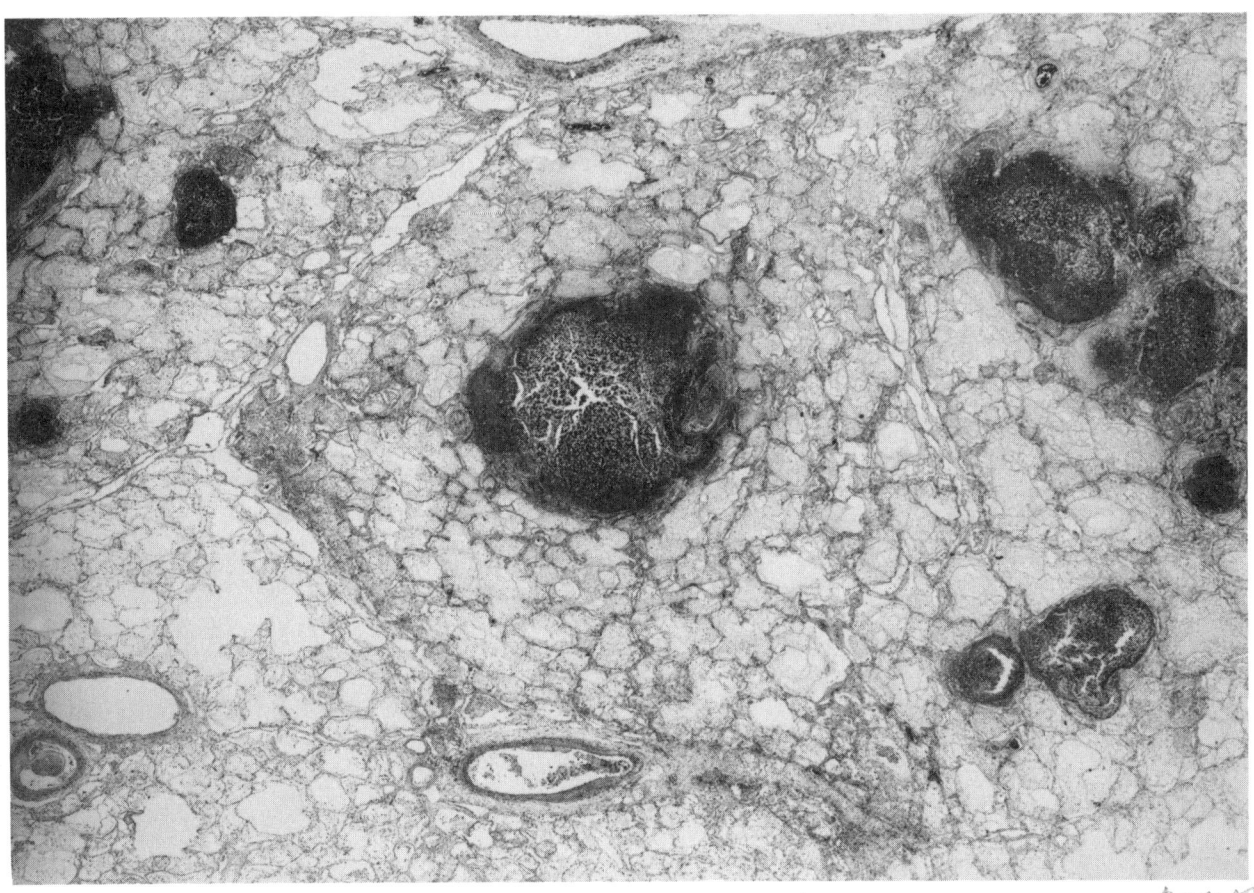

Figures 8–8 and 8–9. Low-power and high-power photomicrographs of lung tissue with several discrete solid areas.

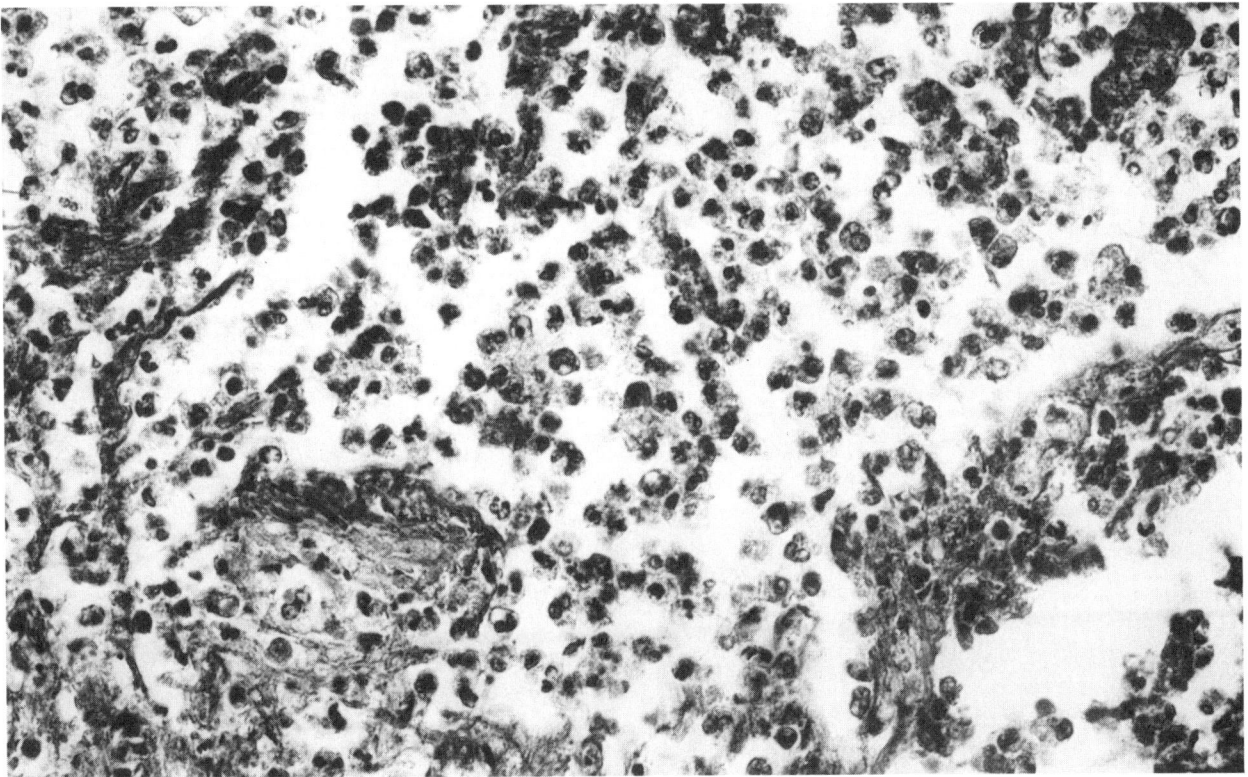

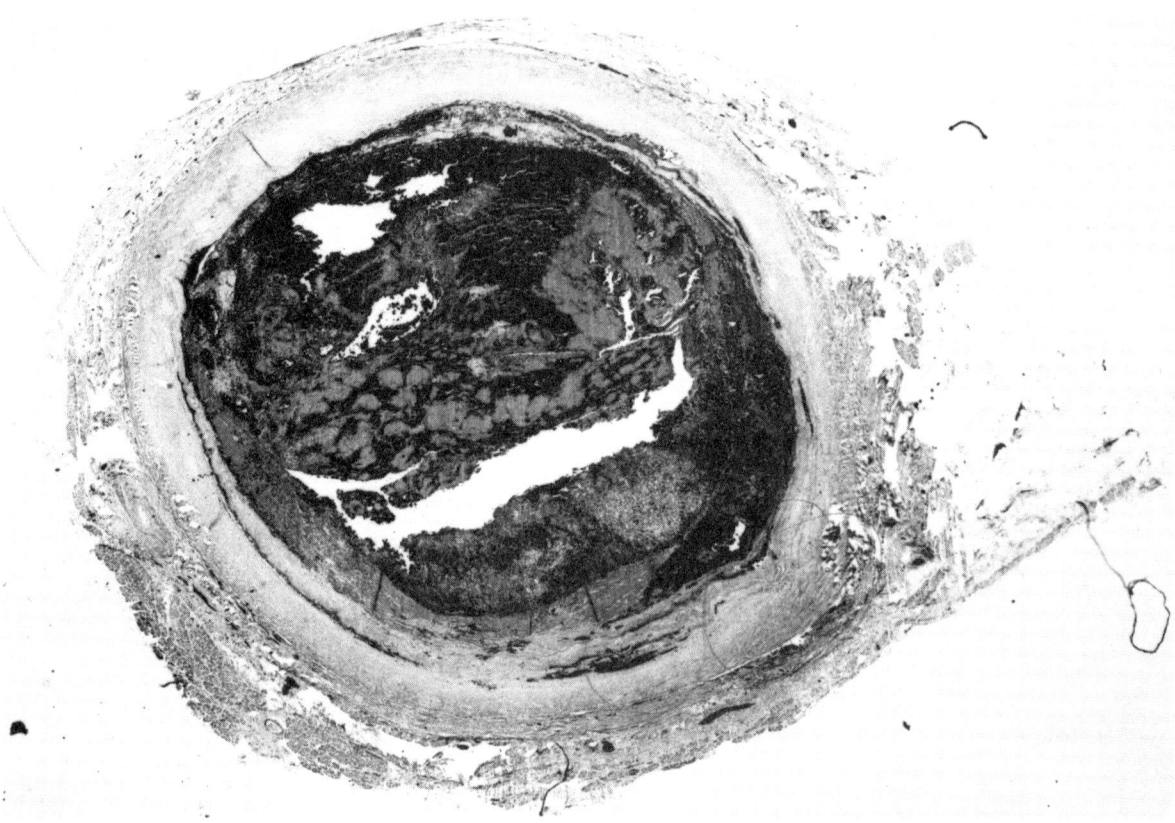

Figures 8–10 and 8–11. The low-power photomicrograph shows blood vessels with filled lumen. The high-power photomicrograph focuses on the occluded material and the adjacent vessel wall.

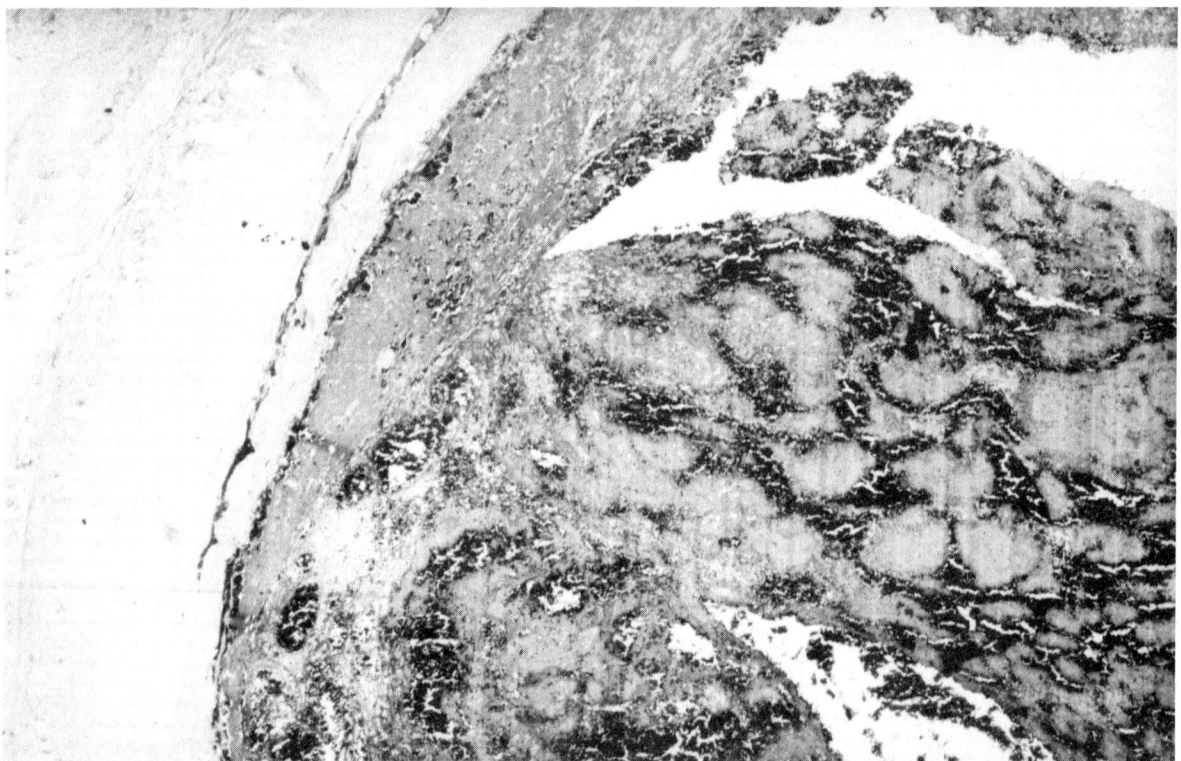

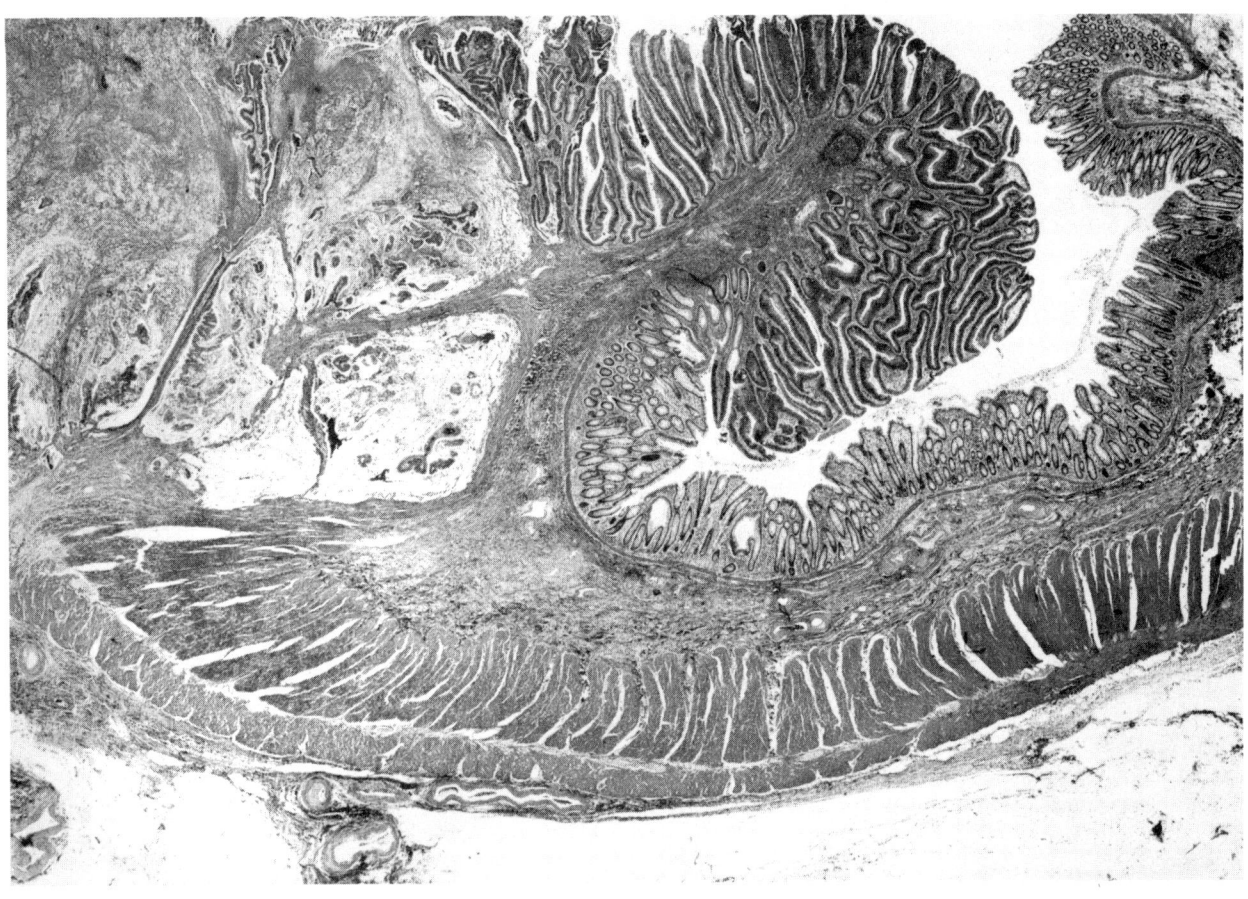

Figures 8–12 and 8–13. The gross specimen is a colon that has been opened. The photomicrograph is a representative section of the lesion.

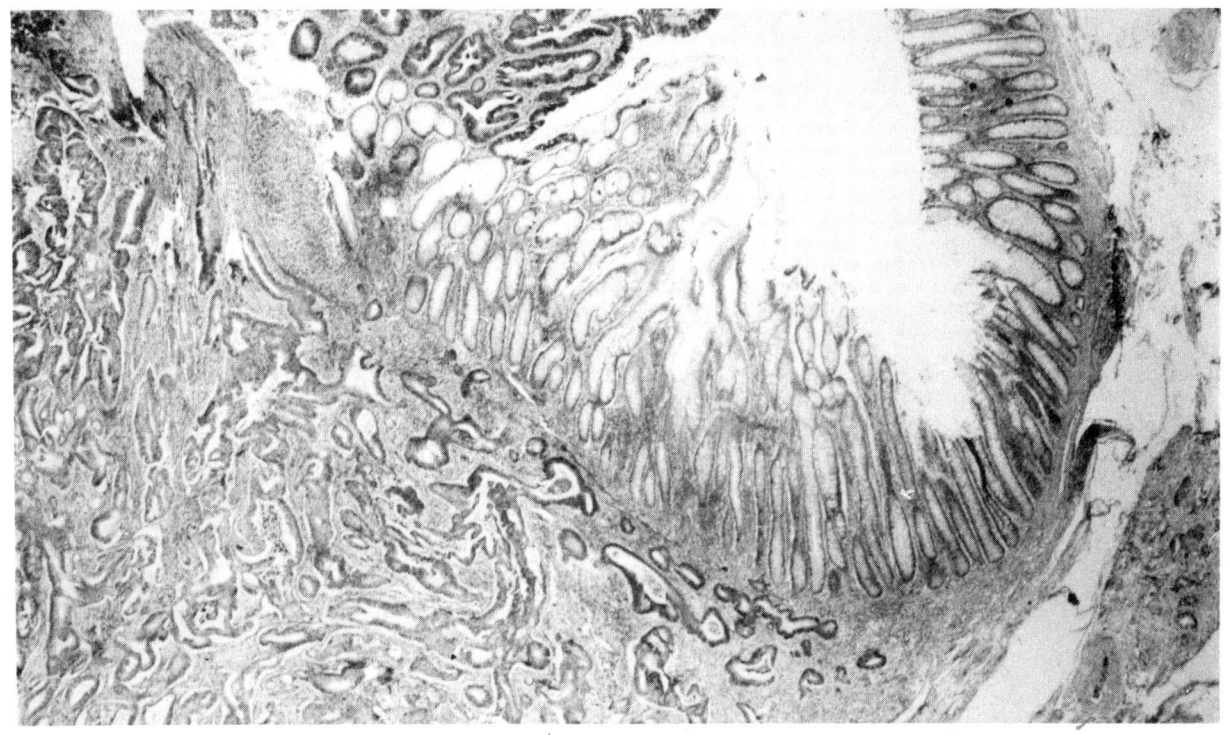

29. Which statement concerning this process is FALSE?

    (A) more often seen in patients over 45 years of age
    (B) arises from gland-forming epithelium
    (C) associated with relatively low-fiber diets
    (D) more common in developed countries
    (E) considered a benign condition

Questions 30 through 33. Refer to Figures 8–14 and 8–15.

30. Which of the following best describes the condition illustrated?

    (A) pulmonary infarct
    (B) lung abscess
    (C) malignant tumor
    (D) benign tumor
    (E) granuloma

31. The microscopic appearance most suggests

    (A) pulmonary infarct
    (B) lung abscess
    (C) epidermoid carcinoma
    (D) adenoma of the bronchus
    (E) tuberculosis

32. Likely complications of this process include all of the following EXCEPT

    (A) pneumonia distal to obstruction
    (B) ulceration
    (C) metastases
    (D) hemorrhage
    (E) spontaneous resolution

33. Which is the most likely etiologic factor?

    (A) low-fiber diet
    (B) hypercoagulate state
    (C) sickle cell anemia
    (D) cigarette smoking
    (E) bacterial infection

Questions 34 through 37. Refer to Figures 8–16 and 8–17.

34. Which of the following best describes the lesion depicted?

    (A) malignant tumor of the breast
    (B) fat necrosis
    (C) benign tumor of the breast
    (D) abscess of the breast
    (E) granuloma

35. The microscopic appearance is most characteristic of

    (A) adenocarcinoma of the breast
    (B) fibroadenoma of the breast
    (C) fat necrosis
    (D) duct obstruction with abscess formation
    (E) tuberculous mastitis

36. Which of the following is the single most important prognostic variable for the depicted process?

    (A) status of progesterone receptors
    (B) status of estrogen receptors
    (C) overexpression of oncogene C-erb
    (D) stage of disease
    (E) high proliferative index

37. Which item is most likely to be associated with this condition?

    (A) low-fat diet
    (B) male sex
    (C) similar condition in older female relatives
    (D) oriental ancestry
    (E) multiparity, late menarche, and early menopause

Questions 38 through 40. Refer to Figures 8–18 and 8–19.

38. Which of the following is the most appropriate description of the condition?

    (A) ectopic pregnancy
    (B) benign tumors of the uterus
    (C) malignant primary tumor of the uterus
    (D) metastatic malignant tumors
    (E) congenital muscular deformity of the uterus

39. Which is the best diagnostic term to describe these lesions?

    (A) benign leiomyomas
    (B) leiomyosarcomas
    (C) adenocarcinoma of endometrium
    (D) squamous cell carcinoma of the cervix
    (E) teratoma of the uterus

40. Which statement concerning this process is FALSE?

    (A) they are the most common neoplasm of the female genital tract
    (B) they are composed of smooth muscle cells from the uterine myometrium
    (C) there is a high incidence of malignant transformation
    (D) they may occur singly or in multiples
    (E) they are benign tumors

Questions: 29–40   159

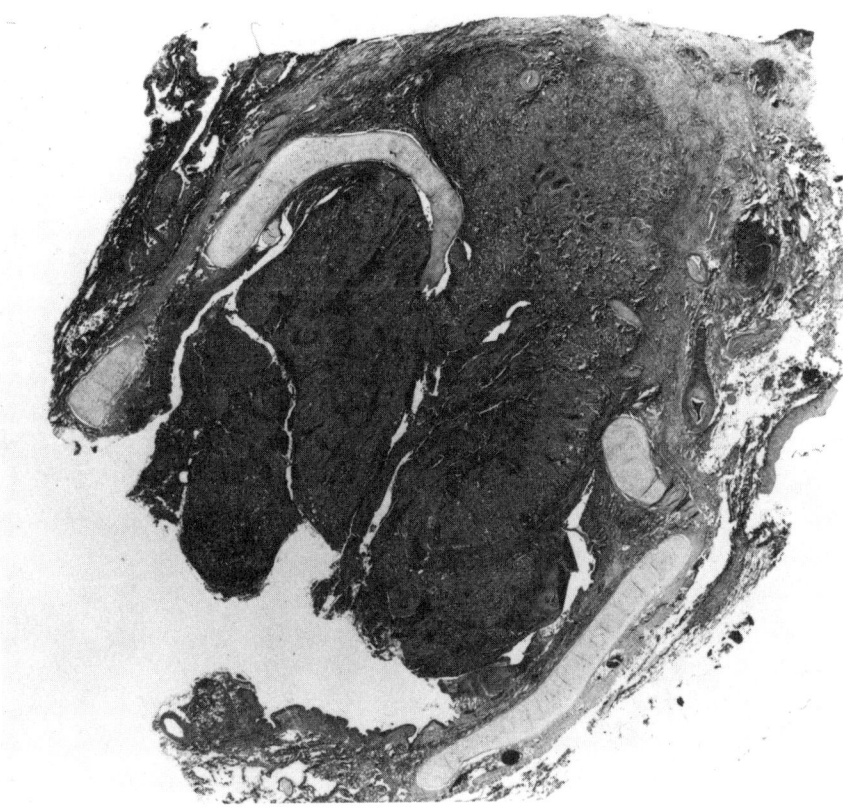

Figures 8–14 and 8–15. The low-power photomicrograph is of a lung, and the high-power photomicrograph is of a section of the abnormality demonstrated. —Bronchogenic Ca

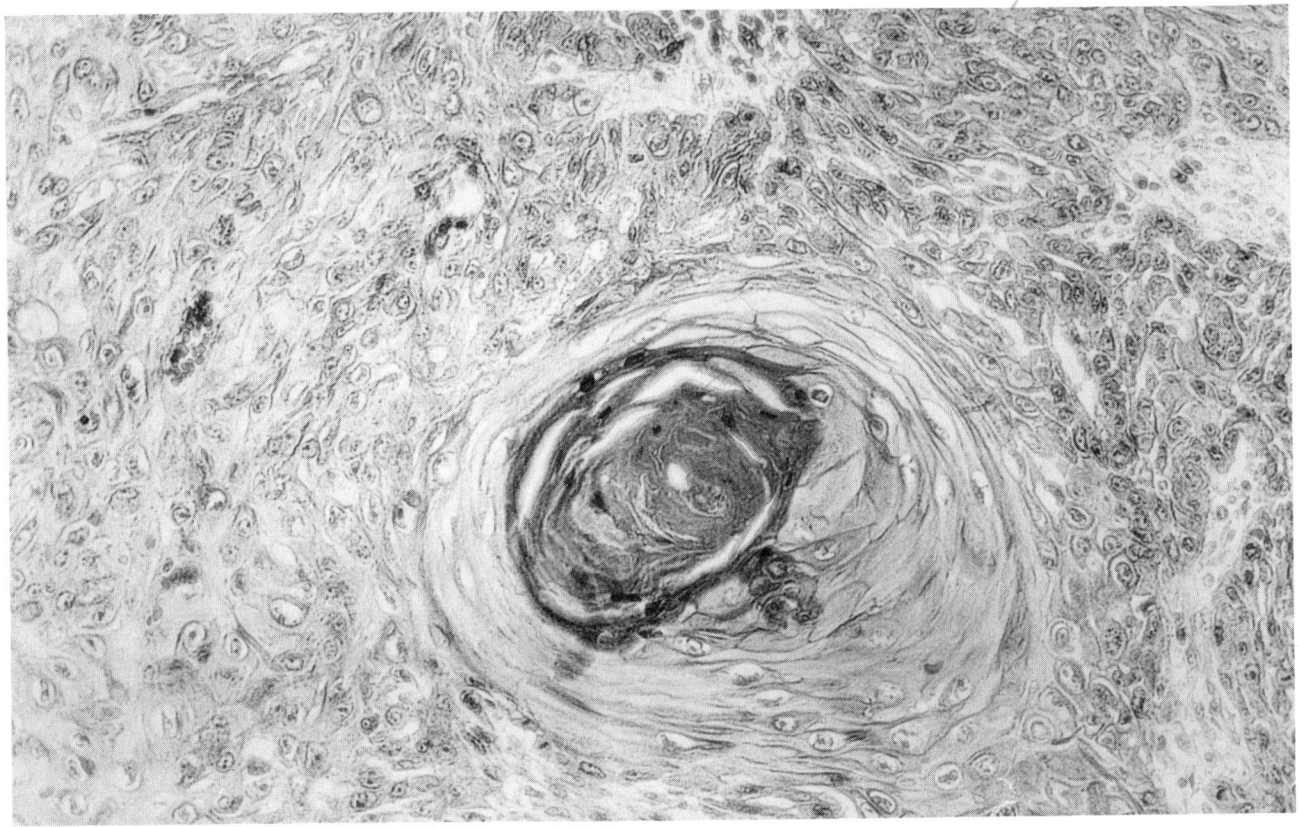

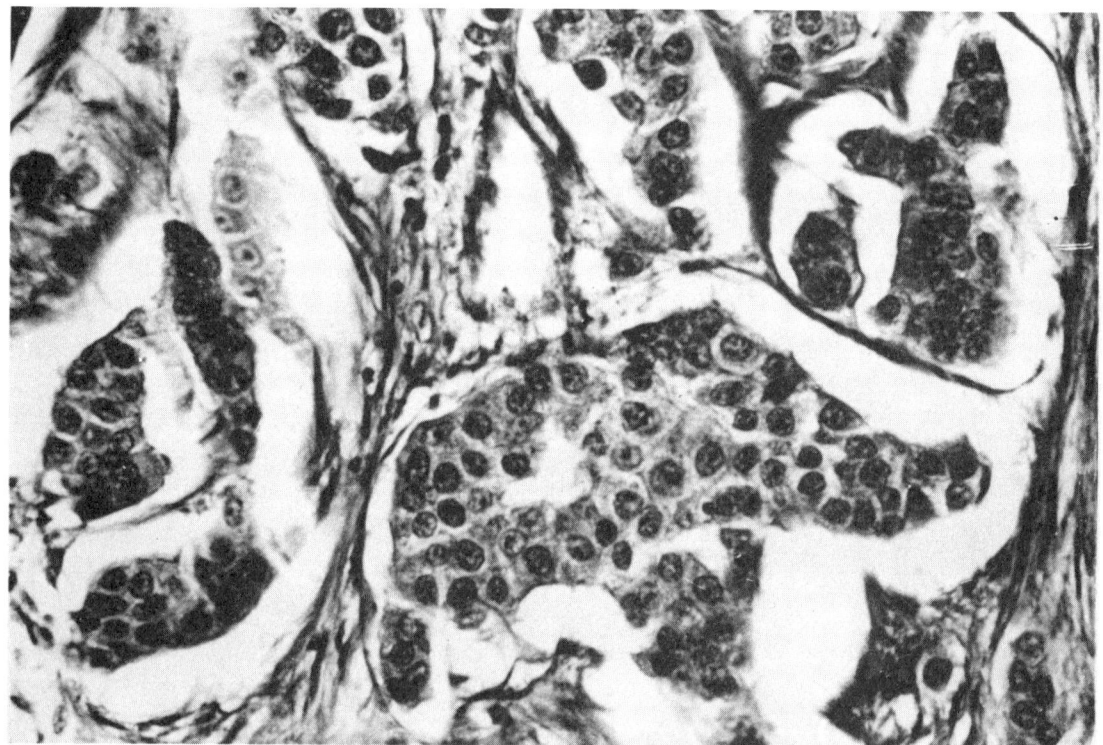

Figures 8–16 and 8–17. The specimen is from a female breast removed surgically for the condition shown. The photomicrograph shows the histologic features of the lesion.

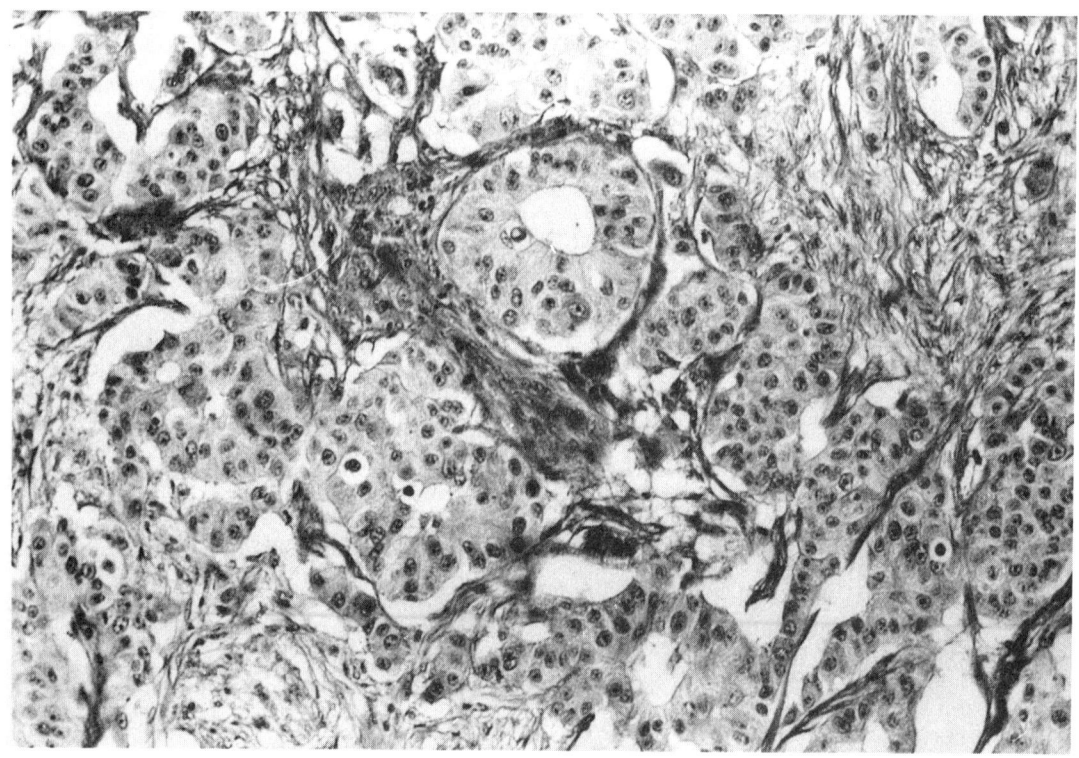

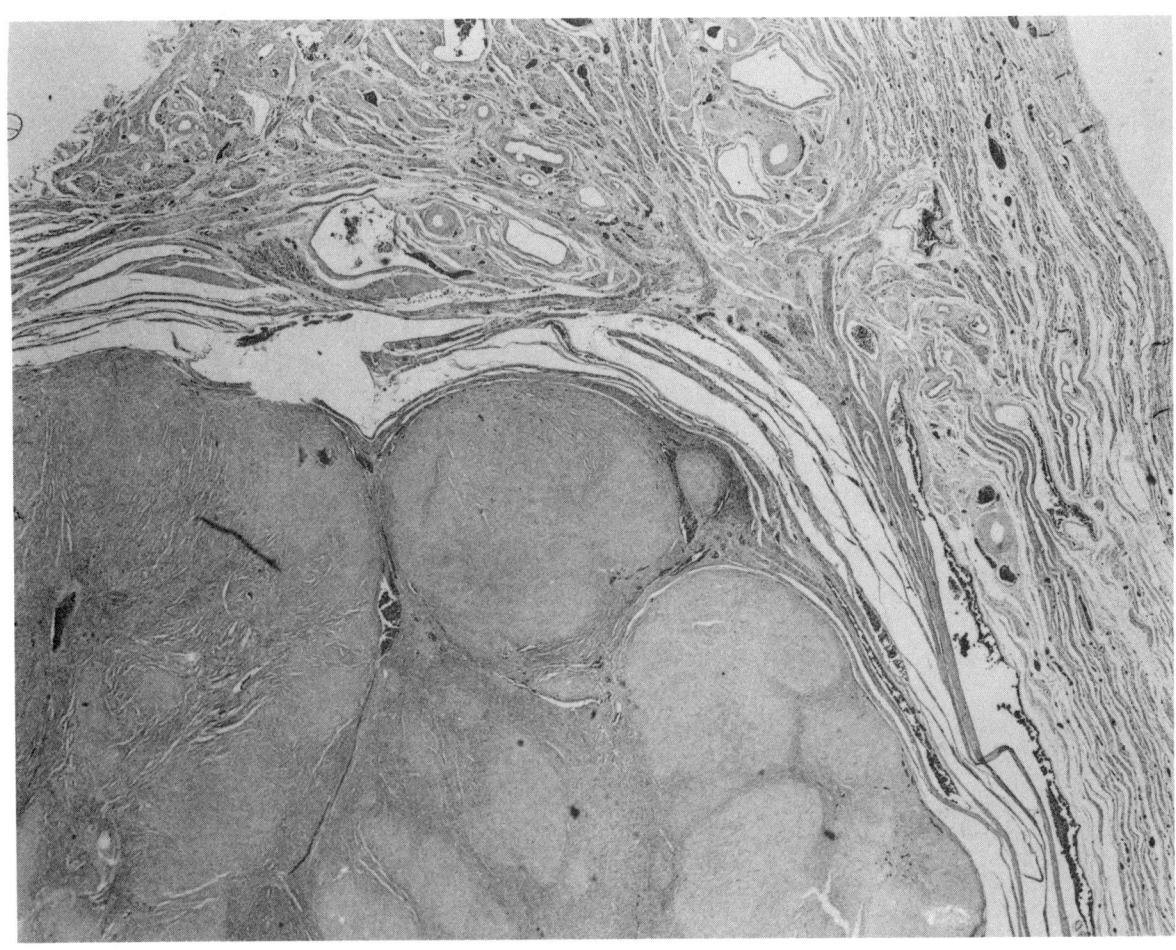

Figures 8–18 and 8–19. A uterus contains multiple, discrete, firm, white nodules. The photomicrograph shows the histologic picture of the lesion.

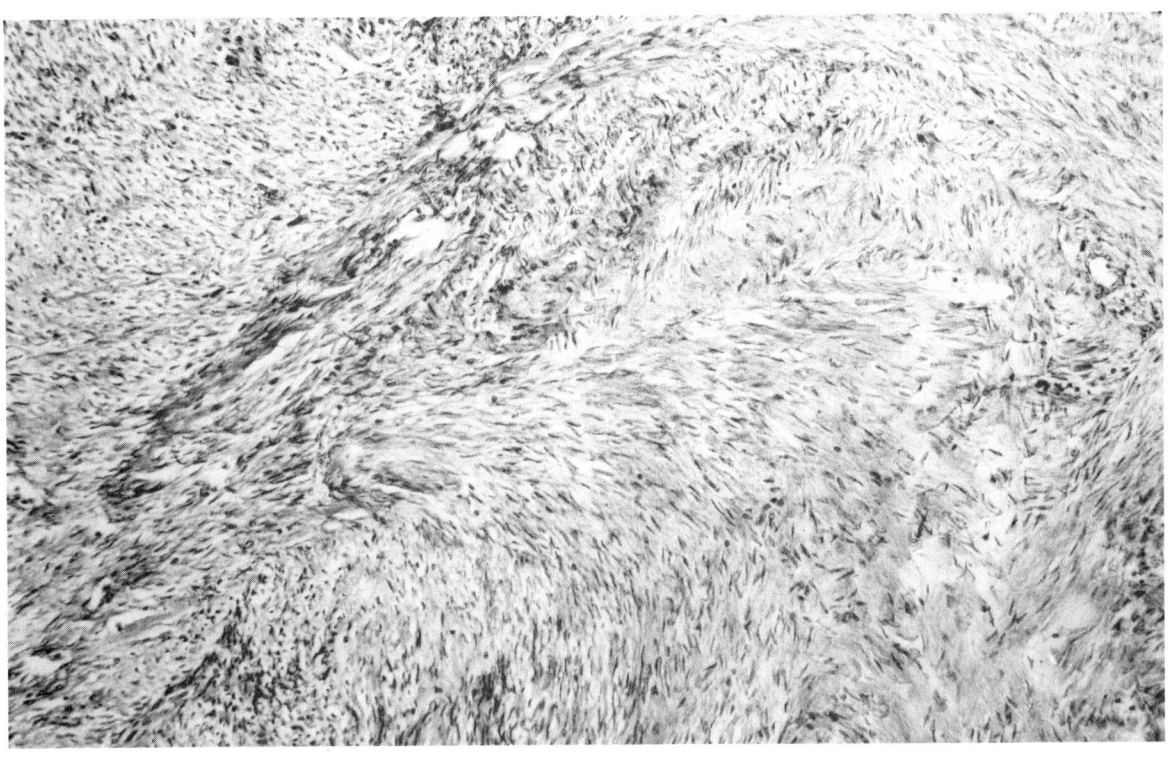

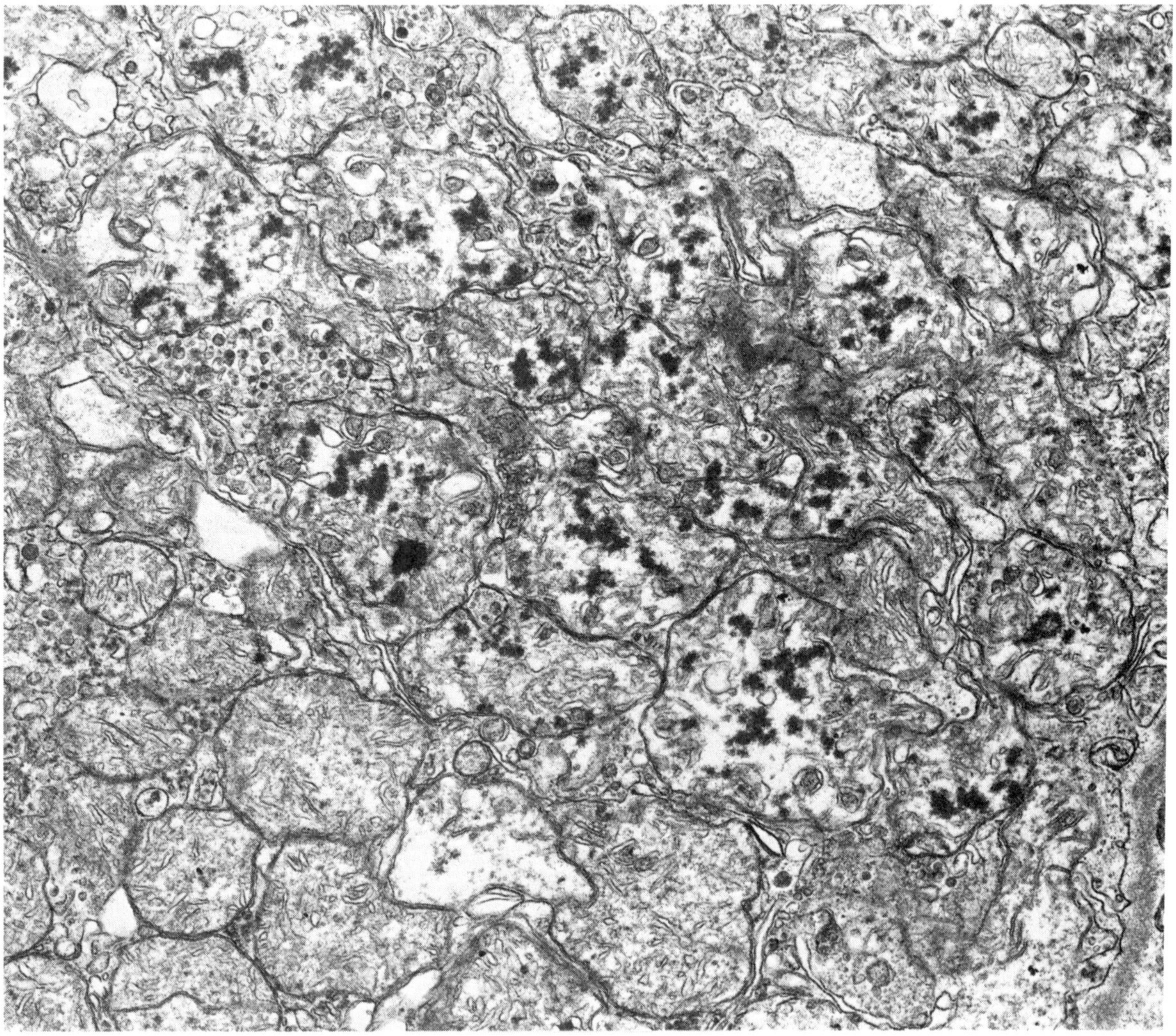

Figure 8–20. Electron micrograph of the cytoplasm of part of a proximal tubule cell of the kidney.

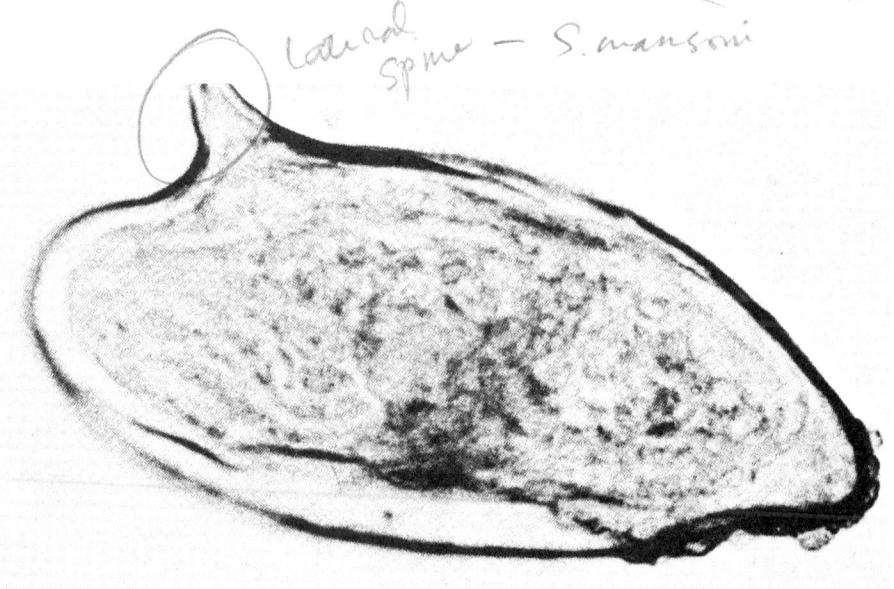

Figure 8–21. Egg seen by microscopy in stool sample.

Questions 41 through 44. Refer to Figure 8–20.

41. The floccular, darkly staining material represents

    (A) apoptosis
    (B) karyolysis
    (C) swollen damaged mitochondria
    (D) viral inclusions
    (E) karyorrhexis

42. Which of the following best describes the condition depicted?

    (A) lipid peroxidation with cell membrane damage
    (B) damage to lysosomes, with cell swelling
    (C) decreased respiration of mitochondria with flocculation
    (D) clumping of chromatin
    (E) damage to endoplasmic reticulum

43. The features are consistent with

    (A) cytoplasmic cloudy swelling
    (B) early ischemic damage or poisoning with mercuric chloride
    (C) cytomegalovirus infection
    (D) saponification
    (E) no alterations present

44. Which of the following best represents the mechanism involved?

    (A) toxic poisoning of the lysosomal system of the cell
    (B) viral transformation of cellular DNA
    (C) abnormality of lipid storage
    (D) disruption of oxidative phosphorylation in the mitochondria
    (E) failure of organogenesis

Questions 45 through 48. Refer to Figure 8–21.

45. The egg pictured is from which parasite?

    (A) *Trichinella spiralis*
    (B) *Trichuris trichiura*
    (C) *Schistosoma mansoni*
    (D) *Ancylostoma duodenale*
    (E) *Ascaris lumbricoides*

46. Which of the following is the most frequent host for the adult forms?

    (A) snail
    (B) fish
    (C) human
    (D) mosquito
    (E) dog

47. The intermediate host in the parasite life cycle is a

    (A) tick
    (B) cow
    (C) fly
    (D) snail
    (E) mosquito

48. Which statement concerning this disorder is FALSE?

    (A) very rarely causes blood loss and anemia
    (B) adult male and female worms copulate in the human host
    (C) common disease infecting millions of people worldwide
    (D) depending on species, the large intestine or the bladder is the site of lodgment of eggs
    (E) cercarial larvae found in contaminated water infects human hosts by penetration of the skin

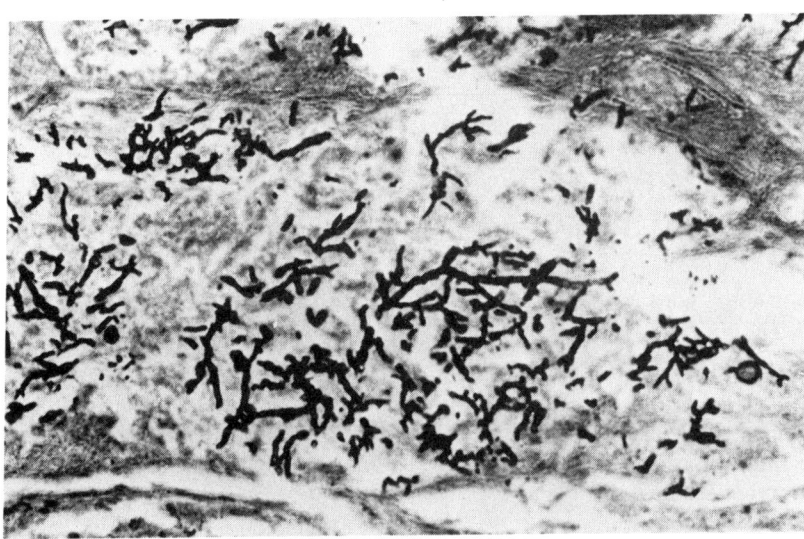

Figure 8–22. Photomicrograph of an area of consolidation in the lung.

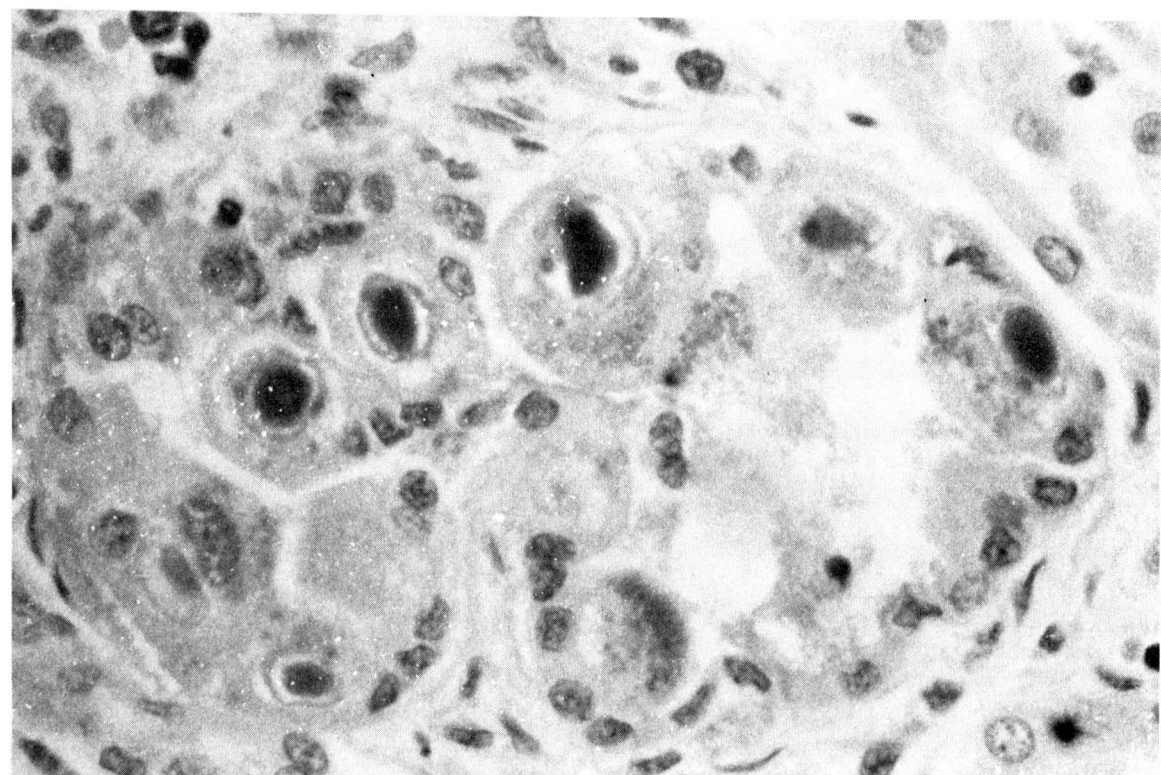

Figure 8–23. Young adult male with acquired immune deficiency syndrome (AIDS). An autopsy showed the changes in the renal tubules shown in the photomicrograph.

Questions 49 through 51. Refer to Figure 8–22.

49. The organisms shown are

    (A) bacteria
    (B) rickettsiae
    (C) fungi
    (D) viruses
    (E) protozoa

50. The organisms depicted are

    (A) Staphylococci
    (B) *Rickettsia burnettii*
    (C) *Aspergillus*
    (D) Epstein-Barr virus
    (E) *Entamoeba histolytica*

51. Which of the following most appropriately describes this condition?

    (A) skin is usual portal of entry
    (B) viral organism of high virulence
    (C) rarely involves lungs or blood vessels
    (D) opportunistic infection seen most commonly in immunocompromised hosts
    (E) only occurs in black males

Questions 52 through 55. Refer to Figure 8–23.

52. Figure 8–23 shows

    (A) storage material
    (B) viral inclusion bodies
    (C) fungal infection
    (D) amyloidosis
    (E) fatty infiltration

53. The most likely cause of the disease is

    (A) chemical poisons
    (B) heredity
    (C) malnutrition
    (D) immune deficiency
    (E) hyperimmune state

54. The clinical and pathologic features best fit

    (A) ganglioside storage disease
    (B) glycogen storage disease
    (C) cytomegalovirus infection
    (D) systemic candidiasis
    (E) thiamine deficiency

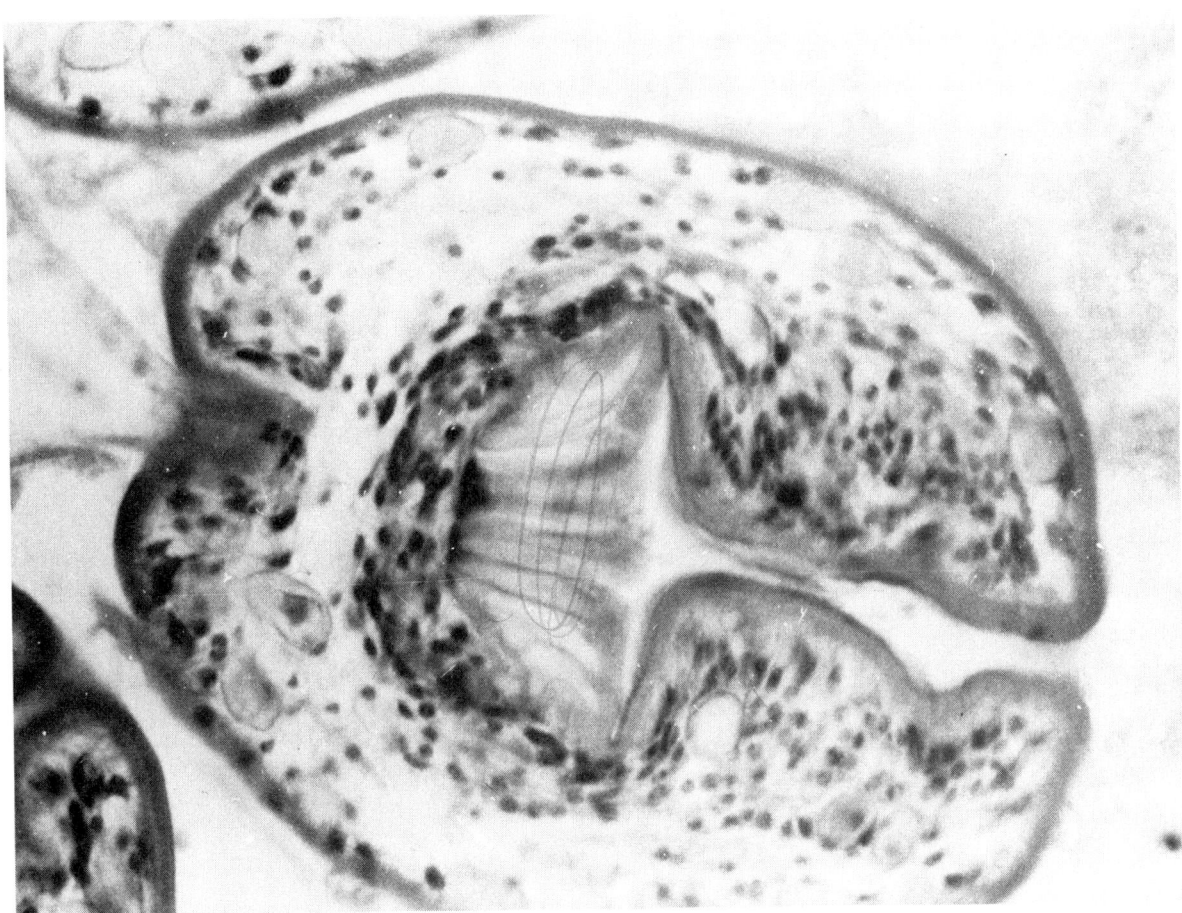

Figure 8-24. A 50-year-old male had a hepatic lobe resected because of a large cyst. The photomicrograph depicts part of the content of the cyst diagnostic of this condition.

55. Which statement concerning this disorder is TRUE?

    (A) epidemic form most common
    (B) seen only in tropics
    (C) never seen in renal transplantation or AIDS
    (D) most commonly seen in immunologically compromised hosts
    (E) bacterial organism is etiologic agent

Questions 56 through 59. Refer to Figure 8-24.

56. The photomicrograph shows a

    (A) group of malignant cells
    (B) colony of bacteria
    (C) portion of a tapeworm
    (D) distorted bile duct
    (E) nidus of future calculus

57. The most likely cause of the cyst is

    (A) hydatid disease
    (B) pyogenic abscess from portal pyemia
    (C) bile duct dilatation
    (D) stasis
    (E) necrosis within the center of a tumor

58. The disease is usually caused by

    (A) congenital abnormalities
    (B) transmission via infected feces
    (C) gallstones
    (D) bacteremia or appendicitis
    (E) unknown etiology

59. Which is a TRUE statement about the depicted disorder?

    (A) disease is always congenital
    (B) sheep are never a secondary host
    (C) humans are the most frequent primary host
    (D) dogs are the most frequent primary host
    (E) ova in dog feces are never infective for humans

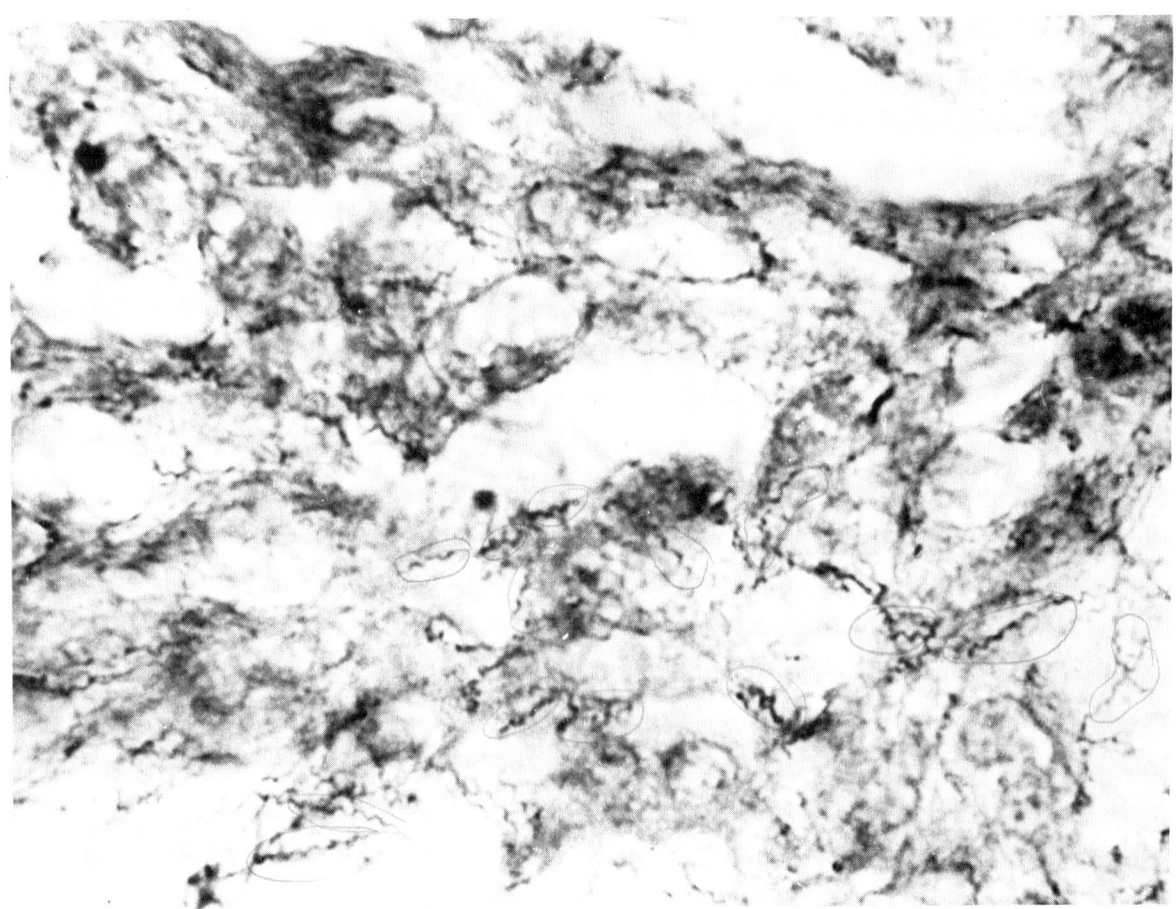

Figure 8–25. Photomicrograph depicting a special stain on a section of a penile ulcer.

Questions 60 through 62. Refer to Figure 8–25.

60. The photomicrograph demonstrates

    (A) gram-positive cocci
    (B) gram-negative bacilli
    (C) *Actinomyces*
    (D) spirochetes
    (E) Donovan bodies

61. The most likely diagnosis is

    (A) chancroid
    (B) granuloma inguinale
    (C) lymphogranuloma venereum
    (D) gonorrhea
    (E) syphilis

62. Which statement is most accurate concerning this disease?

    (A) the organism thrives outside the human body
    (B) the disease is usually transmitted venereally
    (C) the disease is usually transmitted by food contamination
    (D) the organism survives for prolonged periods on dust and debris
    (E) the disease is not seen in sexually active populations

Questions 63 and 64. Refer to Figure 8–26.

63. The photograph demonstrates

    (A) tuberculous pneumonia
    (B) metastatic carcinoma
    (C) disseminated intravascular coagulation
    (D) lung abscess
    (E) pulmonary infarct

64. The source of entry into the lung is

    (A) aspiration of infected material
    (B) infection of contaminated material into the bloodstream
    (C) spread from primary tumor
    (D) penetration injury of lung
    (E) embolism from the deep calf veins

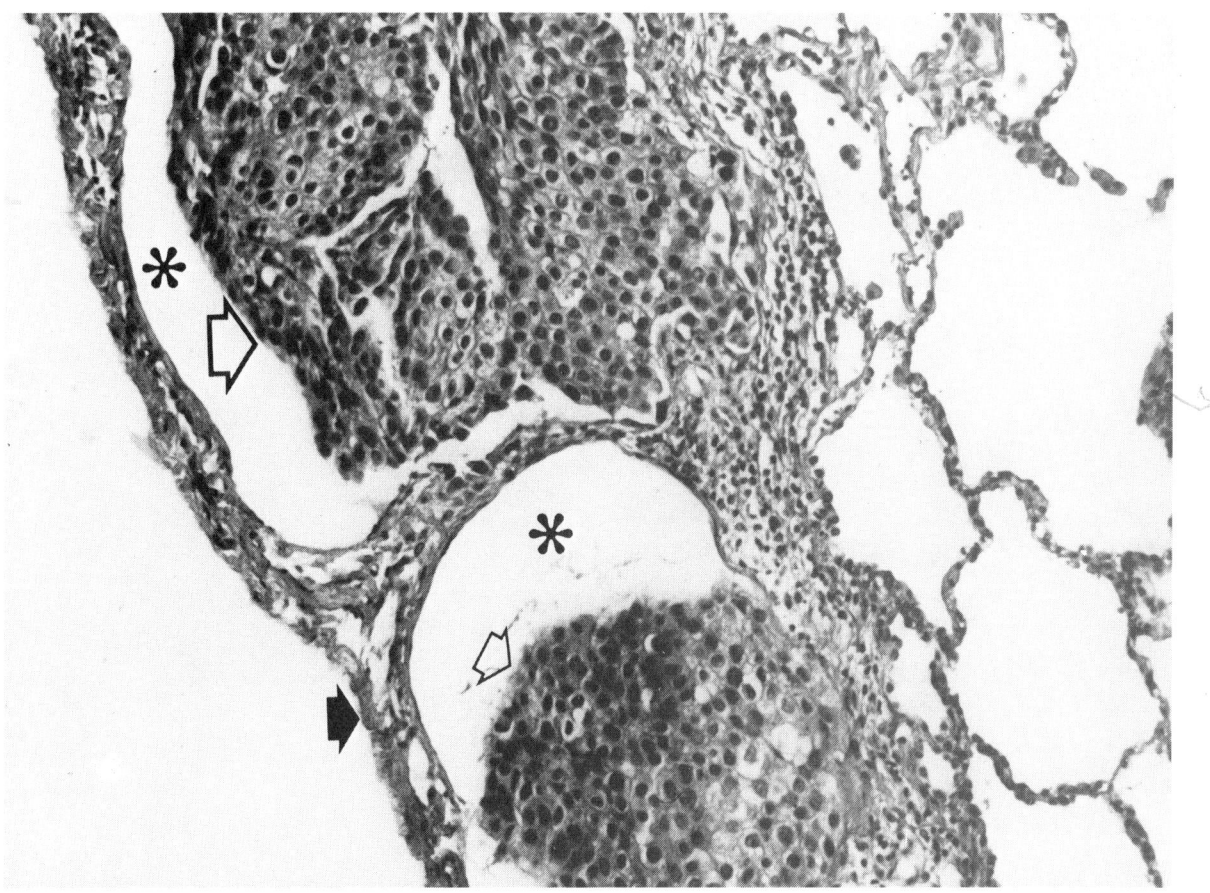

Figure 8–26. Histologic section of the periphery of the lung.

Questions 65 through 68. Refer to Figure 8–27.

65. The process illustrated is best described as

    (A) benign neoplasia
    (B) malignant neoplasia
    (C) healing
    (D) acute suppurative inflammation
    (E) chronic granulomatous inflammation

66. A more precise diagnostic term is

    (A) an osteoid tumor
    (B) osteogenic sarcoma
    (C) healing of fracture
    (D) acute osteomyelitis
    (E) tuberculosis of the bone

67. The dense material extending through the shaft of the bone and continuing onto the periosteal surface is

    (A) osteoid seams in a sarcoma
    (B) hyalinized mature fibrous tissue
    (C) acute suppurative inflammatory exudate
    (D) provisional new bone (callus)
    (E) amyloid

68. Which of the following events is most likely to interfere with proper resolution of the illustrated process?

    (A) high doses of vitamin C
    (B) immobilization of the bone
    (C) foreign material and associated inflammation
    (D) high doses of vitamin D
    (E) high content of calcium in the diet

Questions 69 and 70. Refer to Figures 8–28 and 8–29.

69. Which of the following is the best description of the events illustrated?

    (A) infarction
    (B) lobar pneumonia
    (C) lung abscess
    (D) benign neoplasm
    (E) malignant neoplasm

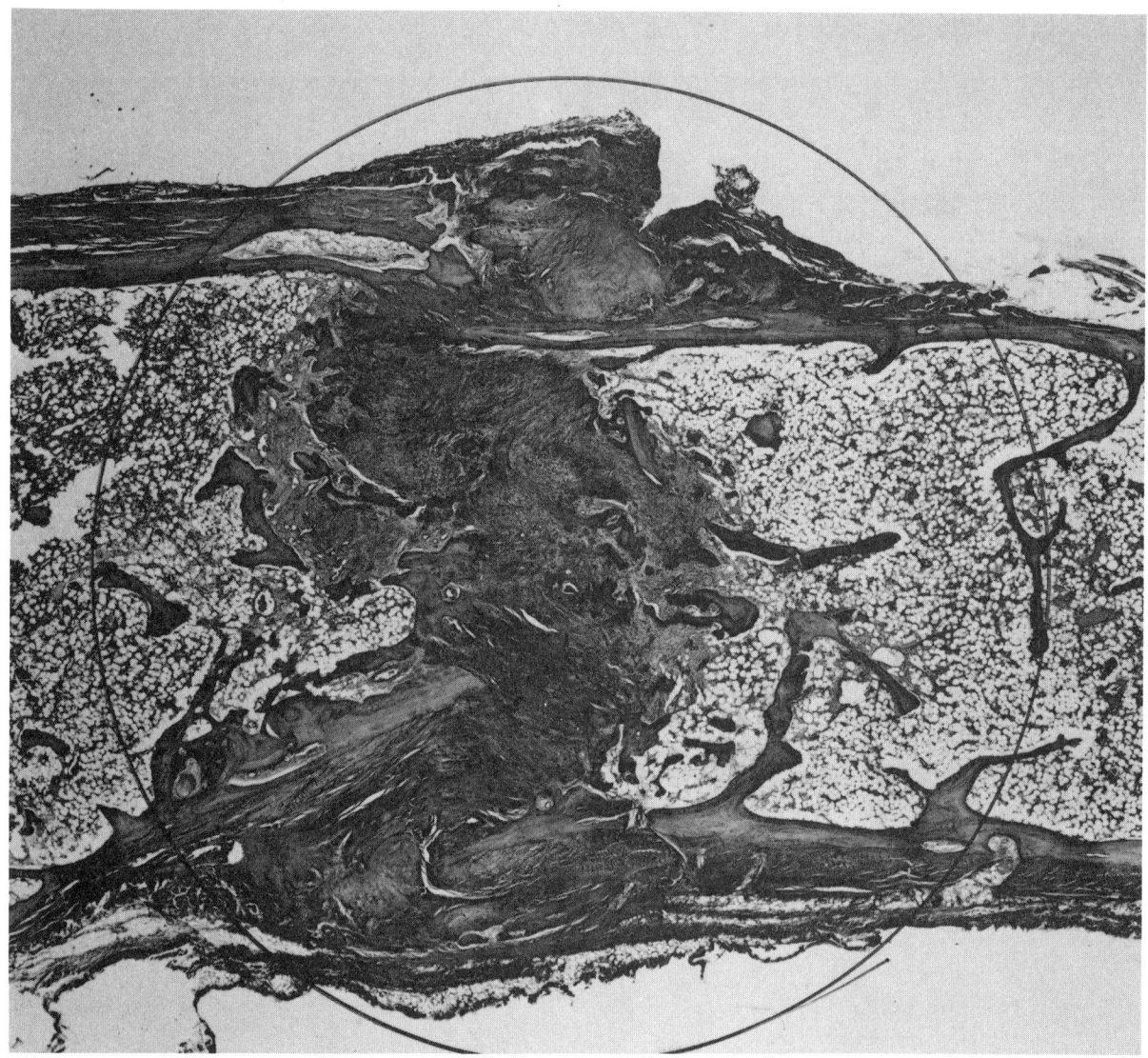

Figure 8–27. Photomicrograph showing section across a long bone.

70. Which of the following is the most likely preceding event?

    (A) cigarette smoking
    (B) asbestos exposure
    (C) deep venous thrombosis with embolus formation
    (D) aspiration of infected materials
    (E) septicemia

Questions 71 through 74. Refer to Figure 8–30.

71. The pale stroma areas are

    (A) metastatic liposarcoma
    (B) lipid accumulation in liver cells
    (C) lipoid granulomas

    (D) viral inclusions in liver cells
    (E) alcoholic hyalin accumulation in liver cells

72. The condition is best described as

    (A) fatty metamorphosis
    (B) hepatocellular carcinoma
    (C) passive venous congestion
    (D) acute viral hepatitis
    (E) miliary tuberculosis of the liver

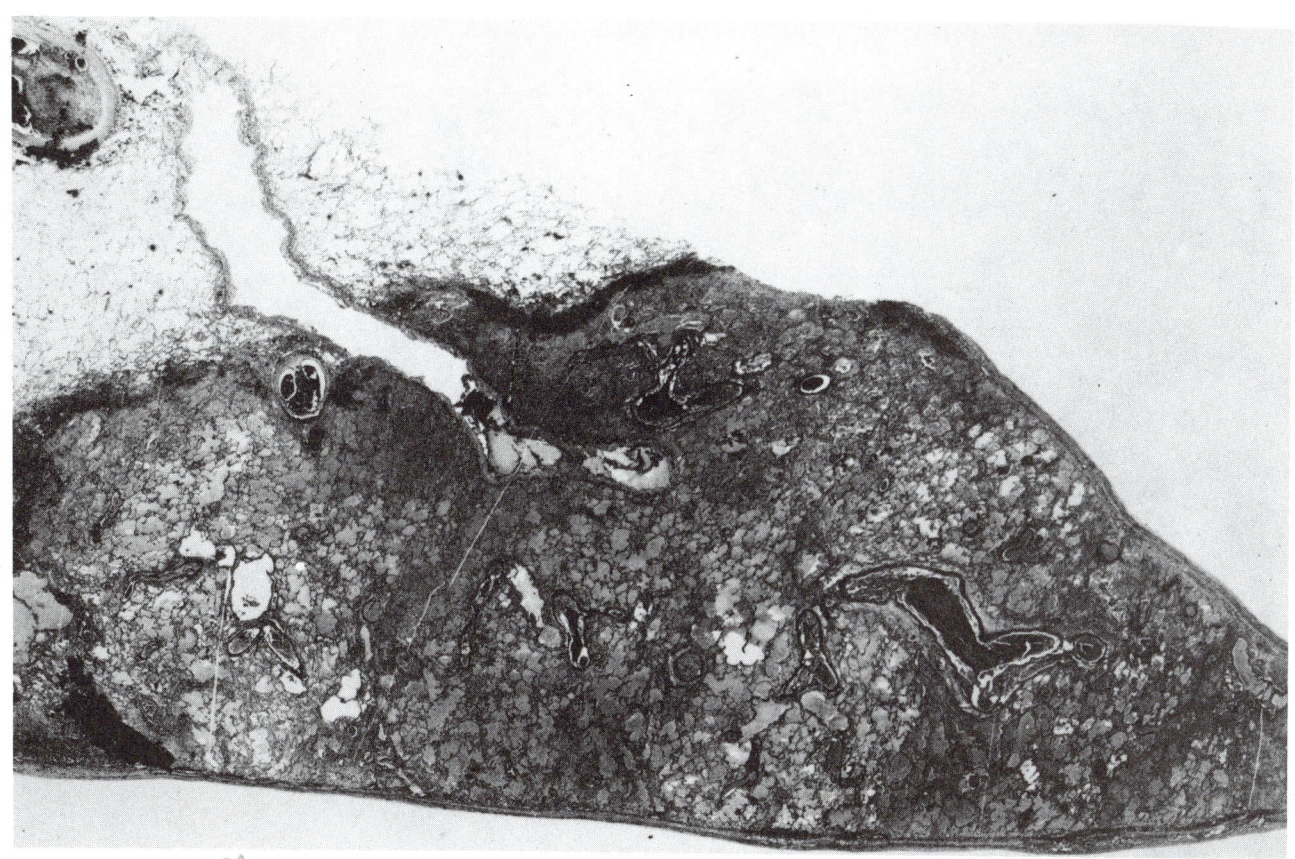

Figures 8–28 and 8–29. A lung shows a form of well-circumscribed consolidation.

INFARCTION   (–) PMN'S

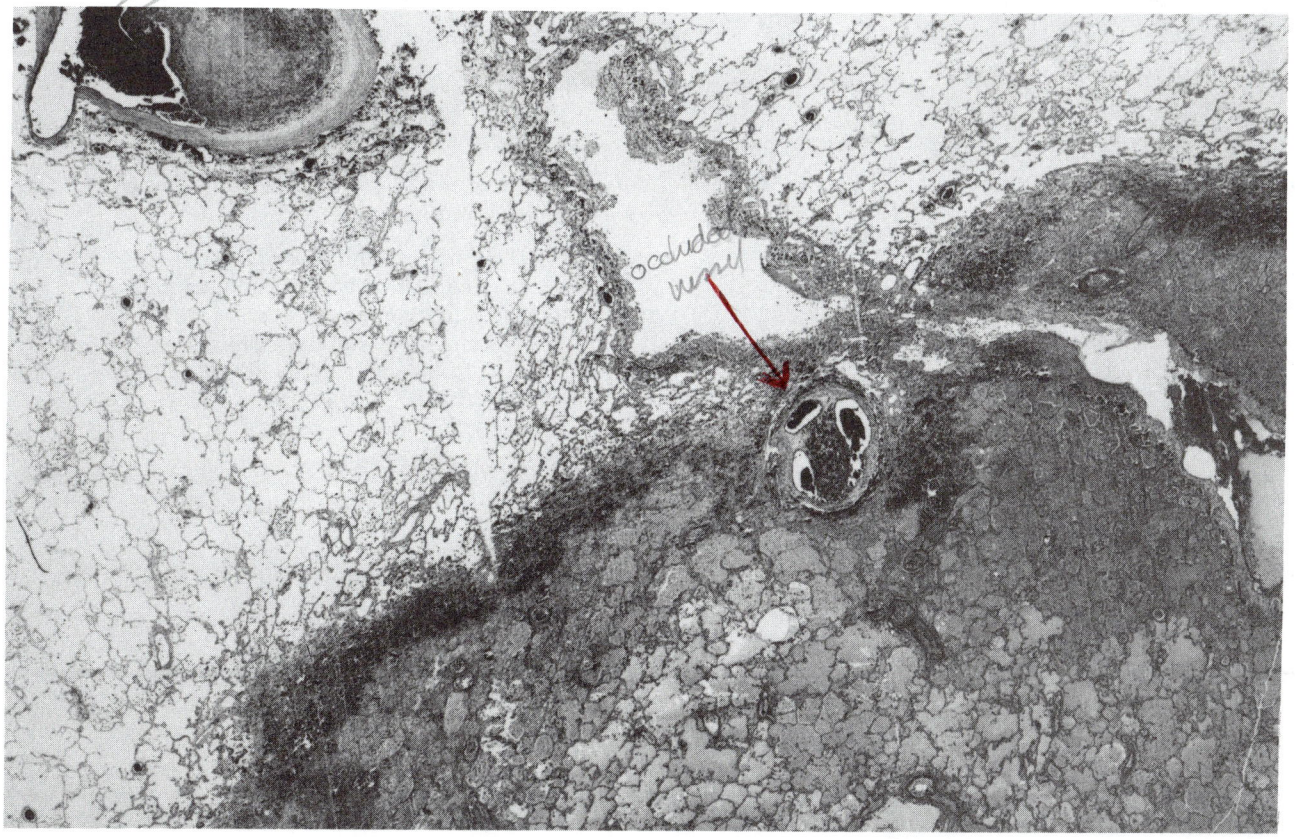

occluded vessel

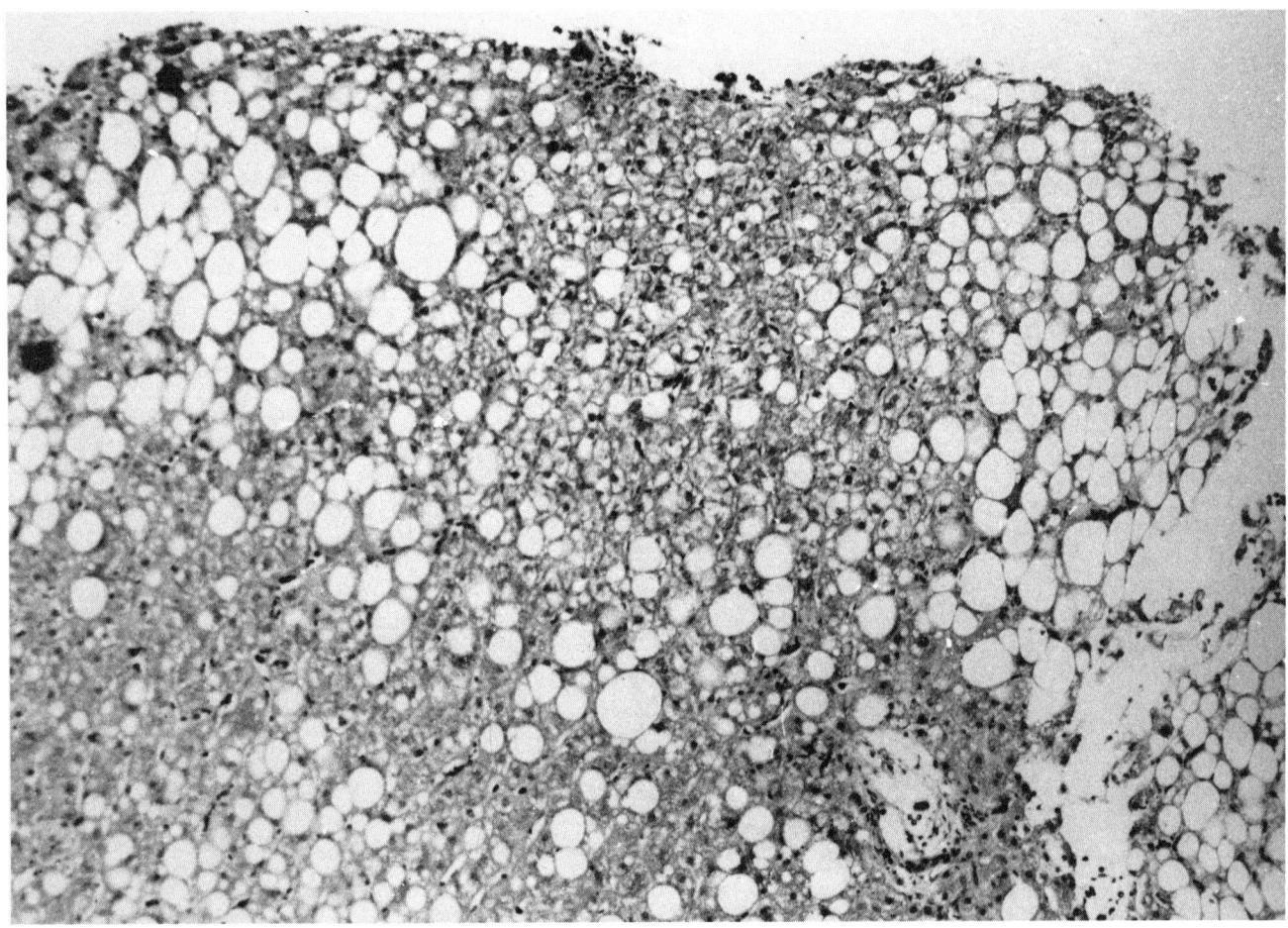

Figure 8-30. Photomicrograph from a liver biopsy.

73. Which one of the following is most likely to produce the depicted changes?

    (A) metastatic carcinoma
    (B) macronodular cirrhosis
    (C) alcoholism
    (D) bile stasis
    (E) miliary tuberculosis

74. Which of the following is FALSE concerning the depicted process?

    (A) there are multiple possible causes
    (B) may be seen in severe malnutrition
    (C) the condition may be seen in children
    (D) the condition is always irreversible
    (E) may be seen in choline deficiency

Answers and Explanations

Figure 8–1 shows a section of stomach with a peptic ulcer.

1. **(B)** Loss of continuity of an epithelial surface is the definition of ulceration. Figure 8–1 illustrates very clearly such a loss of continuity of the epithelium of the gastric mucosa. Therefore, the other listed alternatives are inappropriate. Although atrophic changes may precede or even occur after healing of such an ulcer, in the active stage, there is complete loss of epithelium. *(1:578)*

2. **(B)** The diagnosis that most clearly matches the illustration is peptic ulcer. Hypertrophic gastritis and gastric carcinoma would result in an increase in the amount of cellular material in the epithelium. Intestinal metaplasia of gastric mucosa is not apparent in this case. Although gastric atrophy may occur in the healing phase of a peptic ulcer, congenital gastric atrophy clearly is not applicable in this instance. *(1:578)*

3. **(C)** Peptic ulcers are thought to result from an overproduction of acid and pepsin, with autodigestion and destruction of the mucosa and persistence of the ulcer by the continued effect of such acid and pepsin. Chronic peptic ulcers cause continuous bleeding, often at a relatively low level, that is not apparent clinically but can result in iron deficiency anemia from chronic blood loss. *(1:576–578)*

4. **(C)** The photograph depicts a peptic ulcer, a classic example of the ulcerative inflammation reaction. Chronic peptic ulcers grossly appear as solitary large punched out areas in the gastric mucosa with a smooth surfaced, firm base. The gastric rugae often radiate out from the ulcer bed. Microscopically the ulcer demonstrates necrotic debris, inflammation, fibrin precipitates, and peripheral fibrosis. *(1:578)*

5. **(E)** The potential long-term complications of gastric ulcers include hemorrhage, penetration, perforation, obstruction, and rarely, malignant transformation. Hypertension, pernicious anemia, atrophic gastritis, and gastric leiomyomatosis do not result from gastric peptic ulcers. *(1:578–579)*

Figures 8–2 and 8–3 show gross and microscopic views of an appendix with acute inflammation, or acute appendicitis.

6. **(C)** With acute appendicitis, the inflammation extends through the wall of the appendix where there are many polymorphonuclear leukocytes that break down tissue, often with apparent exudate on the surface and within the lumen. This is, therefore, a good example of acute suppurative inflammation. There is no evidence of peptic ulceration or hyperplasia and chronic inflammation, granulomatous or nongranulomatous, does not produce this kind of picture. *(3:714–715)*

7. **(C)** In most instances, untreated acute appendicitis, particularly if suppuration has taken place, does not heal spontaneously, and resolution certainly does not occur. Atrophy has been seen in the appendix but rarely as the result of an acute inflammation. Malignant transformation is an extremely unlikely event, whereas ischemic necrosis with perforation is a frequently encountered complication because the appendix has an end-artery system. The buildup of pressure resulting from the flow of venous blood increases the engorgement, and obstruction to the arterial supply and gangrene and perforation ensue. *(3:174–715)*

8. **(E)** Acute suppurative appendicitis, as depicted in Figures 8–2 and 8–3, demonstrates luminal suppurative debris, mural neutrophilic infiltration, focal necrosis, edema, vascular congestion, fecalith formation, and serosal exudates. There is no morphologic evidence of malignant mucin-producing cells. *(3:714–715)*

9. **(C)** There is often an obstruction of the lumen of the appendix by a fecalith. This is a hard, inspissated, stonelike area of feces that initially causes irritation or ulceration of the mucosa. This is the portal of entry of intestinal bacteria and, in addition, creates an obstruction, which adds to the problem. Fecaliths occur relatively frequently. Acute appendicitis is much more frequently seen in the

developed countries of the world than in the underdeveloped countries and is thought to be associated with dietary differences. Acute appendicitis rarely if ever resolves without treatment because of the vulnerability of the vasculature described in this answer and in the answer to Question 8. In addition to elderly patients, it is seen frequently in children and young teenagers. *(3:714–715)*

Figures 8–4 and 8–5 are photomicrographs of the lungs. The inflammatory process described extends evenly through all the alveoli with a distribution that is panlobular in type.

10. **(B)** Lobar pneumonia is acute inflammation extending from one alveolus to the other through the pores of Kohn and extending to the interlobar septum and to the pleural surfaces. It differs from the other conditions in that diffuse interstitial pneumonia occurs in the alveolar walls and is usually a monocytic, lymphocytic response. Chronic granulomatous disease produces patchy areas of giant cell granulomas. Pulmonary fibrosis may be diffuse but results from the formation of collagen, not acute inflammatory cells and exudate. Lobular or bronchial pneumonia may be exudate. Lobular or bronchial pneumonia may be confluent, but there usually are some areas of normal alveoli between the consolidated areas that seem to concentrate around the terminal bronchioles and are, therefore, not panlobular as in lobar pneumonia. *(2:782–783)*

11. **(B)** *S. pneumoniae* is by far the most common organism to cause lobar pneumonia. Part of the disease process and the rapidity of spread throughout the entire lobe of the lung are thought to be associated with the immune response to the polysaccharide capsule of these organisms. Adenoviruses are more likely to produce interstitial pneumonia. Coliform organisms and other similar organisms more frequently produce bronchopneumonia. *M. tuberculosis* is characteristically the cause of granulomatous disease of the lungs, or tuberculosis. Asbestos particles may be associated with fibrosis. *(2:782–783)*

12. **(B)** Fibrin and large numbers of PMN in the alveoli are the hallmarks of acute lobular pneumonia, whereas giant cells and lymphocytes are more frequently seen in granulomatous disease. Fibrous tissue would be the end result of these inflammatory conditions, not the acute phase. *(2:782–783)*

13. **(D)** It is of considerable interest that such extensive involvement of the lungs is not a frequently fatal disorder. In fact, it resolves completely, leaving no residual disease providing the alveolar walls have not been destroyed and architectural resolution can take place without fibrosis. Fibrosis does occur but rarely produces the dense fibrosis described here. Gangrene is extremely uncommon in the lungs, and calcification usually occurs as a result of granulomatous disease with fibrosis. *(2:782–783)*

Figures 8–6 and 8–7 are photomicrographs of a lung with a patchy or lobular consolidation characteristic of bronchopneumonia, or lobular pneumonia. There are normal, recognizable alveoli between the areas of consolidation in contrast to Figures 8–4 and 8–5, where there was a diffuse inflammatory process.

14. **(C)** This lobular distribution is different from that of interstitial pneumonia and lobar pneumonia. Under low power, it might be confused with chronic granulomatous disease or patchy pulmonary fibrosis, but high power shows the presence of an acute inflammatory response rather than giant cell granulomas or fibrous tissue. *(2:780–781)*

15. **(C)** *E. coli* is normally an inhabitant of the gastrointestinal tract and may cause aspiration into the lungs, such as a lobular distribution resulting from inflammation commencing around the terminal bronchioles. *S. pneumoniae* usually produces lobar pneumonia. Adenoviruses cause interstitial pneumonia, and *M. tuberculosis* cause granulomatous disease. Asbestos particles are the most likely to produce diffuse pulmonary fibrosis.

16. **(C)** PMNs are the hallmark of acute inflammation, whatever its distribution. The PMNs and their peribronchial and bronchial distribution indicate that the disease is bronchopneumonia. *(2:780–781)*

17. **(D)** Partial resolution with some permanent damage to the bronchi and bronchioles is the most appropriate answer. Gangrene and calcification rarely occur, and complete resolution with no residual disease is very unlikely in bronchopneumonia, since there is usually damage to the terminal bronchioles and the alveolar walls communicating with them. *(2:780–781)*

Figures 8–8 and 8–9 show discrete solid areas that are focal collections of liquefaction necrosis surrounded by polymorphonuclear leukocytes, with some localization characteristic of abscesses.

18. **(D)** These characteristics are those of abscesses. The picture is not diffuse, and, therefore, interstitial pneumonia and lobar pneumonia can be ruled out. The distinction between an abscess and lobular or bronchopneumonia can sometimes be difficult, since breakdown of tissue can complicate bronchopneumonia and produce abscesses. However, the distribution is independent of the terminal bronchioles and scattered through the lungs. Chronic granulomatous disease would produce giant cells and lymphocytes. *(2:785–786)*

19. **(C)** Abscesses can be caused by a number of organisms both aerobic and anaerobic that are pyogenic, ie, they produce pus, which is the hallmark of an abscess. Adenoviruses cause interstitial pneumonitis. *M. tuberculosis* produces granulomas, asbestos particles produce diffuse fibrosis, and *M. pneumoniae* produces mostly interstitial but sometimes a bronchopneumonic type picture, and not characteristically a pyogenic response. *(2:785–786)*

20. **(B)** Abscesses can be caused by aspiration of infected material into the lungs, in which case they usually are associated with the bronchial tree. They can be the result of septicemic spread, a condition known as "pyemia," which is probably the most applicable in this instance. Asbestos and *M. pneumoniae* produce a different pattern in both distribution and the type of inflammatory cells involved. *(2:785–786)*

21. **(D)** Complete resolution is extremely unlikely, since there is liquefaction necrosis and, therefore, loss of tissue that would have to be replaced by fibrous tissue, which could result in pulmonary fibrosis. Abscesses may rupture into the pleural cavity, producing empyema, and may spread further via the bloodstream to produce brain abscess, which is one of the complications of lung abscess. *(2:785–786)*

Figures 8–10 and 8–11 illustrate the process of intravascular coagulation, or thrombosis.

22. **(B)** This is a thrombotic occlusion of a blood vessel and distinctly different from the haphazard arrangement of the elements of the blood seen in a postmortem blood clot. Although acute inflammation may complicate or even precede thrombotic occlusion, there is no evidence in this case, nor is there chronic inflammation or tumor materials in an embolic form present. There is a distinct difference between a blood clot and a thrombus. A thrombus can occur only in a living blood vessel and in blood that is flowing. This creates the structure composed of layers of platelets, fibrin, and red cells in an orderly fashion. Blood may clot haphazardly after death and has no such structure. *(2:93–105)*

23. **(D)** The most probable outcome of thrombotic occlusion of a blood vessel, particularly an artery, is ischemic damage or infarction of the tissue supplied by that artery. Acute suppurative inflammation occasionally may complicate such a procedure but is not the most probable immediate outcome. Dissolution and dissipation of the blood clot may sometimes occur but are not the most probable occurrence. Chronic granulomatous inflammation and metastatic spread of tumor cells are not probable outcomes in this set of circumstances. *(2:93–105)*

24. **(D)** The final outcome of a thrombotic event depends on a complex interplay of a number of factors: the degree of collateral circulation, the type of artery occluded, the state of collateral circulation, the state of tissue oxygenation before the occlusion, the degree and rate of recanalization of the thrombus, and the activity of the fibrinolytic system. The serum osmolality does not directly affect the outcome of a thrombus. *(2:93–105)*

25. **(A)** Alteration of the blood flow, increased coagulability of the blood, and damage to the intima of the vessel wall are the classic Virchow's triad, which is the basis on which thrombosis may occur. A decrease in platelets actually would produce the opposite result by producing a hypocoagulable state. *(2:93–105)*

Figures 8–12 and 8–13 show gross and microscopic characteristics of a neoplasm of the colon, which is a well differentiated adenocarcinoma.

26. **(C)** This is a malignant neoplasm demonstrating invasion of the bowel wall, with a variable degree of involvement of the adjacent mucosa. Hyperplasia would not produce such an invasive process, nor would a benign neoplasm, which in the colon would probably be a polyp. There is no evidence of acute suppurative inflammation. *(1:620–622)*

27. **(C)** This is a malignant neoplasm, since there is lack of encapsulation. It is invasive, and the cells are recapitulating the glandular structure of the colonic mucosa. Therefore, by definition, this is a carcinoma and an adenocarcinoma in type. Ulcerative colitis would produce, as the name implies, multiple areas of ulceration and mucosal inflammation. Crohn's disease of the colon is a granulomatous disease that involves the full thickness of the colonic walls, and adenomatous polyp is a well-defined and not invasive process. Amebic dysentery would produce an inflamed, ulcerated lesion. *(1:620–622)*

28. **(A)** Such tumors will, in fact, grow and produce obstruction to the lumen, ulceration of the mucosa, and subsequent hemorrhage owing to invasion of the blood vessels in the submucosa. Resolution with healing never occurs in such malignant tumors. *(1:620–622)*

29. **(E)** Well differentiated colonic adenocarcinoma is a malignant neoplasm, not a benign tumor. It occurs most frequently in the highly industrialized Western nations, in individuals over 45 years old, in individuals with low-fiber, high-fat diets, in association with chronic ulcerative colitis, and in association with familial polyposis. The malignancy arises from gland-forming epithelium and usually retains at least focal glandular architecture or secretion of mucin by individual tumor cells. *(1:620–622)*

Figures 8–14 and 8–15 show the gross and microscopic appearances of a malignant tumor of the lung, or bronchogenic carcinoma.

30. **(C)** The obvious invasive properties of this tumor and its poorly differentiated state indicate that it is malignant. There is no evidence of infarction, lung abscess, or granuloma, and the tumor does not have the characteristics of a benign lesion. *(1:550–556)*

31. **(C)** The tumor cells appear to be differentiated in the direction of the squamous type of epithelium and, therefore, would be called a "squamous cell" or "epidermoid" carcinoma. An adenoma of the bronchus would be a well differentiated glandular tumor. Tuberculosis would produce the characteristic appearance of giant cell granulomas with caseous necrosis; these are not present. *(1:550–556)*

32. **(E)** This type of tumor can produce obstruction to the bronchial tree, can ulcerate, and can produce hemorrhage. The obstruction will cause collapse and accumulation of materials, with infection and pneumonia distal to the obstruction. It is often these complications that first bring the tumor to the attention of the physician, particularly pneumonia that does not resolve or that recurs after treatment. The hemorrhage often produces the symptoms of hemoptysis or blood in the septum. *(1:550–556)*

33. **(D)** Squamous cell carcinoma of the lung is strongly associated with cigarette smoking. Prior to most frank carcinomas there is squamous metaplasia of the bronchial epithelium with subsequent progressive dysplasia. Other factors that increase the risk for developing lung cancer include inhalation of asbestos, uranium, nickel, chromate, and gold. Low-fiber diets, hypercoagulable states, sickle cell anemia, and bacterial infections are not directly associated with pulmonary squamous cell carcinoma. *(1:550–551)*

Figures 8–16 and 8–17 show aspects of the microscopic findings in a lump removed from the breast of a 45-year-old woman. It has the features of a poorly differentiated malignant tumor, a carcinoma of the breast.

34. **(A)** This is a malignant tumor of the breast. All of the other choices can mimic the gross appearance and the clinical features. Microscopy, therefore, is vital to the correct diagnosis. *(1:823–829)*

35. **(A)** The microscopy shows this to be a tumor, and the similarity to ductal tissue of the breast would classify it as an adenocarcinoma. A fibroadenoma is a distinctly different well-circumscribed combination of duct and fibrous tissue. Fat necrosis produces areas of necrosis of fat, with responding inflammatory changes. Fibrosis and duct obstruction with abscess produce the classic liquefaction necrosis and many polymorphonuclear leukocytes. Tuberculous mastitis is a rare condition in developed countries of the world and produces the typical granulomatous lesion of tuberculosis. *(1:823–829)*

36. **(D)** The stage of the disease is the single most important variable of the listed choices that affects the eventual outcome of breast carcinoma. This is supported by the observation that the 5-year survival rate for stage I, II, III, and IV is 85%, 66%, 41%, and 10%, respectively. In a node-negative patient (all stage I and some stage II), the status of the steroid receptors, DNA ploidy, percent S phase, and oncogene status are additional independent factors affecting prognosis. *(1:823–829)*

37. **(C)** Breast carcinoma is most likely to occur in first- and second-degree female relatives of known breast carcinoma patients. There is a fivefold increased likelihood of breast carcinoma developing in a female whose mother or sister has had breast carcinoma. In addition, there is an independent increased likelihood of breast carcinoma developing in individuals who are nulliparous, those with early menarche, those with late menopause, those who have never breastfed their children, and those whose first pregnancy was at a late age. Breast carcinoma is also more likely to occur in whites than Orientals, and in individuals with high fat diets. *(1:824)*

Figures 8–18 and 8–19 show a uterus with a number of well-defined tumors, which are benign leiomyomas, or tumors arising from the uterine musculature.

38. **(B)** These are well-circumscribed, encapsulated, benign tumors of the uterus. The combination of the gross appearance and the microscopy allows these distinctions to be made. *(3:968–969)*

39. **(A)** The correct diagnostic term is a benign leiomyoma. Leiomyosarcomas are much rarer and produce a more pleomorphic picture, with higher mitotic rate. Adenocarcinoma of the endometrium would have a glandular structure. Squamous cell carcinoma of the cervix or a teratoma of the uterus would be composed of a number of different cell types. *(3:968–969)*

40. **(C)** These tumors are frequently multiple, and there is not a high incidence of malignant transformation, although such malignant changes may occur. They are the most common neoplasm in the adult female genital tract and are benign lesions arising from the uterine myometrium. *(3:968–969)*

Figure 8–20 is an electron micrograph that demonstrates swollen mitochondria with floccular densities that are seen as dense deposits. These are evidence of cell injury and disruption of oxidative phosphorylation.

41. **(C)** The condition is swollen damaged mitochondria. Apoptosis is a nuclear phenomenon, as are karyolysis and karyorrhexis. Viral inclusions have a distinct pattern that is not seen as floccular density as demonstrated. *(3:5–8)*

42. **(C)** The best description of the condition is decreased respiration of the mitochondria with flocculation. Lipid peroxidation with cell membrane damage is not indicated in this instance. Clumping of chromatin is not present, and although there may be damage to the endoplasmic reticulum, it is not as appropriate an answer. Lysosomal changes with cell swelling are not present at this stage. *(3:5–8)*

43. **(B)** Cell injury resulting from mercuric chloride poisoning or early ischemic changes in infarction can produce this kind of mitochondrial damage. Cytomegalovirus produces a characteristic inclusion, and saponification indicates complete disruption of the cell, with soap formation and calcium deposition. *(3:5–8)*

44. **(D)** Disruption of oxidative phosphorylation in the mitochondria is the mechanism involved. Abnormalities of lipid storage would produce a different picture. Viral transformation of the cellular DNA is an unrelated phenomenon, and although toxic poisoning of the lysosomal system may produce similar effects, they occur at different stages in cell damage. *(3:5–8)*

Figure 8–21 depicts an egg with a lateral spine, which is characteristic of Schistosoma mansoni.

45. **(C)** These parasites all produce different shape and size eggs that are clearly distinguishable. *(3:440–443)*

46. **(C)** Humans are the most frequent host for the adult forms, which are the worms that produce eggs. The snail and the fish play a different role in the life cycle of the schistosomes. The mosquito and the dog are not involved at all. *(3:440–443)*

47. **(D)** The intermediate host in the parasitic life cycle of schistosomiasis is the snail. Fertilized eggs exit infected humans via either urine or feces. These eggs develop into miracidium larva in water and infect snails, the intermediate host. Cercaria larva then exit out of the snail into the water and then infect humans by penetrating through the skin. The adult worms come to lodge in either the intestinal or bladder venous plexus, where they copulate and secrete fertilized eggs, repeating the cycle. *(3:440–441)*

48. **(A)** This is, in fact, a very common cause of blood loss in underdeveloped countries or areas where schistosomiasis is frequent. The adult male and female worms copulate either in the veins of the gastrointestinal tract or in the urinary bladder plexus of veins. The eggs are then shed either through the bladder or through the large intestine. Schistosomiasis is a worldwide problem and an extremely common disease for which millions of people carry the parasite. *(3:440–443)*

Figure 8–22 depicts the branching hyphae of a fungus characteristic of Aspergillus.

49. **(C)** The branching hyphae are so characteristic that this is quite distinguishable from bacteria or rickettsia, which are much smaller. Viruses are intracellular, and protozoa have different structures and are separate entities. *(3:422–423)*

50. **(C)** This is characteristic of *Aspergillus,* although other fungi may look similar. *(3:422–423)*

51. **(D)** Aspergillosis rarely is a primary infection but often complicates other infections and is regarded as an opportunistic infection in people with lowered resistance or immune deficiency. It is not of high virulence in normal circumstances, and the portal of entry is usually the respiratory tract. *(3:422–423)*

Figure 8–23 shows a renal tubule with many enlarged tubular epithelial cells and a large nucleus containing intranuclear inclusions with a surrounding halo (the <u>owl eye appearance</u>). This is characteristic of the intranuclear viral inclusions seen in cytomegalovirus infections.

52. **(B)** This is a characteristic representation of viral inclusion bodies and should not be confused with storage material, which would be in the cytoplasm of the cell. *(2:321–323)*

53. **(D)** These viruses are normally of low virulence, and although they may occur in a congenital setting, they are not hereditary diseases. Although malnutrition also can contribute to immune deficiency, the immune deficiency itself appears to be the main problem. *(2:321–323)*

54. **(C)** This condition is characteristic of cytomegalovirus infection. The clinical manifestations of the disease, with hepatosplenomegaly and microcephaly, are characteristic of a congenital infection from transplacental passage of the virus but may be seen in patients with severe immune deficiency. *(2:321–323)*

55. **(D)** The disease is seen most commonly in immunologically compromised hosts, although it may occur because of transplacental passage of the virus. It is not seen in an epidemic form, nor is it confined

to the tropics. It is not transmitted readily from patient to patient, as are the viruses of measles or smallpox. *(2:321–323)*

Figure 8–24 shows the typical scolex of a tapeworm, with many hooklets discernible.

56. **(C)** The photomicrograph demonstrates the mouthparts (scolex) of a tapeworm. These diagnostic structures may be seen in hepatic hydatic cysts caused by *Echinococcus granulosus*. *(3:444–446)*

57. **(A)** Hydatid disease is caused by the dog tapeworm, *E. granulosus*. Accidental ingestion of infected canine feces by humans liberates the larval stage of the organism which may lodge in the liver, bone, brain, or lung. In these sites these larva may evoke a chronic cystic (hydatid cyst) foreign body response. *(3:444–446)*

58. **(B)** The transmission is usually via infected feces that contain the ova of the tapeworm. *(3:444–446)*

59. **(D)** Although humans may be the primary host, this is not the most frequent occurrence. The dog is usually the most frequent primary host of this type of tapeworm, and the sheep is often a secondary host. Humans become a secondary host by ingesting sheep that are infected with the parasite. *(3:444–446)*

Figure 8–25 shows the characteristic corkscrew appearance of multiple spirochetes which require special staining techniques for their demonstration.

60. **(D)** Gram-positive cocci and gram-negative bacilli usually do not show this particular morphology, and although *Actinomyces* may produce a number of different morphologic forms, it is basically different. Donovan bodies occur intracellularly and in a different condition entirely. *(3:353–356)*

61. **(E)** The spirochete of syphilis taken from a penile ulcer is by far the most likely diagnosis in this case. Chancroid, granuloma inguinale, lymphogranuloma venereum, and gonorrhea all are caused by different types of organisms that have different morphology and characteristics. *(3:353–356)*

62. **(B)** Syphilis is largely transmitted venereally, and the organism does not survive long outside the body. It is not transmitted by food contamination and does not survive in dust and debris, as do such organisms as the acid-fast bacillus. *(3:353–356)*

Figure 8–26 shows the periphery of the lung with clusters of malignant cells in what appear to be dilated subpleural lymphatics. This is a metastic carcinoma from a primary carcinoma in the breast.

63. **(B)** This is a characteristic appearance of metastatic carcinoma, in this instance in the subpleural lymphatics of the lung, but it could be seen in lymph nodes or other sites. There is not the granulomatous appearance of tuberculosis, nor is there evidence of intravascular coagulation or the liquefaction necrosis of an abscess or infarction. *(2:803–804)*

64. **(C)** This tumor pattern is very characteristic of a primary source in the breast, with spread to the subpleural lymphatics and to other parts of the lung. Embolization could result in tumor cells in a different, more diffuse metastatic pattern within the lung. *(2:803–804)*

Figure 8–27 shows a section of long bone. The dense material in the center and at the periosteal surface is new bone formation, or callus, characteristic of the healing phase of a fracture.

65. **(C)** This is a form of healing that, in many respects, is very similar to that seen in other tissues, with the exception that the collagen or fibrous tissue is converted into bone. *(3:1323–1326)*

66. **(C)** The healing of a fracture is distinctly different from the appearances of an osteogenic sarcoma or an osteoid osteoma, which are neoplastic transformations of bone. Acute osteomyelitis or tuberculosis of the bone shows the characteristic features of inflammation, which are not present in this illustration. *(3:1323–1326)*

67. **(D)** The appearance of the dense material that extends to the periosteal surface is the new bone, or provisional callus, which is the precursor of the final bone before remodeling occurs in a fracture. Although fibrous tissue may occur as a complication of fractures with non-union, this is not seen in this illustration, and the appearance of osteoid in a sarcoma can sometimes mimic this appearance, although not in its entirety. There is no evidence of inflammation. *(3:1323–1326)*

68. **(C)** A number of factors will retard the normal healing of boney fractures: foreign material in the wound, active inflammation, widely apposed fractured ends, deficiency of vitamin C, deficiency of vitamin D, deficiency of calcium, scar formation, and movement of the fracture ends during healing. High doses of vitamin C or D, a diet high in calcium, and immobilization of the bone would all tend to assist in rapid healing of a fracture. *(3:1323–1326)*

Figures 8–28 and 8–29 show a lung with an area of infarction in which the alveolar walls appear indistinct and the lung is filled with red cells but there is no evidence of inflammatory cells, as seen in pneumonia. The real clue to the condition is the blood vessel leading into the lung, which has a thrombotic occlusion. This is characteristic of infarction.

69. **(A)** Lobar pneumonia would produce many polymorphonuclear leukocytes, as would lung abscesses, with liquefaction necrosis also present. There is no evidence of neoplasm in the photograph. *(3:618–619)*

70. **(C)** Deep venous thrombosis with embolization to the pulmonary vessels is the most likely antecedent. The individual may have had multiple emboli or venous congestion because of right-sided heart failure in addition. Although cigarette smoking and asbestos may contribute to lung disease, they do not in this setting, and there is no evidence of septicemia, although this can in itself produce emboli. Aspiration of infected materials produces a bronchopneumonic type of inflammatory condition. *(3:618–619)*

Figure 8–30 is a photomicrograph of a liver, in which the liver cells appear to be replaced by empty spaces characteristic of fat. The fat is removed during the processing, leaving these circular globules replacing most of the liver cells.

71. **(B)** Lipid accumulation in the liver produces the picture shown. *(3:754–758)*

72. **(A)** This often is described as fatty metamorphosis, although some other terms, such as "fatty infiltration" or "fatty liver," also are used. There is no evidence of hepatocellular carcinoma or of passive congestion, although these may occur in the same liver as fatty metamorphosis. Acute viral hepatitis and tuberculosis, which are inflammatory and destructive processes, also may occur in livers in which fatty metamorphosis is present. *(3:754–758)*

73. **(C)** Hepatic fatty metamorphosis is seen most commonly in alcoholism. Other conditions in which liver cell fatty change may be seen include carbon tetrachloride poisoning, diabetes mellitus, malnutrition, after ingestion of hepatotoxins, after administration of various therapeutic drugs, during pregnancy, and choline deficiency. *(3:754–758)*

74. **(D)** This condition frequently is reversible. In fact, severe protein malnutrition, if corrected, will produce a normal liver with no such accumulations of lipid. There are multiple causes of as similar picture. The condition may well affect children, particularly those with malnutrition, as well as adults with other disorders. Choline deficiency is one of the known causes. *(3:754–758)*

REFERENCES

1. Chandrasoma, P, Taylor CR: Concise Pathology, Norwalk, Appleton and Lange, 1991
2. Cotran RS, Kumar V, Robbins SL: Robbins Pathologic Basis of Disease, 4th edition, Philadelphia, Saunders, 1989
3. Rubin E, Farber JL: Pathology, Philadelphia, Lippincott, 1988

CHAPTER 9

Practice Test

Carefully read the following instructions before taking the Practice Test.

1. This examination consists of 153 questions, covering the subject areas listed in the Table of Contents.
2. The Practice Test simulates an actual examination in question types and integration of subject areas.
3. You should set aside 2 hours and 10 minutes of *uninterrupted,* distraction-free time to take the Practice Test. This averages out to 50 seconds per question.
4. Be sure you have a clock (to time and pace yourself) and an adequate number of No. 2 pencils and erasers.
5. You should tear out and use the answer sheet that is provided on page 199.
6. Be sure to answer all of the questions, and be sure the number on the answer sheet corresponds to the question number in the Practice Test.
7. Use any remaining time to review your answers.
8. After completing the Practice Test, you can check all of your answers on pages 189 to 195. A score of 75% or higher should be considered as a passing score (115 correct answers).
9. After checking your answers and your score, you can analyze your strengths and weaknesses on the Practice Test Subspecialty List on page 197. To do this, you should check off your incorrect Practice Test answers on the Subspecialty List. You may find a pattern developing. For example, you may find you do well on infectious diseases but poorly on immunopathology. In such an instance, you can go back and review the immunopathology section of this book and supplement your review with your texts and with the references cited in that section.

Questions

DIRECTIONS (Questions 1 through 73): Each of the numbered items or incomplete statements in this section is followed by answers or by completions of the statement. Select the ONE lettered answer or completion that is BEST in each case.

1. The severe systemic reactions that occur in diphtheria are caused by

    (A) antihistone autoantibodies
    (B) overwhelming bacterial septicemia
    (C) localized upper respiratory tract infection with release of exotoxin
    (D) anaerobic spore formation within visceral abscesses
    (E) viral septicemia

2. Identify the INCORRECT statement concerning leprosy

    (A) can be found in wild armadillos
    (B) is caused by *Mycobacterium leprae*
    (C) occurs in lepromatous and tuberculoid forms
    (D) organisms show acid-fast staining
    (E) peripheral nerve involvement is rare

3. A kidney from a blood group B donor is transplanted into a group O recipient. What is the expected result?

    (A) acute rejection
    (B) graft-vs-host disease
    (C) successful transplantation
    (D) hyperacute rejection
    (E) chronic rejection

4. Identify the FALSE statement about cell membranes

    (A) portions may be coated by glycocalyx
    (B) membrane-associated particles can include ABO blood groups
    (C) site of oxidative phosphorylation
    (D) composed of complex mixture of lipids, proteins, and carbohydrates
    (E) morphologic pattern is termed "unit membrane"

5. The major extracellular cation is

    (A) calcium
    (B) sodium
    (C) bicarbonate
    (D) potassium
    (E) magnesium

6. Phagocytosis is best defined as

    (A) abnormal mitotic figures in malignancy
    (B) tight junctions on the cell membrane
    (C) collagen deposition in a wound
    (D) engulfment of particulate matter by cells
    (E) enzyme found in ribosomes

7. Identify the INCORRECT statement concerning hydropericardium

    (A) usually contains less than 50 ml
    (B) can produce cardiac tamponade
    (C) is seen with congestive heart failure
    (D) usually is a transudate
    (E) is associated with myxedema

8. A Langhans' giant cell would be an expected finding in

    (A) suppurative inflammation
    (B) granulomatous inflammation
    (C) serous inflammation
    (D) fibrinous inflammation
    (E) purulent inflammation

9. Acetaminophen overdose results in necrosis of which cell type?

    (A) neuron
    (B) smooth muscle
    (C) hepatocyte
    (D) fibroblast
    (E) alveolar macrophage

10. Type I hypersensitivity reactions are mediated by which immunoglobulin?

    (A) IgA
    (B) IgD

- (C) IgE
- (D) IgG
- (E) IgM

11. Identify the INCORRECT statement concerning B lymphocytes
    - (A) express surface immunoglobulin
    - (B) have a receptor for complement 3b (C3b)
    - (C) have a receptor for Fc
    - (D) have receptors for sheep erythrocytes
    - (E) can mature into plasma cells

12. In Gaucher's disease, the lysosomal storage product is
    - (A) sphingomyelin
    - (B) glucocerebroside
    - (C) ceramide trihexoside
    - (D) sulfatide
    - (E) GM2-ganglioside

13. Identify the INCORRECT statement about respiratory distress in newborns
    - (A) prematurity increases risk
    - (B) may have hyaline pulmonary membranes
    - (C) major cause is lack of pulmonary surfactant
    - (D) survivors have no late complications
    - (E) increased risk with diabetic mothers

14. Fat necrosis is most common in fatty tissue next to the
    - (A) ovary
    - (B) testicle
    - (C) heart
    - (D) pancreas
    - (E) skeletal muscle

15. Identify the cell type with the highest radiosensitivity
    - (A) osteocyte
    - (B) fibroblast
    - (C) lymphocyte
    - (D) chondrocyte
    - (E) skeletal muscle cell

16. Gas gangrene is a form of necrosis associated with
    - (A) mycotic infections
    - (B) emphysema
    - (C) tuberculosis
    - (D) clostridial infections
    - (E) genetic disorders

17. Identify the INCORRECT statement about acute cyanide poisoning
    - (A) less than 0.1 g ingested may be lethal
    - (B) at death, blood is cherry red
    - (C) kills by cellular asphyxiation
    - (D) binds to cytochrome oxidase
    - (E) primarily attacks the kidney

18. Identify the FALSE statement about chromoblastomycosis
    - (A) caused by several pigmented fungi
    - (B) involves granulomatous and suppurative reaction
    - (C) also called "tinea capitis"
    - (D) usually occurs in an extremity
    - (E) indolent cutaneous infection

19. Identify the fat-soluble vitamin
    - (A) vitamin B_6
    - (B) vitamin B_{12}
    - (C) niacin
    - (D) vitamin E
    - (E) riboflavin

20. A patient with fever, bradycardia, leukopenia, diarrhea, and lymphoid hyperplasia most likely has
    - (A) staphylococcal meningitis
    - (B) typhoid fever
    - (C) staphylococcal myelitis
    - (D) gonococcal meningitis
    - (E) pneumococcal pneumonia

21. Identify the grade of cancer with the worst prognosis
    - (A) grade I
    - (B) grade II
    - (C) grade III
    - (D) all have the same prognosis
    - (E) cancers are not graded

22. A malignant tumor that produces abundant keratin pearls is
    - (A) choriocarcinoma
    - (B) adenocarcinoma
    - (C) melanocarcinoma
    - (D) epidermoid carcinoma
    - (E) fibroadenoma

23. Identify the infection that *Haemophilus influenzae* is LEAST likely to produce
    - (A) urinary tract infection
    - (B) meningitis
    - (C) upper respiratory tract infection
    - (D) otitis
    - (E) acute epiglottitis

24. Which of the following bacterial pathogens does NOT have toxin production as the major component of its pathogenicity?

    (A) *Corynebacterium diphtheriae*
    (B) *Clostridium tetani*
    (C) *Streptococcus pneumoniae*
    (D) *Clostridium botulinum*
    (E) *Vibrio cholerae*

25. A focal, often circumscribed, overgrowth in improper proportions of tissues normally present in that part of the body is termed a

    (A) hyperdiploid
    (B) metastasis
    (C) hamartoma
    (D) inflammatory response
    (E) abscess cavity

26. Identify the FALSE statement about phenylketonuria

    (A) untreated patients will suffer mental retardation
    (B) usually caused by lack of phenylalanine hydroxylase
    (C) treatment includes phenylalanine-free diet
    (D) inherited in X-linked fashion
    (E) cerebral changes include demyelination

27. An alcoholic is found to have lobar pneumonia. The sputum is purulent and contains abundant pairs of lance-shaped, gram-positive cocci with prominent capsules. The causative organism is

    (A) *Streptococcus pneumoniae*
    (B) *Klebsiella pneumoniae*
    (C) *Neisseria meningitidis*
    (D) *Haemophilus influenzae*
    (E) *Enterobacter aerogenes*

28. A short-term dose of 1000 rad acute whole body irradiation would be expected to produce

    (A) severe nausea, 20% fatality rate
    (B) 100% fatality rate
    (C) mild nausea, 5% fatality rate
    (D) loss of hair, 35% fatality rate
    (E) only minor blood changes, 0% fatality rate

29. Identify the FALSE statement about carbon monoxide poisoning

    (A) carbon monoxide poisons by acting as a systemic asphyxiant
    (B) toxic effects can include mental confusion, unconsciousness, and death
    (C) chronic poisoning may result in degeneration of basal nuclei
    (D) hemoglobin's affinity for carbon monoxide is 200% greater than that of oxygen
    (E) hemorrhage is almost always present

30. Scurvy is caused by a deficiency of

    (A) iron
    (B) thiamine
    (C) niacin
    (D) vitamin D
    (E) vitamin C

31. Diarrhea is uncommon in infections with

    (A) *Shigella* sp.
    (B) *Vibrio cholerae*
    (C) *Campylobacter jejuni*
    (D) *Haemophilus influenzae*
    (E) *Salmonella* sp.

32. Collection of edema fluid in the pleural cavity is termed

    (A) ascites
    (B) hydrothorax
    (C) anasarca
    (D) hydropericardium
    (E) pericardial effusion

33. A man with chronic tuberculosis has deposits of acellular eosinophilic material in his kidney, with apple green birefringence after Congo red staining. This eosinophilic material is

    (A) bilirubin
    (B) amyloid
    (C) hematin
    (D) urate
    (E) hemosiderin

34. All of the following are possible features of herpes simplex type 1, viral infections EXCEPT

    (A) intranuclear inclusions
    (B) keratoconjunctivitis
    (C) latency period in neural ganglia
    (D) shingles
    (E) encephalitis

35. Infections transmitted to humans from an animal host or reservoir are termed

    (A) vertical transmission
    (B) zoonotic
    (C) horizontal transmission
    (D) commensalism
    (E) fomites

36. The process by which the information contained in a molecule of messenger RNA is converted to a protein is known as

    (A) transcription
    (B) translation
    (C) organization
    (D) granulation
    (E) first intention

37. Which would be an unexpected finding in occlusive coronary thrombosis?

    (A) thrombus at the site of abnormal vessel wall
    (B) ischemic necrosis
    (C) myocardial infarct
    (D) coronary arterial atherosclerosis
    (E) thrombocytopenia

38. The occurrence of scrotal carcinoma in chimney sweeps supports which theory for carcinogenesis?

    (A) radiation carcinogenesis
    (B) genetic carcinogenesis
    (C) viral carcinogenesis
    (D) chemical carcinogenesis
    (E) asbestos carcinogenesis

39. An enlarged lymph node is biopsied and found to contain a malignant tumor. Immunoperoxidase stains show that the tumor cells contain kappa-light chains. The most likely diagnosis is

    (A) metastatic adenocarcinoma
    (B) metastatic squamous cell carcinoma
    (C) lymphoma or plasmacytoma
    (D) hepatoma
    (E) melanoma

40. The most common fatal childhood cancer is

    (A) bone cancer
    (B) central nervous system cancer
    (C) leukemia
    (D) kidney cancer
    (E) connective tissue cancer

41. The most common site of cancer other than skin cancers for males in North America is

    (A) prostate
    (B) breast
    (C) bladder
    (D) lung
    (E) lymphomas

42. Acquired immune deficiency syndrome (AIDS) is caused by

    (A) cytomegalovirus
    (B) herpes simplex virus
    (C) human immunodeficiency virus (HIV)
    (D) Epstein-Barr virus
    (E) Kaposi's sarcoma

43. Expected findings in systemic lupus erythematosus (SLE) include all of the following EXCEPT

    (A) antibodies against DNA
    (B) repeated pyogenic infections
    (C) a positive fluorescent antinuclear antibody test
    (D) lesions in skin, joints, and heart
    (E) glomerulonephritis

44. The major chromosomal abnormality in cat's cry syndrome is

    (A) trisomy 18
    (B) deletion of the short arm of chromosome 5
    (C) trisomy 21
    (D) trisomy 13
    (E) 47,XXY

45. Identify an example of hypertrophy from the statements that follow

    (A) low-protein diet causes ascites
    (B) the left cardiac ventricle increases in thickness in systemic hypertension
    (C) a clot in the femoral artery causes gangrene of toes
    (D) vitamin K deficiency predisposes to bleeding
    (E) fibrosis occurs in the pancreas after parenchymal loss

46. The brown granular pigment composed of iron-ferritin complexes present in heart failure macrophages is

    (A) melanin
    (B) hemosiderin
    (C) lipofuscin
    (D) bilirubin
    (E) ceroid

47. Common tumors of infancy and childhood include all of the following EXCEPT

    (A) hepatoblastoma
    (B) Wilms' tumor
    (C) neuroblastoma
    (D) endometrial adenocarcinoma
    (E) retinoblastoma

48. Electron microscopy of brain cells from a deaf infant with rapid mental deterioration reveals abundant whorled membranous bodies in neuronal lysosomes. Which statement is FALSE?

    (A) the disease has a genetic basis
    (B) the disease is probably a lysosomal storage disease
    (C) an enzyme that degrades the membranes may be missing
    (D) the cells will not have any DNA
    (E) the infant's prognosis is poor

49. Identify the LEAST likely symptom of a staphylococcal infection

    (A) furuncle
    (B) caseous necrosis
    (C) carbuncle
    (D) surgical wound abscess
    (E) impetigo

50. Identify the true statement concerning rickettsial diseases

    (A) rickettsiae are obligate intracellular parasites
    (B) rickettsiae usually produce no rash or eschar
    (C) rickettsiae usually have no insect vectors
    (D) rickettsiae cause yaws and pinta
    (E) rickettsiae lack DNA and RNA

51. Carcinoma with a glandular pattern of growth is called

    (A) teratoma
    (B) squamous cell carcinoma
    (C) melanoma
    (D) lymphoma
    (E) adenocarcinoma

52. Arbovirus diseases include all of the following EXCEPT

    (A) yellow fever
    (B) dengue
    (C) cytomegalic inclusion disease
    (D) Eastern encephalitis
    (E) Lassa fever

53. Identify the INCORRECT statement about mumps

    (A) parotid gland swelling is usual
    (B) usually causes diarrhea
    (C) testicular swelling occurs occasionally
    (D) caused by paramyxovirus
    (E) may rarely cause encephalitis

54. Which characteristic is LEAST likely to be seen in malignancy?

    (A) encapsulation
    (B) anaplasia
    (C) invasion of lymphatics
    (D) metastasis
    (E) aneuploidy

55. Chlamydial diseases include all of the following EXCEPT

    (A) nonspecific urethritis
    (B) inclusion conjunctivitis
    (C) lymphogranuloma venereum
    (D) psittacosis
    (E) gonorrhea

56. Bruton's agammaglobulinemia includes all of the following EXCEPT

    (A) X-linked inheritance
    (B) markedly reduced B lymphocytes
    (C) relatively normal delayed hypersensitivity
    (D) increased antibody production
    (E) increased incidence of autoimmune disorders

57. Antibodies against microsomal antigens are commonly seen with

    (A) scleroderma
    (B) mixed connective tissue disease
    (C) Hashimoto's thyroiditis
    (D) dermatomyositis
    (E) systemic lupus erythematosus

58. Type I hypersensitivity reactions usually involve

    (A) anaphylaxis
    (B) cell-mediated reactions
    (C) complement-mediated cytotoxicity
    (D) circulating immune complexes
    (E) delayed hypersensitivity

59. Sphingolipidoses include all of the following EXCEPT

    (A) Tay–Sachs disease
    (B) Pompe's disease
    (C) Krabbe's disease
    (D) Niemann–Pick disease
    (E) Fabry's disease

60. Gummas are associated with
    (A) anthrax
    (B) primary syphilis
    (C) cholera
    (D) tertiary syphilis
    (E) all forms of meningitis

61. Idiopathic arterial medionecrosis is seen frequently in

    (A) Marfan's syndrome
    (B) polycystic kidney disease
    (C) von Willebrand's disease
    (D) thalassemia
    (E) sickle cell anemia

62. The expected karyotype of Klinefelter's syndrome is

    (A) 45,XO
    (B) 46,XX
    (C) 47,XYY
    (D) 46,XY
    (E) 47,XXY

63. A hemorrhagic venous infarct would be most likely in which site?

    (A) small intestine
    (B) heart
    (C) kidney
    (D) spleen
    (E) distal leg

64. Identify the substance critical to wound healing

    (A) chemotactic factors
    (B) myosin
    (C) kinins
    (D) actin
    (E) collagen

65. A localized collection of pus is termed

    (A) caseous necrosis
    (B) ascites
    (C) fibrinous exudate
    (D) abscess
    (E) pseudomembrane

66. A reversible change in which one adult cell type is replaced by another adult cell type is called

    (A) dysplasia
    (B) hypoplasia
    (C) atrophy
    (D) metaplasia
    (E) hyperplasia

67. Intermediate filaments of the cytoskeleton and membrane skeleton include all of the following EXCEPT

    (A) desmin
    (B) vimentin
    (C) actin
    (D) keratins
    (E) neural filaments

68. Identify the irreversible change seen in necrosis

    (A) vacuolar degeneration
    (B) karyorrhexis
    (C) fatty change
    (D) hydropic change
    (E) cellular swelling

69. The microscopic appearance of an occlusive arterial infarct of the spleen is

    (A) coagulative necrosis
    (B) liquefaction necrosis
    (C) enzymatic fat necrosis
    (D) caseous necrosis
    (E) giant cell inflammation

70. Gas embolism is most likely to result from

    (A) hypercoagulable states
    (B) fracture of the femur
    (C) low protein states
    (D) venous stasis
    (E) rapid decompression

71. Identify the factor most likely to oppose thrombus formation

    (A) exposed collagen
    (B) hypercoagulable states
    (C) plasmin
    (D) vascular stasis
    (E) endothelial injury

72. Common causes of edema include all of the following EXCEPT

    (A) hyperproteinemia
    (B) lymphatic obstruction
    (C) increased endothelial permeability
    (D) reduced plasma oncotic pressure
    (E) increased vascular hydrostatic pressure

73. Which is the largest compartment in the body?

    (A) extracellular fluid compartment
    (B) whole blood fluid compartment
    (C) interstitial fluid compartment
    (D) intracellular fluid compartment
    (E) plasma fluid compartment

DIRECTIONS (Questions 74 through 153): Each group of items in this section consists of lettered headings followed by a set of numbered words or phrases. For each numbered word or phrase, select the ONE lettered heading that is most closely associated with it. Each lettered heading may be selected once, more than once, or not at all.

Questions 74 through 77

    (A) rhabdomyosarcoma
    (B) leiomyoma
    (C) hidradenoma
    (D) choriocarcinoma
    (E) lipoma

74. Malignant tumor of trophoblastic cells

75. Malignant tumor of skeletal muscle cells

76. Benign tumor of smooth muscle cells

77. Benign tumor of sweat gland cells

Question 78 through 81

(A) *Mycoplasma pneumoniae*
(B) *Bartonella bacilliformis*
(C) *Yersinia pestis*
(D) *Calymmatobacterium donovani*
(E) *Mycobacterium tuberculosis*

78. Carrion's disease

79. Granuloma inguinale

80. Primary atypical pneumonia

81. Bubonic plague

Questions 82 through 85

(A) *Diphyllobothrium latum*
(B) *Echinococcus granulosus*
(C) *Necator americanus*
(D) *Trichinella spiralis*
(E) *Trichuris trichiura*

82. Hydatid disease

83. Whipworm

84. Raw pork

85. Megaloblastic anemia

Questions 86 through 89

(A) silicosis
(B) asbestosis
(C) byssinosis
(D) anthracosis
(E) amyloidosis

86. Coal worker's pneumoconiosis

87. Multiple fibrotic pulmonary nodules

88. Pleural mesothelioma

89. Cotton fibers

Questions 90 through 93

(A) ribosomes
(B) cell membrane
(C) mitochondria
(D) nucleus
(E) centrioles

90. Site of cellular antigens and glycocalyx

91. Site of translation and protein manufacture

92. Important in cellular division

93. Contains euchromatin

Questions 94 through 97

(A) hemophilia A
(B) albinism
(C) achondroplasia
(D) Tay-Sachs disease
(E) phenylketonuria

94. Autosomal recessive lack of phenylalanine hydroxylase

95. Autosomal dominant dwarfism

96. Autosomal recessive lack of hexosaminidase A

97. Sex-linked deficiency of factor VIII

Questions 98 through 101

(A) Hashimoto's thyroiditis
(B) primary biliary cirrhosis
(C) Goodpasture's syndrome
(D) Addison's disease
(E) vitiligo

98. Anti-adrenal cell antibodies

99. Antimitochondrial antibodies

100. Antithyroglobulin antibodies

101. Antibasement membrane antibodies

Questions 102 through 105

(A) alpha-fetoprotein
(B) acid phosphatase
(C) serotonin
(D) CA 125
(E) cortisol

102. May be elevated with metastatic prostatic carcinoma

103. May be elevated with metastatic ovarian carcinoma

104. May be elevated with carcinoid tumors

105. May be elevated with hepatocellular carcinoma

Questions 106 through 109

(A) gummatous inflammation
(B) foreign body inflammation
(C) acute suppurative inflammation
(D) granulomatous inflammation
(E) coagulative inflammation

106. Usually seen with tuberculosis

107. Usually seen with syphilis

108. Usually seen with staphylococcal infections

109. Usually seen as a reaction to suture material

Questions 110 through 113

    (A) IgA
    (B) IgG
    (C) IgE
    (D) IgD
    (E) IgM

110. Delta heavy chain

111. Most often found as dimers in mucosal secretions

112. Usually constructed as pentamers

113. Serum level frequently elevated with asthma or allergy

Questions 114 through 117

    (A) hydrothorax
    (B) hydroperitoneum
    (C) hematosalpinx
    (D) pyarthrosis
    (E) hematopericardium

114. Ascites

115. Pus in a joint space

116. Watery fluid accumulation in the pleural cavity

117. Collection of blood in the fallopian tube

Questions 118 through 121

    (A) metaplasia
    (B) dysplasia
    (C) atrophy
    (D) karyorrhexis
    (E) hyperplasia

118. Enlargement of individual cells

119. Reversible change of one adult cell type for another

120. Shrinkage in the size of individual cells

121. Irreversible dissolution of the cell nucleus

Questions 122 through 125

    (A) vitamin A
    (B) niacin
    (C) vitamin C
    (D) vitamin D
    (E) vitamin K

122. Deficiency results in scurvy

123. Deficiency results in rickets

124. Deficiency results in pellagra

125. Deficiency results in hypoprothrombinemia

Questions 126 through 129

    (A) plasma cell
    (B) thrombocyte
    (C) neutrophil
    (D) eosinophil
    (E) basophil

126. Often seen with parasitic infections or asthma

127. Secretes immunoglobulin

128. Vital component of thrombosis and coagulation

129. Cell's basophilic granules are rich in histamine

Questions 130 through 133

    (A) granulomas of tuberculosis
    (B) red infarct
    (C) autoimmune hemolytic anemia
    (D) serum sickness
    (E) anaphylaxis

130. Type I hypersensitivity reaction

131. Type II hypersensitivity reaction

132. Type III hypersensitivity reaction

133. Type IV hypersensitivity reaction

Questions 134 through 137

    (A) interleukin-1
    (B) bradykinin
    (C) platelet-activating factor
    (D) myeloperoxidase
    (E) prostacyclin

134. Plasma protease that produces local pain at site of injection

135. Cyclooxygenase pathway member with vasodilatory and antiplatelet aggregating properties

136. Neutrophilic enzyme used for bacterial killing in lysosomes

137. Lymphokine

Questions 138 through 141

(A) Edwards' syndrome
(B) Down's syndrome
(C) Klinefelter's syndrome
(D) Cat's cry syndrome
(E) Turner's syndrome

138. 45,X

139. 47,XXY

140. 47,XX,+21

141. 47,XY,+18

Questions 142 through 145

(A) adenoma
(B) teratoma
(C) hemangioma
(D) lipoma
(E) adenocarcinoma
(F) squamous cell carcinoma
(G) malignant lymphoma
(H) malignant melanoma

142. A 54-year-old woman has noticed a small reddish nodule on her arm for about a year. The nodule blanches with pressure. After surgical excision the nodule is examined microscopically and found to be composed entirely of benign blood vessels. What term most correctly defines this tumor?

143. A 34-year-old woman has an ovary removed. Grossly the ovary has been replaced by a solid and cystic tumor composed of hair, teeth, skin, and other benign elements. Microscopically there are organoid constructions of various benign ectodermal, endodermal, and mesenchymal elements. What term most correctly describes this tumor?

144. A 77-year-old man has an enlarged lymph node removed. Grossly the nodal architecture is effaced by a solid tan "fish flesh" tumor. Microscopically there is a monomorphic population of large malignant lymphoid cells. What term most correctly defines this tumor?

145. A 65-year-old man complains to his doctor of increasing fatigue. On examination the man is found to be anemic and have a mass in his right colon. The colonic tumor is excised and found to be composed of malignant cells which form numerous gland-like structures. What term most correctly identifies this tumor?

Questions 146 through 149

(A) anaerobic bacteria
(B) aerobic bacteria
(C) spirochete
(D) mycobacterium
(E) rickettsia
(F) virus
(G) protozoan
(H) nematode

146. A 13-year-old male with sore throat, fever, and enlarged tonsils has a throat culture performed. The laboratory reports that *Streptococcus pyogenes* has been isolated. What type of organism has been isolated?

147. A 23-year-old sexually active male suddenly develops painful vesicles on his penis. A culture of vesicle fluid is reported as containing herpes simplex. What kind of organism is this?

148. A 34-year-old female camper develops diarrhea. An examination of her feces reveals *Giardia lamblia*. What type of organism is this?

149. A 43-year-old male hiker develops a rash, headache, and malaise. A diagnosis of Rocky Mountain spotted fever is made. What type of organism causes this disease?

Questions 150 through 153

(A) tophus
(B) ceroid
(C) borate
(D) bilirubin
(E) amyloid
(F) cholesterol
(G) carbon
(H) asbestos

150. A 55-year-old female with chronic osteomyelitis develops congestive heart failure. A rectal biopsy demonstrates abundant eosinophilic acellular material that has apple green birefringence after Congo red staining. What is this material?

151. A hilar lymph node is removed from an urban dweller who also smokes. The nodal macrophages contain abundant black particulate material. What is this material most likely to be?

152. An end-stage alcoholic is admitted to the hospital. He is jaundiced and in particular, his sclerae have a yellowish discoloration. What is this yellowish pigment?

153. A 47-year-old male with gout notices numerous subcutaneous nodules along the extensor tendons of his arm. One of these nodules is removed and demonstrates abundant positively birefringent needle-shaped crystals. What are these nodules?

Answers and Explanations

1. **(C)** Diphtheria is caused by *Clostridium diphtheriae,* an organism that causes a localized upper respiratory tract infection. The release of exotoxin produces the severe systemic changes that accompany the disease. *(2:351–352)*

2. **(E)** Leprosy is caused by *M. leprae,* an acid-fast bacillus. Clinically, the disease is divided into tuberculoid and lepromatous forms. Armadillos in the wild can harbor leprosy. The peripheral nerves are almost always involved in leprosy. *(2:380–382)*

3. **(D)** Hyperacute rejection involves preformed circulating antibodies, such as the blood group O recipient's anti-A and anti-B. Kidney cells will contain the donor's B antigen, and a hyperacute rejection will occur. *(1:120–122)*

4. **(C)** The site of oxidative phosphorylation is mitochondria. The other statements about cell membranes are true. *(1:3–5)*

5. **(B)** Cations are positively charged ions and include all the listed choices except bicarbonate (anion). The major intracellular cation is potassium. Sodium is the major extracellular cation. *(1:28)*

6. **(D)** Phagocytosis is the engulfment of particulate matter by cells. These cells can be of two classes, fixed tissue cells (Kupffer cells in liver) and migrating cells (neutrophils). *(3:54–57)*

7. **(A)** The normal pericardial sac contains about 5 to 50 ml of fluid. Accumulation of 100 ml or more of transudative fluid is a hydropericardium. The term "hydropericardium" is not applied to exudative expansions of the pericardium as seen in pericarditis. Hydropericardium can occur in most edematous states, including heart failure and myxedema. An accumulation of fluid can distend the pericardial sac to as great as 1000 ml if there is no associated pericardial disease offering resistance to gradual expansion. *(2:648–649)*

8. **(B)** Langhans' giant cells are the hallmarks of granulomatous inflammation. *(2:65–68)*

9. **(C)** Acetaminophen is a hepatotoxin. Toxic metabolites bind to the macromolecules of hepatocellular protein, with resultant coagulative necrosis of hepatocytes. *(2:487)*

10. **(C)** Type I hypersensitivity reactions are anaphylactic and require IgE (cytotropic antibody) to trigger release of vasoactive amines from basophils and mast cells. *(1:107–108)*

11. **(D)** T lymphocytes, not B lymphocytes, have receptors for sheep erythrocytes. *(3:98–101)*

12. **(B)** The lysosomal storage product in Gaucher's disease is glucocerebroside. The diseases in which sphingomyelin, ceramide trihexoside, sulfatide, and GM-2 ganglioside accumulate are Niemann–Pick, Fabry's, metachromatic leukodystrophy, and Tay-Sachs, respectively. *(1:240–242)*

13. **(D)** Respiratory distress in newborns results in large part from lack of pulmonary surfactant. Diabetic mothers and prematurity increase the risk. Pulmonary histopathologic changes usually include hyaline membranes. Survivors have an increased risk of patent ductus arteriosus, intraventricular hemorrhage and necrotizing enterocolitis. *(1:247, 513–514)*

14. **(D)** Fat necrosis is common in adipose tissue contiguous to the pancreas as a result of leakage of lipase after acute injury to pancreatic acinar tissue. Grossly, minute firm yellowish-white deposits occur. Microscopically, the necrotic fat cells have pale outlines and are filled with fine basophilic soap material. *(2:18–19)*

15. **(C)** The more radiosensitive a cell is, the more likely it is that the cell will be damaged or killed by a given dose of radiation. Lymphocytes are highly radiosensitive. The other listed choices have low radiosensitivity. *(1:175–176)*

16. **(D)** In gas gangrene, the tissues become discolored and foul, with microscopic evidence of cellular disruption. Leukocytes are scarce. This pattern of necrosis is seen in association with clostridial toxins and infections. *(2:358–360)*

17. **(E)** Acute cyanide poisoning is caused by cyanide's ability to bind to cytochrome oxidase and produce cellular asphyxia. Less than 0.1 g of ingested inorganic salt may be fatal. At death, the blood is cherry red, and a pungent bitter-almond smell may be present. The kidney is affected no more so than other organs in the body. *(1:190)*

18. **(C)** Tinea capitis is a superficial fungal infection of the hair of the scalp, eyebrows, and eyelashes. *(2:1309–1310)*

19. **(D)** Of the listed choices, only vitamin E is fat-soluble. The other choices are water-soluble vitamins. *(1:156–164)*

20. **(B)** The triad of fever, leukopenia, and bradycardia should suggest the diagnosis of typhoid fever, particularly in association with diarrhea and lymphoid hyperplasia. Typhoid fever is caused by *Salmonella typhi*. *(2:353–355)*

21. **(C)** Cancers are graded into three or four grades by their microscopic appearance. Increasing anaplasia and dedifferentiation are seen with increasing grades from I (well differentiated) to grade III or IV (poorly differentiated). With most tumors, the highest grades are associated with the poorest prognoses. *(1:311)*

22. **(D)** Epidermoid carcinoma, alternatively called "squamous cell carcinoma," usually produces keratin products, including keratin pearls. None of the other listed choices routinely produces keratin. The fibroadenoma is a benign tumor. *(3:143–146)*

23. **(A)** All of the listed choices, except urinary tract infections, are common forms of *H. influenzae* infection. Other forms are bronchiolitis, laryngotracheobronchitis, and pneumonia. *(3:363–364)*

24. **(C)** The virulence of the pneumococcus is caused by a thick polysaccharide coat and an M protein. *(3:567–568)*

25. **(C)** A hamartoma is a focal, often circumscribed overgrowth in improper proportions of tissue normally present in that part of the body. Hamartomas arise in many organs and locations. One of the most common sites for hamartomas is the lungs. *(2:537–538)*

26. **(D)** Phenylketonuria is an autosomal recessive disorder, not X-linked. *(3:231)*

27. **(A)** The only organism of the five listed that is gram positive is *S. pneumoniae*. *K. pneumoniae* and *E. aerogenes* pneumonias also occur in alcoholics but are caused by gram-negative, rod-shaped bacteria. *(3:385–391)*

28. **(B)** A 1000-rad acute whole body irradiation is a devastating amount of radiation, and after a few days, the fatality rate would be 100%. *(1:173–178)*

29. **(E)** Hemorrhage is not a feature of carbon monoxide poisoning. All the other statements are true. *(2:495)*

30. **(E)** Scurvy is caused by a lack of vitamin C. Lack of iron, thiamine, niacin, and vitamin D result in microcytic anemia, beriberi, pellagra, and rickets, respectively. *(1:156–164)*

31. **(D)** *H. influenzae* usually causes meningitis and respiratory infections, not diarrhea. The other choices classically produce acute gastroenterocolitis with diarrhea. *(3:363–364)*

32. **(B)** Edema fluid that accumulates in the pleural cavity is hydrothorax. Ascites are edema fluid collections in the abdominal cavity. Anasarca is severe generalized edema, particularly noticeable in the subcutaneous tissues. Hydropericardium is a pericardial effusion. *(2:87–88)*

33. **(B)** The positive Congo red stain is characteristic of amyloid deposition. Hemosiderin, hematin, and bilirubin are brownish pigments. Urate is eosinophilic but does not have Congo red birefringence. *(2:24–26,210–220)*

34. **(D)** Herpes simplex type I (HSV 1) infections are caused by a DNA virus. The most common infection is the fever blister or cold sore. Less common infections include keratoconjunctivitis, aphthous stomatitis, and a latency of virus in ganglia. Herpes zoster shingles is a reactivation of the varicella virus not HSV 1. *(3:334–340)*

35. **(B)** Zoonotic infections are transmitted to humans from animal hosts or reservoirs. Examples include arboviruses and rickettsial diseases. *(2:308–310)*

36. **(B)** Translation involves the production of protein molecules from messenger RNA. Transcription is the production of RNA from DNA. Organization, first intention, and granulation are terms used with wounds and healing. *(1:7)*

37. **(E)** An occlusive arterial thrombus, such as coronary thrombosis, is almost always at the site of a vessel abnormality. The most common abnormality is atherosclerosis. Rarer abnormalities would include arteritis and trauma. An expected finding in

coronary thrombosis is infarction of the myocardium with ischemic (coagulative) necrosis. Thrombocytopenia is not expected in coronary thrombosis, since platelets must be present in adequate numbers and function to initiate a thrombus. A low platelet count would make thrombus formation unlikely. *(2:99–105)*

38. **(D)** Sir Percival Pott astutely related an increased incidence of scrotal skin cancer in chimney sweeps to chronic exposure to soot. After institution of the practice of daily bathing, the rate of cancer dropped dramatically. Many polycyclic and heterocyclic aromatic hydrocarbons are chemical carcinogens and are present in high concentration in soot. *(1:286)*

39. **(C)** The malignant tumor is derived from lymphocytes, resulting from an immunologic kappa-chain marker. Malignant tumors of lymphocytes are termed "lymphoma" or "plasmacytoma" depending on the degree of cellular maturation. The other choices do not contain kappa light chains. *(3:1091–1108)*

40. **(C)** Leukemia is the most common fatal malignancy in children 15 years old and younger. The other choices are the four next most common causes of childhood fatal cancers. *(1:275–276)*

41. **(D)** After skin cancer, lung carcinoma is the most frequent cancer in North American males. Lung cancer is followed in frequency by prostate cancer, colorectal cancer, bladder cancer, and lymphomas, respectively. *(1:274–277)*

42. **(C)** AIDS is caused by HIV, formerly called HTLV III. The other listed choices are commonly found with AIDS but are not the direct cause of the disease. *(1:98–103)*

43. **(B)** SLE is an autoimmune disorder characterized by autoantibodies against numerous nuclear components. Repeated pyogenic infections are not a feature of SLE. *(1:123–125)*

44. **(B)** Cat's cry syndrome involves the deletion of the short arm of chromosome 5. Trisomy 18, trisomy 21, trisomy 13, and 47,XXY are Edward's syndrome, Down's syndrome, Patau's syndrome, and Klinefelter's syndrome, respectively. *(1:233–237)*

45. **(B)** Hypertrophy is an increase in the size of cells and, with such a change, an increase in the size of the organ. A classic example of hypertrophy is left ventricular cardiac hypertrophy seen in systemic hypertension. *(2:31–32)*

46. **(B)** Hemosiderin is the iron–ferritin complexes seen in heart failure macrophages. The other listed choices have black to brown coloration but are not composed of iron–ferritin complexes. *(2:24–26)*

47. **(D)** Endometrial adenocarcinoma is a tumor of adulthood. The other choices are common malignant neoplasms of childhood and infancy. *(2:1150–1151)*

48. **(D)** The electron microscope pattern describes a lysosomal storage disease. These are genetic and usually result from an absence of a specific degradative enzyme. The infant's prognosis is poor. DNA is still present in the affected cells, however. *(3:226)*

49. **(B)** Most staphylococcal infections result in abundant pus formation, termed "suppuration." Staphylococcal skin infections include furuncles, carbuncles, surgical wounds, and impetigo. Caseous necrosis is not a pattern of reaction as seen in staphylococcal infections. *(3:381–385)*

50. **(A)** Rickettsiae are obligate intracellular parasites that contain DNA and RNA and usually produce rashes and eschars. Insect vectors are necessary for transmission of all the rickettsial diseases except Q fever. Spirochetes cause yaws and pinta. *(3:349–351)*

51. **(E)** Gland-forming carcinomas are called "adenocarcinomas." Squamous cell carcinoma, melanoma, and lymphoma are malignant tumors derived from squamous cells, melanocytes, and lymphocytes, respectively. *(2:240–243)*

52. **(C)** Cytomegalic inclusion disease is caused by a herpes family double-strand DNA virus. All the other choices are arthropod-borne viruses (arbovirus) of the single-strand RNA type. *(3:337–338)*

53. **(B)** Mumps is an acute contagious childhood disease caused by a paramyxovirus that usually is acquired by respiratory droplet infection. Parotitis, orchitis, and encephalitis occur. Diarrhea is unusual. *(3:341–342,1275–1276)*

54. **(A)** Common features of malignancy include invasiveness, metastases, aneuploidy, elevated mitotic rate, abnormal mitoses, and anaplasia. Encapsulation usually is seen with benign tumors. *(1:266–270)*

55. **(E)** Gonorrhea is caused by a bacterium, not a chlamydial organism. *(3:389–391)*

56. **(D)** Bruton's agammaglobulinemia is a sex-linked disorder characterized by virtual absence of B cells. Antibody production is, therefore, essentially nil. The T cell functions, such as delayed hypersensitivity, are normal. An increased incidence of autoimmune disorders occurs with Bruton's agammaglobulinemia. *(2:221)*

57. **(C)** Antimicrosomal and antithyroglobulin antibodies characterize Hashimoto's thyroiditis. The other listed autoimmune diseases principally have antibodies against nuclear fractions. *(1:123–126)*

58. **(A)** Type I hypersensitivity reactions are anaphylactic. Complement-mediated cytotoxicity and circulating immune complexes are type II and III hypersensitivity reactions, respectively. Type IV reactions are those of cell-mediated or delayed hypersensitivity. *(1:107–117)*

59. **(B)** Pompe's disease is a glycogenosis caused by a buildup of glycogen in skeletal muscle, cardiac muscle, and liver. The other choices are sphingolipidoses caused by an inherited inability to degrade sphingolipids. *(2:151–152)*

60. **(D)** Gummas are circumscribed, rubbery lesions measuring from a few millimeters to several centimeters in diameter. Microscopically, the central portion has coagulative necrosis, which is surrounded by a peripheral wall of epithelial cells, lymphocytes, and plasma cells. Gummas are the characteristic lesion of tertiary syphilis. *(3:356)*

61. **(A)** Marfan's syndrome (arachnodactyly) usually has cardiovascular dissolution termed "cystic medionecrosis." The other choices are also hereditary diseases but are not associated with cystic medionecrosis. *(3:222)*

62. **(E)** Klinefelter's syndrome (testicular atrophy, eunuchoid habitus, mental retardation, gynecomastia) usually has a 47,XXY karyotype. The 46,XX and 46,XY karyotypes are normal female and male karyotypes, respectively. Turner's syndrome is 45, XO. The double-Y male is 47,XYY. *(1:230–237)*

63. **(A)** Hemorrhagic venous infarcts are most likely to occur with occlusive venous thromboses, in loose tissues, tissues with a double circulation, and tissues previously congested. These criteria usually are present in the small intestine. The other choices usually experience pale arterial infarcts. *(2:111–114)*

64. **(E)** Collagen provides the critical framework for wound healing. Actin and myosin are contractile proteins. Chemotactic factors and kinins are important in acute inflammatory reactions but are not critical components of wound healing. *(2:78–82)*

65. **(D)** An abscess is a localized collection of pus. *(2:69)*

66. **(D)** Metaplasia is the reversible change in which one adult cell type is replaced by another. *(2:34)*

67. **(C)** Intermediate filaments include keratins, desmin, vimentin, glial filaments, and neural filaments. Actin (6–8 nm) is a thin contractile protein, not an intermediate filament. Identification of intermediate filaments in a tumor tissues permits more precise histologic diagnoses. *(2:301)*

68. **(B)** Cell death, necrosis, is best identified by nuclear changes, such as karyorrhexis, the dissolution of the nucleus. Vacuolar degeneration, hydropic change, and cellular swelling are interchangeable terms describing nonlethal, reversible intracellular water accumulation. Fatty change is a nonlethal, reversible change, usually occurring in hepatocytes. *(2:16–17)*

69. **(A)** The hallmark of ischemic infarcts is coagulative necrosis. Liquefaction necrosis, enzymatic necrosis, and caseous necrosis are seen with brain infarcts, acute pancreatitis, and tuberculosis, respectively. Giant cells are seen in a number of nonspecific reactions and with tumors. They are not usually associated with ischemic necrosis. *(2:17–19)*

70. **(E)** Gas embolism (caisson disease) usually results from rapid decompression, eg, scuba divers who ascend too rapidly to the surface. Less common causes include traumatic pneumothorax or uterine manipulation. The other choices have no relation to gas embolism. *(2:109–110)*

71. **(C)** Thrombus formation is most likely with endothelial damage (exposure of collagen), hypercoagulable states, and alterations in blood flow, such as stasis. Activated plasmin is a key component of the fibrinolytic system and is likely to oppose thrombus formation. *(2:99–105)*

72. **(A)** Edema can be caused by increased vascular hydrostatic pressure, reduced oncotic plasma pressure, lymphatic obstruction, increased sodium retention, or increased endothelial permeability. Hyperproteinemia would increase the vascular oncotic pressure, making edema less likely. *(2:80–87)*

73. **(D)** The body is about 65% water. Of that, two thirds is intracellular water, and one third is extracellular water. The extracellular compartment is further subdivided as 80% interstitial water and 20% plasma water. Whole blood volume is only about twice the plasma volume. *(2:87–88)*

74. **(D)**

75. **(A)**

76. **(B)**

77. **(C)**

74 through 77. The nomenclature of tumors is complex. The suffix *oma* implies a tumor. Benign tumors usually are named by adding the suffix to the name of the cell type involved, such as leiomyoma (smooth muscle cells) and hidradenoma (sweat gland cells). Malignant tumors of mesenchyme are sarcomas. This suffix can be added to the cell type, eg., rhabdomyosarcoma (skeletal muscle cells). Malignant tumors of epithelium are called "carcinomas," which can be added as a suffix to the cell type, eg., choriocarcinoma (trophoblastic cells). *(2:240–243)*

78. **(B)**

79. **(D)**

80. **(A)**

81. **(C)**

78 through 81. Each of the listed diseases has only one causative organism. *(3:328–449)*

82. **(B)**

83. **(E)**

84. **(D)**

85. **(A)**

82 through 85. All of the organisms listed are helminths. *(3:328–449)*

86. **(D)**

87. **(A)**

88. **(B)**

89. **(C)**

86 through 89. The four disease states are all pneumoconioses, pulmonary diseases caused by inhaled substances. Inhaled cotton fibers and coal dust characterize byssinosis and coal workers' pneumoconiosis, respectively. Pleural mesotheliomas occur with increased frequency with exposure to asbestos. Inhaled silica particles characteristically caused nodular pulmonary fibrosis. *(2:472–484)*

90. **(B)**

91. **(A)**

92. **(E)**

93. **(D)**

90 through 93. The nucleus of the cell contains interphase chromosomes that are relatively uncoiled, called "euchromatin." The cell membrane, a unit membrane, is the site of glycocalyx and numerous cellular antigens. The centrioles direct cellular division. The ribosomes, either free or attached to the endoplasmic reticulum, are the site of protein synthesis, or translation. *(2:4–9)*

94. **(E)**

95. **(C)**

96. **(D)**

97. **(A)**

94 through 97. Phenylketonuria is an autosomal recessive disorder caused by a hereditary lack of the enzyme phenylalanine hydroxylase. Affected neonates suffer from mental retardation unless fed a diet deficient in phenylalanine. Dwarfism, also termed "achondroplasia," is an autosomal dominant disorder of abnormal cartilage growth with resultant short stature. A genetic absence of the enzyme hexosaminidase A produces Tay-Sachs disease. Mental retardation and blindness occur because of an accumulation of ganglioside in lysosomes. Hemophilia A is a sex-linked hemorrhagic disorder due to a lack of factor VIII. *(3:233–234,229,231,1315–1316)*

98. **(D)**

99. **(B)**

100. **(A)**

101. **(C)**

98 through 101. Autoantibodies characterize a number of diseases. In Addison's disease there are usually antibodies directed against adrenal cells. Antimitochondrial antibodies are seen in primary biliary cirrhosis. Antibodies against thyroglobulin and basement membrane material are seen with Hashimoto's thyroiditis and Goodpasture's syndrome, respectively. With vitiligo there may be autoantibodies against melanocytes. *(1:124)*

102. **(B)**

103. **(D)**

104. **(C)**

105. **(A)**

102 through 105. A number of tumor cell products are manufactured by neoplasms. The detection of these products may assist in diagnosis and in directing therapy. Metastatic prostate cancer may produce elevations of serum-acid phosphatase and prostate-specific antigen. Ovarian carcinomas may secrete CA 125. Carcinoid tumors can be associated with elevations of serotonin and its urinary metabolite, 5-HIAA. Elevations in serum alpha-fetoprotein can be seen with hepatocellular carcinoma and with gonadal germ cell tumors. *(1:300–301)*

106. (D)

107. (A)

108. (C)

109. (B)

106 through 109. The specific pattern of inflammation is orchestrated by both the immune state of the host and the type of challenge presented to it. With tubercle bacilli a granulomatous reaction characteristically develops. In chronic syphilitic infections a gummatous reaction is seen. Staphylococcal infections produce acute suppuration and abscess formation. Suture material usually causes a foreign body inflammatory reaction. *(3:54–62)*

110. (D)

111. (A)

112. (E)

113. (C)

110 through 113. The delta heavy chain is present in IgD immunoglobulin molecules. IgA is most frequently encountered as dimers in mucosal secretions. The pentameric form of IgM is the most common variant of the IgM molecule. Elevated serum levels of IgE may be seen with asthma or with other allergic states. *(1:61–63)*

114. (B)

115. (D)

116. (A)

117. (C)

114 through 117. Watery accumulations of fluid in the peritoneum and pleural cavities are termed "hydroperitoneum" (ascites) and "hydrothorax," respectively. An accumulation of pus in a joint space is called a "pyarthrosis." A dilated, blood-filled fallopian tube is called a "hematosalpinx." *(2:87,1172)*

118. (E)

119. (A)

120. (C)

121. (D)

118 through 121. Hyperplasia is an enlargement of individual cells, such as cardiac ventricular hyperplasia due to essential hypertension. The reversible change of one adult cell type for another is metaplasia. Metaplasia is usually a protective adaptation of cells to noxious environmental stresses. Atrophy can be defined as the shrinkage of individual cells. Karyorrhexis is the irreversible dissolution of the cell nucleus associated with cell death. *(2:30–34)*

122. (C)

123. (D)

124. (B)

125. (E)

122 through 125. Deficiencies of vitamin C and vitamin D produce scurvy and rickets, respectively. Niacin-deficient diets can produce a disease state termed "pellagra" characterized by diarrhea, dermatitis, and dementia. Deficiency of vitamin K, a fat-soluble vitamin, can result in a hemorrhagic diathesis due to an inability of the liver to synthesize sufficient prothrombin and other vitamin K dependent blood clotting factors. *(1:158–163)*

126. (D)

127. (A)

128. (B)

129. (E)

126 through 129. Eosinophils may be seen in increased numbers in parasitic and allergic reactions. Plasma cells manufacture and secrete immunoglobulins. Platelets, also called "thrombocytes," are an integral part of coagulation and thrombosis. The basophil has abundant histamine containing granules that are strikingly basophilic when stained with the routinely employed hematology dyes. *(3:38–62)*

130. (E)

131. (C)

132. (D)

133. (A)

130 through 133. Anaphylaxis is an example of a type I hypersensitivity reaction. Autoimmune hemolytic anemia is an example of a cytotoxic hypersensitivity reaction (type II). Serum sickness serves as an example of generalized immune complex disease. Immune complex reactions with or without complement activation are type III hypersensitivity reactions. Granulomatous inflammation with tuberculosis is a type IV hypersensitivity reaction of the cell-mediated variety. *(1:107–117)*

134. **(B)**

135. **(E)**

136. **(D)**

137. **(A)**

134 through 137. Bradykinin is a plasma protease that produces local pain if injected into the skin and elicits reversible edema. Prostacyclin is a cyclooxygenase-derived prostaglandin with vasodilatory and antiplatelet aggregating properties. Myeloperoxidase is an enzyme manufactured by neutrophils. It is used for bacterial killing in phagolysosomes. Interleukin-1 is a lymphokine with the ability to produce fever and stimulate prostaglandin synthesis. *(3:42–48,55,62–63)*

138. **(E)**

139. **(C)**

140. **(B)**

141. **(A)**

138 through 141. Turner's syndrome may include short stature, web neck, cardiac abnormalities, and streak gonads. The karyotype is 45,X or a mosaic 45,X/46,XX. The karyotype for Klinefelter's syndrome is 47,XXY. Down's syndrome and Edward's syndrome are trisomies of chromosomes 21 and 18, respectively. *(1:230–237)*

142. **(C)**

143. **(B)**

144. **(G)**

145. **(E)**

142 through 145. Hemangiomas are benign tumors composed of blood vessels. A benign teratoma of the ovary, also called a "dermoid," is usually constructed by organoid ectoderm, endoderm, and mesenchyme. Malignant lymphomas are composed of clonal proliferations of lymphoid cells. The degree of cellular anaplasia and differentiation vary from case to case. Malignant tumors of glandular epithelium are termed "adenocarcinomas." *(2:240–243)*

146. **(B)**

147. **(F)**

148. **(G)**

149. **(E)**

146 through 149. The organism, *Streptococcus pyogenes*, is an aerobic bacterium. It is the usual cause of strep throat. Infection with herpes simplex, a virus, may result in painful genital vesicles. *Giardia lamblia* is a protozoan organism that frequently causes diarrhea. The infectious agent of Rocky Mountain spotted fever is a rickettsial organism. *(1:193–212)*

150. **(E)**

151. **(G)**

152. **(D)**

153. **(A)**

150 through 153. Amyloid is acellular eosinophilic material that may accumulate throughout the body. It is seen with chronic infections and lymphoproliferative disorders. Amyloid material demonstrates apple green birefringence after staining with Congo red. Carbon particles, also termed "anthracotic pigment," are commonly seen in the hilar lymph nodes of smokers, urban dwellers, and coal miners. The yellowish pigment that causes jaundice is bilirubin. Uric acid crystals form tophi in many individuals with chronic gout. *(2:24–26,210–220,1358–1359)*

REFERENCES

1. Chandrasoma P, Taylor CR: Concise Pathology, Norwalk, Appleton & Lange, 1991
2. Cotran RS, Kumar V, Robbins SL: Robbins Pathologic Basis of Disease, 4th ed. Philadelphia, Saunders, 1989
3. Rubin E, Farber JL: Pathology, Philadelphia, Lippincott, 1988

Practice Test Subspecialty List

CELL INJURY AND DEATH

4, 36, 46, 67, 68, 69, 90, 91, 92, 93, 118, 119, 120, 121, 150, 151, 152, 153

INFLAMMATION, HEALING, AND REPAIR

6, 8, 14, 45, 60, 64, 65, 66, 114, 115, 116, 117, 126, 127, 128, 129, 134, 135, 136, 137

FLUID BALANCE, HEMODYNAMICS, COAGULATION, AND ACID-BASE

5, 7, 13, 32, 37, 63, 70, 71, 72, 73

IMMUNOPATHOLOGY

3, 10, 11, 33, 42, 43, 56, 57, 58, 98, 99, 100, 101, 110, 111, 112, 113, 130, 131, 132, 133

INFECTIOUS DISEASES

1, 2, 16, 18, 20, 23, 24, 27, 31, 34, 35, 49, 50, 52, 53, 55, 78, 79, 80, 81, 82, 83, 84, 85, 94, 95, 96, 97, 106, 107, 108, 109, 146, 147, 148, 149

GENETIC, METABOLIC, AND ENVIRONMENTAL PATHOLOGY

9, 12, 15, 17, 19, 26, 28, 29, 30, 44, 48, 59, 61, 62, 86, 87, 88, 89, 122, 123, 124, 125, 138, 139, 140, 141

NEOPLASIA AND ABNORMALITIES OF GROWTH

21, 22, 25, 38, 39, 40, 41, 47, 51, 54, 74, 75, 76, 77, 102, 103, 104, 105, 142, 143, 144, 145

NAME _____
         Last   First   Middle

ADDRESS _____
              Street

_____
      City   State   Zip

SOCIAL SECURITY NUMBER

	0 1 2 3 4 5 6 7 8 9
	0 1 2 3 4 5 6 7 8 9
	0 1 2 3 4 5 6 7 8 9
	0 1 2 3 4 5 6 7 8 9
	0 1 2 3 4 5 6 7 8 9
	0 1 2 3 4 5 6 7 8 9
	0 1 2 3 4 5 6 7 8 9
	0 1 2 3 4 5 6 7 8 9
	0 1 2 3 4 5 6 7 8 9

DIRECTIONS

MAKE ERASURES COMPLETE

Mark your social security number from top to bottom in the appropriate boxes on the right. Refer to the section " HOW TO TAKE THE PRACTICE TEST" in the introduction to the book for more information. PLEASE USE NO. 2 PENCIL ONLY.

1 Ⓐ Ⓑ Ⓒ Ⓓ Ⓔ
2 Ⓐ Ⓑ Ⓒ Ⓓ Ⓔ
3 Ⓐ Ⓑ Ⓒ Ⓓ Ⓔ
4 Ⓐ Ⓑ Ⓒ Ⓓ Ⓔ
5 Ⓐ Ⓑ Ⓒ Ⓓ Ⓔ
6 Ⓐ Ⓑ Ⓒ Ⓓ Ⓔ
7 Ⓐ Ⓑ Ⓒ Ⓓ Ⓔ
8 Ⓐ Ⓑ Ⓒ Ⓓ Ⓔ
9 Ⓐ Ⓑ Ⓒ Ⓓ Ⓔ
10 Ⓐ Ⓑ Ⓒ Ⓓ Ⓔ
11 Ⓐ Ⓑ Ⓒ Ⓓ Ⓔ
12 Ⓐ Ⓑ Ⓒ Ⓓ Ⓔ
13 Ⓐ Ⓑ Ⓒ Ⓓ Ⓔ
14 Ⓐ Ⓑ Ⓒ Ⓓ Ⓔ
15 Ⓐ Ⓑ Ⓒ Ⓓ Ⓔ
16 Ⓐ Ⓑ Ⓒ Ⓓ Ⓔ
17 Ⓐ Ⓑ Ⓒ Ⓓ Ⓔ
18 Ⓐ Ⓑ Ⓒ Ⓓ Ⓔ
19 Ⓐ Ⓑ Ⓒ Ⓓ Ⓔ
20 Ⓐ Ⓑ Ⓒ Ⓓ Ⓔ
21 Ⓐ Ⓑ Ⓒ Ⓓ Ⓔ
22 Ⓐ Ⓑ Ⓒ Ⓓ Ⓔ
23 Ⓐ Ⓑ Ⓒ Ⓓ Ⓔ
24 Ⓐ Ⓑ Ⓒ Ⓓ Ⓔ
25 Ⓐ Ⓑ Ⓒ Ⓓ Ⓔ

26 Ⓐ Ⓑ Ⓒ Ⓓ Ⓔ
27 Ⓐ Ⓑ Ⓒ Ⓓ Ⓔ
28 Ⓐ Ⓑ Ⓒ Ⓓ Ⓔ
29 Ⓐ Ⓑ Ⓒ Ⓓ Ⓔ
30 Ⓐ Ⓑ Ⓒ Ⓓ Ⓔ
31 Ⓐ Ⓑ Ⓒ Ⓓ Ⓔ
32 Ⓐ Ⓑ Ⓒ Ⓓ Ⓔ
33 Ⓐ Ⓑ Ⓒ Ⓓ Ⓔ
34 Ⓐ Ⓑ Ⓒ Ⓓ Ⓔ
35 Ⓐ Ⓑ Ⓒ Ⓓ Ⓔ
36 Ⓐ Ⓑ Ⓒ Ⓓ Ⓔ
37 Ⓐ Ⓑ Ⓒ Ⓓ Ⓔ
38 Ⓐ Ⓑ Ⓒ Ⓓ Ⓔ
39 Ⓐ Ⓑ Ⓒ Ⓓ Ⓔ
40 Ⓐ Ⓑ Ⓒ Ⓓ Ⓔ
41 Ⓐ Ⓑ Ⓒ Ⓓ Ⓔ
42 Ⓐ Ⓑ Ⓒ Ⓓ Ⓔ
43 Ⓐ Ⓑ Ⓒ Ⓓ Ⓔ
44 Ⓐ Ⓑ Ⓒ Ⓓ Ⓔ
45 Ⓐ Ⓑ Ⓒ Ⓓ Ⓔ
46 Ⓐ Ⓑ Ⓒ Ⓓ Ⓔ
47 Ⓐ Ⓑ Ⓒ Ⓓ Ⓔ
48 Ⓐ Ⓑ Ⓒ Ⓓ Ⓔ
49 Ⓐ Ⓑ Ⓒ Ⓓ Ⓔ
50 Ⓐ Ⓑ Ⓒ Ⓓ Ⓔ

51 Ⓐ Ⓑ Ⓒ Ⓓ Ⓔ
52 Ⓐ Ⓑ Ⓒ Ⓓ Ⓔ
53 Ⓐ Ⓑ Ⓒ Ⓓ Ⓔ
54 Ⓐ Ⓑ Ⓒ Ⓓ Ⓔ
55 Ⓐ Ⓑ Ⓒ Ⓓ Ⓔ
56 Ⓐ Ⓑ Ⓒ Ⓓ Ⓔ
57 Ⓐ Ⓑ Ⓒ Ⓓ Ⓔ
58 Ⓐ Ⓑ Ⓒ Ⓓ Ⓔ
59 Ⓐ Ⓑ Ⓒ Ⓓ Ⓔ
60 Ⓐ Ⓑ Ⓒ Ⓓ Ⓔ
61 Ⓐ Ⓑ Ⓒ Ⓓ Ⓔ
62 Ⓐ Ⓑ Ⓒ Ⓓ Ⓔ
63 Ⓐ Ⓑ Ⓒ Ⓓ Ⓔ
64 Ⓐ Ⓑ Ⓒ Ⓓ Ⓔ
65 Ⓐ Ⓑ Ⓒ Ⓓ Ⓔ
66 Ⓐ Ⓑ Ⓒ Ⓓ Ⓔ
67 Ⓐ Ⓑ Ⓒ Ⓓ Ⓔ
68 Ⓐ Ⓑ Ⓒ Ⓓ Ⓔ
69 Ⓐ Ⓑ Ⓒ Ⓓ Ⓔ
70 Ⓐ Ⓑ Ⓒ Ⓓ Ⓔ
71 Ⓐ Ⓑ Ⓒ Ⓓ Ⓔ
72 Ⓐ Ⓑ Ⓒ Ⓓ Ⓔ
73 Ⓐ Ⓑ Ⓒ Ⓓ Ⓔ
74 Ⓐ Ⓑ Ⓒ Ⓓ Ⓔ
75 Ⓐ Ⓑ Ⓒ Ⓓ Ⓔ

76 Ⓐ Ⓑ Ⓒ Ⓓ Ⓔ
77 Ⓐ Ⓑ Ⓒ Ⓓ Ⓔ
78 Ⓐ Ⓑ Ⓒ Ⓓ Ⓔ
79 Ⓐ Ⓑ Ⓒ Ⓓ Ⓔ
80 Ⓐ Ⓑ Ⓒ Ⓓ Ⓔ
81 Ⓐ Ⓑ Ⓒ Ⓓ Ⓔ
82 Ⓐ Ⓑ Ⓒ Ⓓ Ⓔ
83 Ⓐ Ⓑ Ⓒ Ⓓ Ⓔ
84 Ⓐ Ⓑ Ⓒ Ⓓ Ⓔ
85 Ⓐ Ⓑ Ⓒ Ⓓ Ⓔ
86 Ⓐ Ⓑ Ⓒ Ⓓ Ⓔ
87 Ⓐ Ⓑ Ⓒ Ⓓ Ⓔ
88 Ⓐ Ⓑ Ⓒ Ⓓ Ⓔ
89 Ⓐ Ⓑ Ⓒ Ⓓ Ⓔ
90 Ⓐ Ⓑ Ⓒ Ⓓ Ⓔ
91 Ⓐ Ⓑ Ⓒ Ⓓ Ⓔ
92 Ⓐ Ⓑ Ⓒ Ⓓ Ⓔ
93 Ⓐ Ⓑ Ⓒ Ⓓ Ⓔ
94 Ⓐ Ⓑ Ⓒ Ⓓ Ⓔ
95 Ⓐ Ⓑ Ⓒ Ⓓ Ⓔ
96 Ⓐ Ⓑ Ⓒ Ⓓ Ⓔ
97 Ⓐ Ⓑ Ⓒ Ⓓ Ⓔ
98 Ⓐ Ⓑ Ⓒ Ⓓ Ⓔ
99 Ⓐ Ⓑ Ⓒ Ⓓ Ⓔ
100 Ⓐ Ⓑ Ⓒ Ⓓ Ⓔ

101	Ⓐ Ⓑ Ⓒ Ⓓ Ⓔ	131	Ⓐ Ⓑ Ⓒ Ⓓ Ⓔ
102	Ⓐ Ⓑ Ⓒ Ⓓ Ⓔ	132	Ⓐ Ⓑ Ⓒ Ⓓ Ⓔ
103	Ⓐ Ⓑ Ⓒ Ⓓ Ⓔ	133	Ⓐ Ⓑ Ⓒ Ⓓ Ⓔ
104	Ⓐ Ⓑ Ⓒ Ⓓ Ⓔ	134	Ⓐ Ⓑ Ⓒ Ⓓ Ⓔ
105	Ⓐ Ⓑ Ⓒ Ⓓ Ⓔ	135	Ⓐ Ⓑ Ⓒ Ⓓ Ⓔ
106	Ⓐ Ⓑ Ⓒ Ⓓ Ⓔ	136	Ⓐ Ⓑ Ⓒ Ⓓ Ⓔ
107	Ⓐ Ⓑ Ⓒ Ⓓ Ⓔ	137	Ⓐ Ⓑ Ⓒ Ⓓ Ⓔ
108	Ⓐ Ⓑ Ⓒ Ⓓ Ⓔ	138	Ⓐ Ⓑ Ⓒ Ⓓ Ⓔ
109	Ⓐ Ⓑ Ⓒ Ⓓ Ⓔ	139	Ⓐ Ⓑ Ⓒ Ⓓ Ⓔ
110	Ⓐ Ⓑ Ⓒ Ⓓ Ⓔ	140	Ⓐ Ⓑ Ⓒ Ⓓ Ⓔ
111	Ⓐ Ⓑ Ⓒ Ⓓ Ⓔ	141	Ⓐ Ⓑ Ⓒ Ⓓ Ⓔ
112	Ⓐ Ⓑ Ⓒ Ⓓ Ⓔ	142	Ⓐ Ⓑ Ⓒ Ⓓ Ⓔ
113	Ⓐ Ⓑ Ⓒ Ⓓ Ⓔ	143	Ⓐ Ⓑ Ⓒ Ⓓ Ⓔ
114	Ⓐ Ⓑ Ⓒ Ⓓ Ⓔ	144	Ⓐ Ⓑ Ⓒ Ⓓ Ⓔ
115	Ⓐ Ⓑ Ⓒ Ⓓ Ⓔ	145	Ⓐ Ⓑ Ⓒ Ⓓ Ⓔ
116	Ⓐ Ⓑ Ⓒ Ⓓ Ⓔ	146	Ⓐ Ⓑ Ⓒ Ⓓ Ⓔ
117	Ⓐ Ⓑ Ⓒ Ⓓ Ⓔ	147	Ⓐ Ⓑ Ⓒ Ⓓ Ⓔ
118	Ⓐ Ⓑ Ⓒ Ⓓ Ⓔ	148	Ⓐ Ⓑ Ⓒ Ⓓ Ⓔ
119	Ⓐ Ⓑ Ⓒ Ⓓ Ⓔ	149	Ⓐ Ⓑ Ⓒ Ⓓ Ⓔ
120	Ⓐ Ⓑ Ⓒ Ⓓ Ⓔ	150	Ⓐ Ⓑ Ⓒ Ⓓ Ⓔ
121	Ⓐ Ⓑ Ⓒ Ⓓ Ⓔ	151	Ⓐ Ⓑ Ⓒ Ⓓ Ⓔ
122	Ⓐ Ⓑ Ⓒ Ⓓ Ⓔ	152	Ⓐ Ⓑ Ⓒ Ⓓ Ⓔ
123	Ⓐ Ⓑ Ⓒ Ⓓ Ⓔ	153	Ⓐ Ⓑ Ⓒ Ⓓ Ⓔ
124	Ⓐ Ⓑ Ⓒ Ⓓ Ⓔ		
125	Ⓐ Ⓑ Ⓒ Ⓓ Ⓔ		
126	Ⓐ Ⓑ Ⓒ Ⓓ Ⓔ		
127	Ⓐ Ⓑ Ⓒ Ⓓ Ⓔ		
128	Ⓐ Ⓑ Ⓒ Ⓓ Ⓔ		
129	Ⓐ Ⓑ Ⓒ Ⓓ Ⓔ		
130	Ⓐ Ⓑ Ⓒ Ⓓ Ⓔ		